THERAPY IN NUCLEAR MEDICINE

Front cover: The University of Connecticut Health Center, the host for the symposium on *Therapy in Nuclear Medicine,* is depicted inside an atom.

Therapy in Nuclear Medicine

Editor

Richard P. Spencer, M.D., Ph.D.

Professor and Chairman
Department of Nuclear Medicine
University of Connecticut Health Center
Farmington, Connecticut

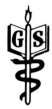

Grune & Stratton
A Subsidiary of Harcourt Brace Jovanovich, Publishers
New York   San Francisco   London

Library of Congress Cataloging in Publication Data
Main entry under title:

Therapy in nuclear medicine.

    Based on a symposium held Mar. 17–19, 1977, Hartford.
    Includes bibliographical references and index.
    1. Radioisotopes—Therapeutic use—Congresses.
I. Spencer, Richard P. [DNLM: 1. Radioisotopes—
Therapeutic use—Congresses. 2. Nuclear medicine—
Congresses. WN450 T398 1977]
RM858.T38   615'.8424
ISBN 0-8089-1070-1   78-7384

Grune & Stratton, Inc.
111 Fifth Avenue
New York, New York 10003

Distributed in the United Kingdom by
Academic Press, Inc. (London) Ltd.
24/28 Oval Road, London NW1

Library of Congress Catalog Number 78-7384
International Standard Book Number 0-8089-1070-1
Printed in the United States of America

Contents

Preface

The excellent and rapid advances in diagnostic aspects of nuclear medicine have perhaps made us lose sight of steady progress in the therapeutic use of radionuclides. In an effort to bring together the past history of such therapeutic applications, their present use, and emerging areas which have clinical implications, a symposium was held in Hartford, Connecticut (March 17–19, 1977).

By means of formal presentations, questions and answers, a round table discussion, and individual interactions, the extent of present information was probed. It became clear that this meeting, and its resultant publication, marked but an early step in exploring the clinical radiation biology of therapeutic radionuclides. The enthusiasm generated at the meeting suggested that others might follow. We are appreciative of the commercial support that aided in funding the symposium, and of the assistance of the sponsoring organizations: University of Connecticut Health Center, Hartford County Medical Association, American College of Nuclear Medicine, Society of Nuclear Medicine, and the Connecticut Division of the American Cancer Society.

Richard P. Spencer

List of Contributors

Mohammed A. Antar, M.D., Ph.D., University of Connecticut Health Center, Farmington, Connecticut

Irving M. Ariel, M.D., Pack Medical Group, New York, New York

Harold L. Atkins, M.D., Brookhaven National Laboratory, Upton, New York

Philip A. Bardfeld, M.D., Montefiore Hospital, New York, New York

Stephen P. Bartok, M.D., Food and Drug Administration, Rockville, Maryland

William H. Beierwaltes, M.D., University Hospital, Ann Arbor, Michigan

Robert E. Belliveau, M.D., Salem Hospital, Salem, Massachusetts

Rodney E. Bigler, Ph.D., Memorial Sloan-Kettering Cancer Center, New York, New York

R. J. Blanchard, M.D., University of Manitoba, Winnipeg, Manitoba, Canada

William D. Bloomer, M.D., Harvard Medical School, Boston, Massachusetts

Gordon L. Brownell, Ph.D., Massachusetts General Hospital, Boston, Massachusetts

Gerald A. Bruno, Ph.D., Squibb Institute for Medical Research, New Brunswick, New Jersey

H. Donald Burns, Ph.D., Johns Hopkins Medical Institutions, Baltimore, Maryland

Gerard N. Burrow, M.D., Toronto General Hospital, Toronto, Ontario, Canada

Tuhin K. Chaudhuri, M.D., University of Texas, San Antonio, Texas

Rashid A. Fawwaz, M.D., Ph.D., Columbia University, College of Physicians and Surgeons, New York, New York

Arnold M. Friedman, Ph.D., Argonne National Laboratory, Argonne, Illinois

Edgar D. Grady, M.D., Georgia Institute of Technology, Atlanta, Georgia

Joel I. Hamburger, M.D., Northland Thyroid Laboratory, Southfield, Michigan

Thomas P. Haynie, M.D., M. D. Anderson Hospital, Houston, Texas

Tapan Hazra, M.D., Medical College of Virginia, Richmond, Virginia

Fazle Hosain, Ph.D., University of Connecticut Health Center, Farmington, Connecticut

Ervin Kaplan, M.D., Veterans Administration Hospital, Hines, Illinois

Klaus Mayer, M.D., Memorial Sloan-Kettering Cancer Center, New York, New York

I. Ross McDougall, Ph.D., Stanford University Medical Center, Stanford, California

Robert E. O'Mara, M.D., Strong Memorial Hospital, Rochester, New York

Savita Puri, M.D., University of Connecticut Health Center, Farmington, Connecticut

Leonard Rosenthall, M.D., Montreal General Hospital, Montreal, Quebec, Canada

Richard P. Spencer, M.D., Ph.D., University of Connecticut Health Center, Farmington, Connecticut

Larry A. Spitznagle, Ph.D., University of Connecticut Health Center, Farmington, Connecticut

Henry N. Wagner, Jr., M.D., Johns Hopkins Medical Institutions, Baltimore, Maryland

Niel Wald, M.D., Graduate School of Public Health, University of Pittsburgh, Pittsburgh, Pennsylvania

Joseph T. Witek, M.D., St. Elizabeth's Hospital, Brighton, Massachusetts

SECTION I

Background

Richard P. Spencer

1

Nuclear Medicine and Therapy:
A Reorientation to Specificity
and Beta Ray Generators

The field we refer to as nuclear medicine has come full circle. It began with a combination of diagnostic studies and therapeutic applications. Indeed ^{32}P and ^{131}I were the mainstays of the discipline for many years and they found employment in several therapeutic schemes. As the imaging applications of short-lived radionuclides were recognized and developed, nuclear medicine became primarily a diagnostic specialty. Yet we can ask a fundamental question: how have we benefited the patient if we establish the diagnosis of an incurable disorder? We view this volume as recognition of the immediacy of that question, and of the potential role of radioactive pharmaceuticals in the therapy for certain human diseases. The full circle has been traversed for we again notice that radioactive materials have a role to play in both diagnosis and therapy. We are at an early stage in understanding the microdosimetry of the therapeutic agents employed, and progress is needed in this fundamental area as well as in clinical applications.

The development of diagnostic radiopharmaceuticals was spurred both by their clinical usefulness and by the appreciation that there was no host reaction routinely expected. In other words, they were diagnostic agents, and were not given in pharmaceutical amounts or to elicit a pharmaceutical effect. By way of contrast, when we utilize radionuclides (R*) in therapy, we must reorient our thinking. The entire reason for using these materials is to elicit a therapeutic response; more particularly, we are relying on a response to radiation. There are thus the considerations shown in Table 1-1.

The list is by no means all inclusive, but it does illustrate the wide variety of considerations. We can perhaps make this concrete by mapping out some basic concepts in the therapeutic application of radionuclides (Table 1-2). As knowledge of these basic topics increases, we may be able to better design and utilize radiopharmaceuticals for therapeutic purposes.

Supported by U.S. Public Health Service Grant CA 17802 from the National Cancer Institute.

3

Table 1-1
Considerations in the Response to Radiation by a Radionuclide

1. Time course of R* deposition in the lesion.
2. Radiation to the lesion by R*.
3. Release of R* from the lesion.
4. Whole-body irradiation by R*.
5. Radiobiology of events within the lesion.
6. Abscopal effects (possibly by release of antigenic and other components).
7. Objective and subjective patient response.

CHOICE OF RADIONUCLIDES FOR THERAPY

There are two basic considerations in the selection of a radionuclide for a specific therapeutic purpose:

1. Chemical or physical properties required for localization in the lesion.
2. Type of radiation, and time course of irradiation (a combination of physical decay and biological turnover).

Five types of radionuclides useful in therapy can be identified (Table 1-3). In addition to pure beta ray emitters, we can also utilize beta ray emitting radionuclides which additionally give off positrons or gamma rays (both of which will somewhat contribute to the radiation dose in the region, and which can also be imaged, thus allowing a check on the uniformity of distribution). We presently have access to gamma ray emitters with conversion or Auger electrons. Additionally, alpha ray emitters and radionuclides which undergo fission might be used in therapy. The list is thus extensive and more choices are available than ^{131}I, ^{32}P, and ^{148}Au which have been the standbys in the past.

In a way this requires a reorientation of our thinking. Certain parallels with diagnostic nuclear medicine are apparent—for example, a high target to nontarget ratio. However, a marked reversal of viewpoints also occurs. Consider, for example, the use of radioiodide (^{131}I). When a scanner was passed over the neck, gamma rays were utilized and the presence of beta rays was deplored. When ^{131}I

Table 1-2
Some Basic Aspects of the Biological Effects of Radionuclide Delivery of
Radiation*

1. "Added" effects of chemical interaction and irradiation. Example: enhanced tumoricidal effect of ^{125}I-iododeoxyuridine over iododexoyuridine.
2. "Radiation sensitizers." Example: adriamycin as an inhibitor of postirradiation proliferation.
3. Time-dose effects.
    a. Destruction of "repair mechanisms."
    b. Differential sensitivity, and recovery, of normal and malignant tissues.
    c. Role of anoxia.

*These effects are currently under investigation.

Table 1-3

Five Types of Radionuclides Potentially of Use in Therapy

---

1. Pure beta ray emitters
2. Beta ray emitters also having gamma and/or positron emissions
3. Gamma ray emitters with Auger or conversion electrons
4. Alpha ray emitters (administered, or produced internally)
5. Radionuclides which undergo fission

---

was employed in therapy, the beta rays were the essential contributors and the gamma rays had but a minor role to play. It was the same radioiodide. Only the perspective and intended use had changed. A comparison of views on beta and gamma rays from therapeutic and diagnostic viewpoints, is given in Table 1-4.

We can carry this to the next logical step by examining two groups of known antitumor chemicals (Table 1-5). The compound *cis*-diamminedichloroplatinum (II) has been synthesized with ^{193m}Pt or ^{195m}Pt for imaging.[1,2] If the radiolabeled compound were to be used in therapy, then ^{197}Pt might be the radionuclide of choice (this substance emits a 670-kev beta ray as well as a gamma emission). Similarly, purine and pyrimidine analogues can be labeled with ^{123}I, ^{18}F, or ^{77}Br for imaging. For therapeutic applications, radionuclides which deposited much energy locally would be employed. These include ^{125}I (Auger electrons), ^{131}I (beta particles in addition to the gamma rays; ^{82}Br and ^{83}Br are also in this class), and the pure beta emitters ^{3}H, ^{14}C, and ^{35}S. The choice of radionuclide is largely dictated by its intended purpose—diagnosis or therapy. The next extension is to ask if various radionuclides can be incorporated *into* an aliphatic chain or aromatic ring in order to gain the needed specificity of the molecule (Table 1-6). There are several apparent choices here (and the list will likely grow with time). Some of these are monoseleno and diseleno compounds,[3] mono- and diarseno chemicals,[4] rings carrying a positively charged iodine,[5] and those carrying both phosphorus and iodine in the ring.[6] Indeed, if a molecule were cleaved in vivo, it might be possible to deliver two or more labeled atoms into the tissue, so that each (or the selected portion) would carry a therapeutic radionuclide.

Table 1-4

Comparison of Views on Beta and Gamma Rays

Therapy	Diagnosis
Beta rays are useful since they deliver ionizing radiation to the limited area that is to be treated.	Beta rays can not be visualized externally and only increase tissue radiation exposure.
Gamma rays are of little therapeutic value (except those of very low energy) since they distribute the radiation exposure over a wide area.	Gamma rays are of primary importance in imaging (except those of low energy, which do not penetrate the tissue).
There may be a role for longer lived radionuclides if the radiation has to be delivered over a period of time.	Short-lived radionuclides are preferred since they do not have to be present after the initial images are obtained.

Table 1-5

Imaging and Therapeutic Radionuclides Which Might Be Employed in the Antitumor Agent
cis-Diamminedichloroplatinum and in Purine and Pyrimidine Analogues

	Imaging			Therapy		
cis-diamminedichloroplatinum	^{193m}Pt	4.4 days	x-rays	^{197}Pt	0.75 days	670 kev $\beta-$ plus gamma
	^{195m}Pt	4.1 days	x-rays			
Purine and pyrimidine analogues	^{123}I	13 hr	159 kev gamma	^{125}I	57 days	E.C.
				^{131}I	8.1 days	600 kev $\beta-$ plus gamma
	^{18}F	1.7 hr	positron	^{3}H	12.5 years	18.6 kev $\beta-$
				^{14}C	5,700 years	156 kev $\beta-$
				^{35}S	88 days	167 kev $\beta-$
	^{77}Br	2.4 days	positron	^{82}Br	1.5 days	444 kev $\beta-$ many gammas
				^{83}Br	2.4 hr	930 kev $\beta-$ 1% gamma

In some instances we have a plethora of radionuclides which might do the task for us. Consider the therapy of lesions in bone (Table 1-7). In addition to ^{32}P (with its energetic beta particle), ^{33}P has a slightly longer physical half-life, but a less energetic beta particle. However, ^{89}Sr has also been used in the therapy of lesions in bone.[7] Moreover, ^{91}Sr has an even more energetic beta emission and also gives off gamma rays. There are, in addition, two radionuclide pairs that might be used in therapy as "internal" or "in situ" or "in vivo" radionuclide generators. That is, the parent localizes in bone and emits a beta particle. The daughter radionuclide produced is also a beta particle emitter.

$$^{140}\text{Ba} \longrightarrow {}^{140}\text{La}$$
$$^{47}\text{Ca} \longrightarrow {}^{47}\text{Sc}$$

The use of such internal radionuclide generators still awaits biological exploration.

Table 1-6

Noncarbon Atoms that Can Be Inserted into
Aliphatic or Aromatic Molecules and Radiolabeled

Grouping	Example
—C—Se—C—	Selenomethionine
—C—Se—Se—C—	Diselenodibutyric acid
—C—As—	Arsonoacetic acid
—C—As≡As—C—	Diarsono compounds
—C—I$^+$—C—	Diphenyleneiodonium
—P—I—	Iodophosphorus ring compounds

Table 1-7

Radionuclides Potentially of Use in Therapy for Bone Lesions*

	T½	Beta Ray (mev max.)	Comments
^{32}P	14.3 days	1.71	No gamma
^{33}P	24.5 days	0.248	No gamma
^{89}Sr	52 days	1.463	Gamma in less than 0.01%. Has been used in therapy at 30 μCi/kg body weight.
^{91}Sr	9.7 hr	2.67	Gamma rays of 0.645, 0.748 mev (and others).
^{140}Ba	12.8 days	1.02	La x-rays emitted. There is also radiation from: ^{140}Ba $-\!\!\!\longrightarrow$ ^{140}La (T½ = 1.7 days) "Internal radionuclide generator." "In situ generator."

Also: ^{47}Ca is a beta ray emitter, which decays to ^{47}Sc (also an emitter of a beta ray).

*From ref. 7. Assumptions: 2/3 dose stored in skeleton; skeleton is 10 percent of body weight. Administer 30 μCi ^{89}Sr/kg body weight = 300 μCi/kg skeleton = uptake of 200 μCi/kg skeleton.

What "selection rules" do we wish to employ in choosing a beta ray emitter? Several are possible. First, we might seek a radionuclide that emits a very energetic beta particle. Table 1-8 lists some of the most energetic beta particles known. It can be observed that several of these are from radionuclides that can be made from parent-daughter pairs (radionuclide generators). For example, we have described a ^{144}Ce $\longrightarrow$ ^{144}Pr generator, for obtaining the 17.3 minute radiopreasodymium with its nearly 3-mev beta particle.[8] Recently, another ^{144}Ce $\longrightarrow$ ^{144}Pr generator, based on an alumina base, has been described.[9] Such radionuclide generators allow us a wide choice as to the rate at which we wish the radiation dose delivered (and the energy of the beta particle). Observe that we are selecting on the basis of beta ray energy, and are not concerned with any accompanying gamma emissions.

Table 1-8

Some Radionuclides that Emit Energetic Beta (Minus) Rays

Beta Energy mev (max.)	Radionuclide	T½	Comment
3.9–4.2	^{66}Ga	9.4 hr	Also γ
	^{112}Ag	3.2 hr	^{112}Pd $-\!\!\!\longrightarrow$ ^{112}Ag
3.5–3.7	^{42}K	12.5 hr	Also γ
	^{106}Rh	0.5 min	^{106}Ru $-\!\!\!\longrightarrow$ ^{106}Rh
3.1–3.5	^{72}Ga	14.1 hr	^{72}Zn $-\!\!\!\longrightarrow$ ^{72}Ga; also γ
	^{214}Bi	19.7 min	Daughters; γ in 0.01%
2.9–3.1	^{76}As	26.5 hr	Also γ
	^{144}Pr	17.3 min	^{144}Ce $-\!\!\!\longrightarrow$ ^{144}Pr; also γ
2.7–2.9	^{93}Y	10.2 hr	Also γ

A second selection mechanism might be the choice of beta particles (which come from radionuclides produced via generators) which have beta ray energies of *over* 2 mev. Some of these are listed in Table 1-9. These radionuclides have half-lives principally in the range of minutes (but some are longer lived, for example, ^{90}Y).[10] A third selection criterion might be that we wish beta ray emitting radionuclides of elements (generator produced) which have interesting chemical or physical properties. Several of these are shown in Table 1-10. Some of these of course duplicate those shown in the previous table.

Another selection rule is more demanding. We might wish a beta ray emitter *without* any appreciable accompanying gamma rays. There are not many radionuclides which meet this criterion. We have listed some of these in four tables, based on their half-lives. Table 1-11 lists those whose half-lives are on the order of minutes. In the Tables (1-12 through 1-14) are given the pure beta ray emitters with half-lives on the order of hours, days, and years. Some of these

Table 1-9
Radionuclide Generators Giving Species with Beta (Minus) Rays of Over 2 mev Energy

	Parent		Daughter		
		T½	T½	mev β–max	Comment
1.	^{28}Mg 12	21 hr	^{28}Al 13	2.3 min	2.85	γ
2.	^{38}S 16	2.9 hr	^{38}Cl 17	37 min	4.91	γ
3.	^{42}Ar 18	3.5 yr	^{42}K 19	12.5 hr	3.52	γ
4.	^{66}Ni 28	2.3 days	^{66}Cu 29	5.2 min	2.63	γ
5.	^{72}Se 34	8.5 days	^{72}As 33	1.1 day	3.34	γ, β+
6.	^{90}Sr 38	28 years	^{90}Y 39	2.7 days	2.27	Also ^{89}Y (n, γ)
7.	^{112}Pd 46	21 hr	^{112}Ag 47	3.2 hr	3.94	γ, β+
8.	^{122}Xe 54	20 hr	^{122}I 53	3.5 min	3.1	γ, β+
9.	^{128}Ba 56	2.4 days	^{128}Cs 55	3.4 min	2.9	γ, β+
10.	^{144}Ce 58	290 days	^{144}Pr 59	17.2 min	2.99	γ
11.	^{188}W 74	69 days	^{188}Re 75	17 hr	2.12	γ
12.	^{194}Os 76	2 years	^{194}Ir 77	18 hr	2.24	γ
13.	^{200}Pt 78	11.5 hr	^{200}Au 79	48 min	2.2	γ

Table 1-10
Radionuclide Generators that Produce Species Emitting Beta Particles*

	Parent			Daughter				End Product
	Radionuclide	T½	Decay	Radionuclide	T½	β− mev (max)	mev Other	
1.	^{28}Mg 12	0.9 days	$\beta-$	^{28}Al 13	2.3 min	2.85	1.78γ	^{28}Si (stable) 14
2.	^{47}Ca 20	4.5 days	$\beta-$	^{47}Sc 21	3.4 days	0.65	0.160γ	^{47}Ti (stable) 22
3.	^{66}Ni 28	2.3 days	$\beta-$	^{66}Cu 29	5.1 min	2.63	1.04γ	^{66}Zn (stable) 30
4.	^{90}Sr 38	28 yr	$\beta-$	^{90}Y 39	2.7 days	2.27	Also from 89 γ (n, γ)	^{90}Zr (stable) 40
5.	^{106}Ru 44	368 days	$\beta-$	^{106}Rh 45	30 sec	3.54	γ	^{106}Pd (stable) 46
6.	^{112}Pd 46	0.9 days	$\beta-$	^{112}Ag 47	3.2 hr	3.94	γ	^{112}Cd (stable) 48
7.	^{115}Cd 48	2.2 days	$\beta-$	^{115m}In 49	4.5 hr	0.83	In x-rays	^{115}In (10^{14} yr) 49
8.	^{132}Te 52	3.2 days	$\beta-$	^{132}I 53	2.3 hr	2.12	Many γ	^{132}Xe (stable) 54
9.	^{140}Ba	12.8 days	$\beta-$	^{140}La 57	1.7 days	2.1, other	occ. γ	^{140}Ce (stable) 48
10.	^{144}Ce 58	284 days	$\beta-$	^{144}Pr 57	17 min	2.99	occ. γ	^{144}Nd (stable) 60
11.	^{194}Os 76	6 yr	$\beta-$	^{194}Ir 77	18 hr	2.24	0.328 γ + others	^{194}Pt (stable) 78

*Some have implications for "in situ" or "in vivo" generators.

Table 1-11

"Pure" Beta Ray Emitters with T½ on the
Order of Minutes*

Radionuclide	T½ (min)	Max. Beta Minus (mev)
^{49}Sc	57	2.01 (0.03%)
^{55}Cr	3.6	2.59
^{69}Zn	52	0.90
^{70}Ga	21	1.65 (0.66% γ)
^{91}Rb	1.2	4.6
^{102}Mo†	11	1.2
^{121}In‡	3.1	3.7
^{144}Pr	17.3	3.0 (2.5% γ)
^{176}Tm	1.5	4.2
^{178}Lu	30	2.25
^{180}Lu	2.5	3.3
^{195}Os	6.5	2.
^{206}Tl	4.2	1.52
^{241}Np§	16	1.4

*Decay products may be radioactive. The radionuclide ^{144}Pr can be
readily produced from ^{144}Ce.
†Decays to ^{102}Tc, a gamma ray emitter.
‡May be one of an isomer pair.
§Decays to ^{241}Am, an alpha particle emitter.

radionuclides are produced from generators. A few may be ruled out since they
themselves produce daughters that emit gamma rays. It can be seen that there are
a number of selection criteria that can be utilized; more precise delineation awaits
better biological data as to compound specificity for various tissues and the desired range and ionization of the emission.

ROLE OF GAMMA RAYS

In order to obtain chemical or physical specificity, it may be necessary to
utilize radionuclides which have gamma ray emissions as well as beta particles.

Table 1-12

"Pure" Beta Ray Emitters with T½ on the
Order of Hours*

Radionuclide	T½ (hr)	Max. Beta Minus (mev)
^{31}Si	2.6	1.48 (0.07% γ)
^{83}Br†	2.4	0.93 (1.4% γ)
^{127}Te	9.4	0.70 (0.65% x-rays)
^{209}Pb	3.3	0.63

*Decay products may be radioactive.
†Daughter radiations from ^{83m}Kr.

Table 1-13

"Pure" Beta Ray Emitters with T½ on the Order of Days*

Radionuclide	T½ (days)	Max. Beta Minus (mev)
^{32}P	14.3	1.71
^{33}P	25.2	0.25
^{35}S	87.2	0.17
^{45}Ca	165	0.252
^{89}Sr	52	1.46 (0.01% γ)
^{90}Y	2.7	2.27
^{91}Y	58	1.54
^{121}Sn	1.1	0.38
^{143}Pr	13.6	0.93
^{185}W	75	0.43
^{210}Bi	5.0	1.16 (5×10^{-5}% γ, Po x-rays)

*Decay products may be radioactive.

Table 1-14

"Pure" Beta Ray Emitters with T½ on the Order of Years

Radionuclide	T½ (years)	Max. Beta Minus (mev)
^{3}H	12.5	0.0186
^{10}Be	2.5×10^{6}	0.555
^{14}C	5600	0.156
^{32}Si†	700	0.21
^{36}Cl	$3 \ \times 10^{5}$	0.714
^{39}Ar	269	0.565
^{63}Ni	92	0.067
^{79}Se	6.5×10^{4}	0.16
^{85}Kr‡	10	0.67 (0.41% γ)
^{90}Sr§	27	0.546
^{93}Zr‖	1.5×10^{6}	0.060
^{99}Tc	2.1×10^{5}	0.292
^{107}Pd	$7 \ \times 10^{6}$	0.04
^{113m}Cd	14	0.58 (0.1% x-rays)
^{147}Pm	2.6	0.224
^{171}Tm	1.9	0.097 (x-rays)
^{204}Tl	3.8	0.766 (x-rays)

*Decay products may be radioactive.
†Daughter is ^{32}P.
‡One of isomer pair.
§Daughter is ^{90}Y.
‖Daughter radiations from ^{93m}Nb.

The gamma component can of course contribute to local irradiation. It has been estimated that in the treatment of hyperthyroidism with ^{131}I, the beta particles contribute about 90 percent of the radiation dose to the thyroid, and the gamma rays about 10 percent. Gamma rays contribute to radiation of sites away from the area of interest. From the viewpoints of both diagnosis and therapy, the "bad actors" are the gamma ray emitters with a high output (an elevated gamma ray constant). Some of these are listed in Table 1-15. These materials of course may have use as external sources of gamma radiation.

In selected instances, a gamma ray component may be useful in tracing the distribution and turnover of a beta particle emitter. Indeed, it might be desirable in the future to admix a gamma ray emitter with a beta particle emitter in order to follow location while obtaining the desired therapeutic effect. Weissleder and coworkers[11] have pointed out the potential use of an admixture of ^{131}I-triolein in oil with ^{32}P-tri-n-octyl-phosphate for intralymphatic therapy. Difficulties with counting the beta ray of ^{32}P in the presence of ^{131}I were noted.

CONVERSION AND AUGER ELECTRONS

Lathrop and coworkers[12] noted that radioactive species "...decaying by electron capture or isomeric transition...produce greater lethality...than predicted from the energy released." Internal conversion liberates electrons from atoms undergoing this event (Table 1-16) and delivers a high radiation flux locally. During electron capture with subsequent atomic rearrangement, Auger electrons can be ejected, contributing to local radiation. Bloomer and Adelstein[13] have

Table 1-15

Gamma Radiation Constants, Arranged by Decreasing Values, for Selected Radionuclides

Value of Gamma Ray Constant	Radionuclide	T½	
18.6	[52]Mn	5.6	days
18.4	[24]Na	15	hr
17.6	[56]Co	77	days
15.7	[28]Mg	21	hr
15.6	[48]V	16	days
14.6	[82]Br	35	hr
14.3	[110m]Ag	253	days
14.1	[88]Y	106	days
13.2	[60]Co	5.2	years
12.4	[140]Ba	12.8	days
12.0	[22]Na	2.6	years
11.8	[132]I	2.3	hr
11.6	[72]Ga	14.1	hr
11.3	[140]La	40.2	hr
10.9	[46]Sc	84	days

Table 1-16
Internal Conversion Coefficients for Several
Radionuclides*

Radionuclide	T½ (days)	Gamma Ray energy (kev)	$^eK/\gamma$
^{141}Ce	33	145	0.38
^{203}Hg	47	279	0.16
^{113}Sn	115	391	0.44
^{198}Au	2.7	412	0.03

*By $^eK/\gamma$ is meant the number of K-shell electrons converted per gamma ray. Common values range from over 1 (for ^{109}Cd) to 10^{-4} for ^{65}Zn, and lower.

shown that Auger electrons (from ^{125}I) can be used to deliver significant radiation to tumors. This is an evolving and important area, since it adds a significant number of radionuclides to the list of therapeutic possibilities. Some of these radionuclides can be produced from parent-daughter pairs. One of these, which is highly internally converted, is ^{103m}Rh (Table 1-17).

ALPHA PARTICLES

Although they are usually not considered as useful in the therapeutic use of radionuclides, alpha particles may have a distinct role to play. Most alpha emitters are bone seekers, and many are long lived. However, if the proper selection criteria are applied, then alpha ray emitting radionuclides should be considered. These selection rules are three in number.

Alpha particles in therapy
1. If produced within the lesion: B (n,α) That is, boron in the lesion is irradiated with neutrons, producing an alpha particle.

Table 1-17
Production of ^{103m}Rh, a Radionuclide with Significant Internal Conversion

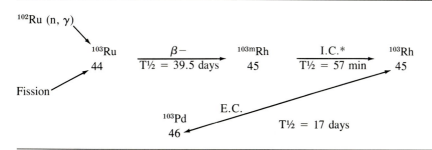

*I.C. = emissions that are highly internally converted during the isomeric transition; 17- and 37-kev conversion electrons are emitted. A 40-kev x-ray occurs in 0.4%.

Table 1-18
Some Energetic Alpha Particles Emitted by
Radionuclides

Radionuclide	T½	Energy of Alpha Particle (mev)
^{254}Fm	3.2 days	7.2
^{253}Es	20.4 days	6.6
^{254}Es	276 days	6.4
^{242}Cm	163 days	6.1
^{211}At	7.2 hr	5.9
^{222}Rn	3.8 days	5.5

2. If appropriately lesion directed and of short half-life (example: astatine radionuclides ^{209}At, ^{210}At, ^{211}At).
3. If rapidly eliminated, so that whole-body exposure is low. For example, all known forms of astatine are alpha particle emitters. Since they are short-lived, they have potential use in therapy (and this is discussed in a later chapter). By analogy to beta ray therapy, we might select alpha rays by energy (Table 1-18). Recognize, however, that the alpha rays are densely ionizing, and often produce a "chain" of daughter products which can also be ionizing.

NEUTRONS

These uncharged particles may also have a role in the therapy for certain lesions.[14] They can be used in four ways.

1. External neutron beam (as from a neutron generator).
2. External neutron beam bombarding an internally delivered stable nuclide, such as $B(n,\alpha)$.
3. External neutron beam with gamma ray component (as from nuclear reactor).
4. Internal (sealed or given parenterally) neutron emitter such as Californium-252.

These particles of course produce a radiation dose in part from the induced radioactivity.

SUMMARY

The key considerations of physicochemical specificity and the time course and type of radiation can be met by a variety of radionuclides. In addition to radiation from beta rays, we can utilize that from weak gamma rays, conversion and Auger electrons, alpha particles, and neutrons. The role to be played by in vivo and in vitro radionuclide generators in this area is likely very considerable.

REFERENCES

1. Lange, R. C., Spencer, R. P., Harder, H. C.: Synthesis and distribution of a radiolabeled antitumor agent: cis-diamminedichloroplatinum (II). J. Nucl. Med. 13:328–330, 1972.
2. Lange, R. C., Spencer, R. P., Harder, H. C.: The antitumor agent cis-pt $(NH_3)2C12$; distribution studies and dose calculations for [193m]Pt and [195m]Pt. J. Nucl. Med. 14:191–195, 1973.
3. Spencer, R. P., Brody, K. R.: ^{75}Se-diselenodibutyric acid: parent compound for a series of gamma-labeled lipids. J. Nucl. Med. 9:349–350, 1968.
4. Palmer, C. S.: Arsono- and arsenoacetic acids. Organic Syntheses. Collective I:73–75, 1921.
5. Spencer, R. P., Brody, K. R.: Distribution of a hypoglycemic agent: ^{131}I-diphenyleneiodonium. Fed. Proc. 35:685, 1976.
6. Leffler, J. E., Jaffe, H.: Orthoiodosophenyl phosphoric acid. J. Org. Chem. 38:2719–2720, 1973.
7. Firusian, N., Mellin, P., Schmidt, C. G.: Results of [89]Strontium therapy in patients with carcinoma of the prostate and incurable pain from bone metastases: a preliminary report. J. Urol. 116:764–768, 1976.
8. Lange, R. C., Spencer, R. P.: [144]Ce- [144]Pr radionuclide generator: possible use in blood-flow studies. J. Nucl. Med. 11:340, 1970.
9. Bhattacharyya, D. K., Basu, S.: Use of alumina as an ion exchanger in the separation of carrier-free [144]Pr from [144]Ce. Separation Sci. 11:503–508, 1976.
10. Bhattacharyya, D. K., Basu, S.: Use of alumina as ion exchanger in the separation of carrier free ^{90}Y from [90]Sr. J. Indian Chem. Soc. 53:850–852, 1976.
11. Weissleder, H., Pfannenstiel, P., Peters, P. E.: Distribution pattern of radioactive labelled Lipiodol-UF following intralymphatic application for therapy. Lymphology 9:122–126, 1976.
12. Lathrop, K. A., Gloria, I. V., Harper, P. V.: Some effects of radiation from Tc-99m on the in utero and neonatal mouse and its progeny. J. Nucl. Med. 16:544, 1975.
13. Bloomer, W. D., Adelstein, S. J.: 5-^{125}I-iododeoxyuridine as prototype for radionuclide therapy with Auger emitters. Nature 265:620–621, 1977.
14. Barschall, H. H.: The production and use of neutrons for cancer treatment. Am. Sci. 64:668–673, 1976.

Rodney E. Bigler

2

Relationship of External Radiation Doses to Internal Dosimetry

OVERVIEW

It has long been recognized, especially in the area of external fractionated radiotherapy, that differing radiation dose, time, and fractionation patterns influence the effect of radiation on normal tissues. The nominal standard dose (NSD) concept was introduced to provide radiotherapists with a method for planning treatments utilizing a variety of radiotherapy delivery patterns which result in equal biological effects on normal tissues. This concept has been extended to implant brachytherapy and to nuclear medicine therapy with internally deposited radionuclides and labeled compounds. This chapter presents computational procedures needed to evaluate the effects of treatments by the three therapy methods either alone or in combination, and the results of calculations using these procedures to estimate the hazard to marrow associated with the internal use of ^{131}I and ^{125}I-sodium iodide; ^{32}P and ^{33}P-EHDP; and ^{35}S-sulfate. The theory of Douglas and Fowler is shown by a procedure suggested by them to be consistent with the empirical normalization used to quantitatively compare the effects of fractionated and continuous radiotherapy.

INTRODUCTION

A major problem in the use of radiation for therapy or diagnostic purposes is the development of predictive relationships between radiation-absorbed dose and the effects on normal tissues during such procedures. Ellis suggested such a relationship, based on radiobiologic studies[1] and clinical radiotherapy results,[2] for fractionated external beam radiotherapy termed the nominal standard dose (NSD)

This research supported in part by U.S. Energy Research and Development Administration Contract E(11-1)-3521 and by National Cancer Institute Grant CA 08748-11B.

concept. The NSD has been used extensively to plan treatments having equal effects on normal tissues where wide differences in time and dose fractionation patterns are utilized.

Kirk et al.[3,4] and Orton[5] devised procedures for assessing damage from fractionated and continuous radiation treatments in unified systems. Both methods use data from clinical observations based on ^{226}Ra treatments varying in dose rate from about 30 to 150 rads/hour to provide an empirical bridge between fractionated and continuous therapy. Douglas and Fowler[6] have recently developed a theoretical method for accounting for the effects of dose fractionation. It is possible by their method to extrapolate the effects of fractionation down to the level of continuous dose delivery. Further evidence supporting the Douglas and Fowler theory is provided in this chapter by demonstrating that it theoretically predicts the empirical normalization used to extend the effects of fractionated radiotherapy to implant brachytherapy.

Bigler[7] extended the work of Orton[5] to radiation delivered by radionuclides and labeled compounds distributed within the body by biologic processes. This extension may prove useful in more accurately evaluating and predicting the effects of one or more nuclear medicine therapy or diagnostic procedures on normal tissues.

The primary purpose of this chapter is to present the formulas with definitions needed to estimate the biologic effects on normal tissues of radiation delivered by external beam radiotherapy, brachytherapy, and nuclear medicine procedures either separately or in combination. Essentials of radiation dosimetry required for analysis of nuclear medicine procedures will be presented following methods developed by the Medical Internal Radiation Dose Committee (MIRD) of the Society of Nuclear Medicine. The results of calculations illustrating the application of this method to the effects on normal marrow brought about by ^{131}I-sodium iodide, ^{32}P-EHDP (ethane-1-hydroxy-1, 1-diphosphonate), and ^{35}S-sulfate therapies are shown, where a single administration of the radioactive material has been assumed. The ^{35}S calculations are extended to the situation where multiple isotope administrations are performed.

FRACTIONATED RADIOTHERAPY

The equation defining the NSD concept of Ellis[1] in fractionated external beam radiotherapy is

$$D = NSD \cdot N^{0.24} \cdot T^{0.11} \tag{1}$$

where D is the dose in rads of cobalt-60 gamma rays, N is the number of fractions, and T is the overall time of the course of treatment in days. With these definitions the unit for the NSD is termed *rad equivalent therapy* (ret). The dose required for radiations other than cobalt 60 can be determined by multiplying the dose by the ratio of the cobalt 60 relative biological effect (RBE) to the RBE of the other radiation.[3,8] The RBE of a ^{60}Co beam is considered clinically to be 0.9. According to Ellis,[8] the NSD concept applies to acute radiation reactions given in the same total time or to late effects occurring after 100 days or more.

In order to evaluate complex protocols in which several distinct treatments have been or are proposed for combination, one can calculate a partial tolerance (PT) for each treatment and then add the PTs for each treatment. This sum will equal the NSD for all equivalent protocols. The expression for the PT is

$$PT = NSD \cdot \frac{n}{N} \tag{2}$$

where N is the number of fractions known to result in full tolerance and n is the number of such dose fractions actually given. It has been shown that partial tolerance calculations can be simplified by writing the PT equation in the following form:[9,10]

$$PT = (NSD)^{-0.538} (TDF) \cdot 10^3 \tag{3}$$

where TDF is the time, dose, and fractionation factor

$$TDF = C\frac{n}{N} \tag{4}$$

and

$$C = (NSD)^{1.538} \cdot 10^{-3} \tag{5}$$

If rest periods are interposed between treatments, the effectiveness of the earlier part or parts will diminish. Multiplying the earlier parts by the following recovery factor will account for this decrease:[11]

$$\text{Recovery factor} = \left(\frac{T}{T+R} \right)^{0.11} \tag{6}$$

where the duration of the first part of the split course is T days, and the rest period is R days. Tables of recovery factors and TDF factors designed for convenient use are contained in ref. 10.

IMPLANT BRACHYTHERAPY

The basis for the use of the NSD concept in interstitial implant therapy is the clinical judgment that 6000 rads of treatment with ^{226}Ra gamma rays in 7 days produces the same maximum mucous membrane reaction as do 18 fractions of 300 rads given 3 times weekly.[12] Recently Douglas and Fowler[6] investigated both experimentally and theoretically the $N^{0.24}$ factor in the NSD relationships in Equation 1. The NSD formula matched to their data and theory at 30 dose fractions agrees also at 4 fractions but not elsewhere. The maximum disagreement between 4 and 30 fractions is 5 percent less dose for the NSD value at midrange. When the Douglas and Fowler data and theory are plotted on an inverse dose versus dose per fraction plot, a straight line results, which can presumably be extrapolated

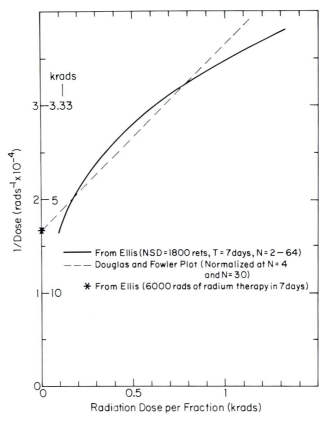

Fig. 2-1. Graph of inverse dose versus dose per fraction of the NSD formula for a constant time period of 7 days. The straight line drawn through 4 and 30 fractions intersects the vertical axis at 6000 rads.

down to zero dose per fraction. Zero dose per fraction is equivalent to continuous delivery of radiation dose. In Figure 2-1 a straight line drawn through the 4 and 30 fraction positions on the curve derived from Equation 1 for a constant time period of 7 days intersects the vertical axis at 6000 rads. Apparently the method of Douglas and Fowler could have been used to predict the empirically derived normalization between fractionated and continuous radiation treatment. This analysis suggests it may be possible to provide a theoretical basis for the empirical method used to normalize the effects of fractionated and continuous radiotherapies.

Orton[5] showed how a TDF for brachytherapy could be defined in which clinically equivalent continuous and fractionated radiotherapy treatments result in identical TDF values. By this definition treatment protocols combining both methods can be analyzed by a sum of the TDF values for each. The following definition was proposed as equivalent to Equation 4:[5]

$$\text{TDF} = \text{K} \frac{t}{T_{tol}} \text{ (rad)} \tag{7}$$

where K is the TDF at full tolerance; T_{tol} is the time of application at a chosen dose rate which would result in full tolerance; and t is the actual treatment time at that dose rate. The general equation which allows TDFs to be calculated is the following:[5]

$$\text{TDF} = 4.76 \times 10^{-3} \int_{t_i}^{t_f} R(t)^{1.35} \, dt \ (\text{rad}) \tag{8}$$

where R(t) is the dose rate integrated over the time period t, ranging from the initiation of therapy at time t_i, to the completion of therapy at time t_f. Tables of TDF factors for implant brachytherapy designed for convenient use are contained in ref. 5.

NUCLEAR MEDICINE THERAPY AND DIAGNOSTIC PROCEDURES

Time and dose factors for radionuclides and labeled compounds distributed within the body by biologic processes can be evaluated by the use of Equation 8. An estimate of the time-dependent dose rate, R(t), can be obtained by methods based on the basic schema proposed by Loevinger and Berman in MIRD Pamphlet No. 1.[13] The procedures covered here show how to estimate $\bar{R}(t)$ which is the mean dose to the target organ of interest. If the activity contained within the target organ is not distributed uniformly on a scale appropriate to the range of the emissions of the particular radionuclide, e.g., Auger electrons, conversion electrons, x-rays, and low-energy gamma rays, more microscopic calculations of the radiation dose rate to the sensitive sites within the tissue should be carried out. Knowledge of the kinetics of activity incorporation and clearance from the total body and other tissues are needed, including the target tissue, tissues which due to their positioning within the body with respect to the target tissue modify significantly the target tissue dose, and other tissues where a risk estimate is desired. Gonad data for genetic risk estimates are especially important.

Activity kinetics $A_r(t)$ for each tissue r can be expressed using the formula:

$$A_r(t) = A_o e^{-\lambda t} F_r(t) \quad (\mu\text{Ci}) \tag{9}$$

where A_o is the administered activity in microcuries (μCi), λ is the physical decay constant (h^{-1}), and $F_r(t)$ is a fraction of the administered activity retained within the tissue r at time t in hours (h). This equation serves as the starting point for radiation dose or dose-rate estimations when $F_r(t)$ can be or has been measured directly. Total-body retention, $F_{tb}(t)$, is obtained either by the difference between activity administered and activity excreted or by quantitative total-body counting. A quantitative, noninvasive method for measuring tissue distribution data in vivo using tracer doses pretreatment and with confirmation studies during treatment for each patient is preferred where possible. Radioiodine treatment for thyrotoxicosis is an example where external scanning procedures can be used for this purpose.

When noninvasive methods cannot be applied for measuring activity distributions within body tissues, less direct methods are used, such as using data obtained from autopsy of cadavers or animals. Investigations of any new radionuclide or labeled compound considered for use in humans are generally carried out in animal systems, and this information should be in the literature. Unfortunately, data from both animal and human studies are often reported in terms of percent dose per gram of tissue. The desirability of expressing data in terms of dose fraction per whole organ[14] and in relative concentrations[15,16] has been previously discussed. The use of indirectly obtained data often leads to large errors in dose estimates due to interspecies and interpatient biological variations. In such cases one or more tissue samples made available by biopsy are obtained at times considered best suited for activity concentration confirmation. These data should be expressed in terms of relative concentrations (RCs) defined as:

$$RC = \frac{\text{Administered dose fraction}}{\text{Tissue weight}} \cdot \text{Body weight} \tag{10}$$

where both weights are expressed in identical units. The administered dose fraction retained, $F_r(t)$, then becomes:

$$F_r(t) = \frac{m_r}{m_{tb}} \cdot RC \tag{11}$$

where m_r and m_{tb} are masses of the target volume and total body used in the model calculation. For the purposes of the discussion here and for the calculations to illustrate these methods contained in a later section of this chapter, the model used will be the heterogeneous standard phantom defined by the MIRD Committee.[17] Individual differences in organ size are often important in calculations performed for patients. Such data may often be obtained by palpation, radiograph, sonography, computed transaxial tomography or by other means. Further refinement of dosimetry calculations will include allowance for any tissue shrinkage and/or alterations in isotope uptake and retention due to radiation damage effects on tissues.[18]

The mean dose rate ($\bar{R}$) in rads per hour from a specified radionuclide or labeled compound to a target volume (v) from as many identified source regions (r) as desired can be calculated using the equation:

$$\bar{R}_v = \frac{A_v}{m_v} \Sigma \Delta_{np} \phi_{np} + \sum_{r=a}^{v} \frac{A_r}{m_v} \Sigma \Delta \phi_{v \leftarrow r} + \frac{A_{rem}}{m_v} \Sigma \Delta \phi_{v \leftarrow rem} \tag{12}$$

where

$$\phi_{v \leftarrow rem} = \frac{m_{tb}}{m_{rem}} \left(\phi_{v \leftarrow tb} - \sum_{r=a}^{v} \frac{m_r}{m_{tb}} \phi_{v \leftarrow r} \right)$$

$$A_{rem} = A_{tb} - \sum_{r=a}^{v} A_r,$$

$$m_{rem} = m_{tb} - \sum_{r=a}^{v} m_r,$$

A is the activity defined in Equation 9, m is the organ mass (g), Δ is the equilibrium dose constant (g-rad/μCi-h), ϕ is the absorbed fraction, np designates nonpenetrating radiations, tb designates the total body, and the subscript rem designates the remainder of the body. The unspecified sum (Σ) in the first term should be taken over all nonpenetrating radiations. The unspecified sums in the other terms are overall penetrating radiations. The first term of Equation 12 includes the nonpenetrating radiation within the target organ. The second term includes the penetrating radiation exposing the target organ from activity contained within itself (r = v in the summation) and from activity in separately identified organs. The third term includes the penetrating radiation exposing the target organ from the remainder (rem) of activity which is assumed to be uniformly distributed throughout the remainder of the body. Dillman and Von der Lage[19] have produced a computer code from which the usual nuclear decay scheme data found in the literature have been reduced to the equilibrium dose constants needed for evaluating Equation 12. Absorbed fractions for the MIRD adult phantom can be found in publications by Snyder et al.[20,21]

Dose-rate calculations are simplified for some purposes by the introduction of a quantity termed the S factor:[17,20]

$$S_{v \leftarrow r} = \frac{1}{m_v} \Sigma \Delta \phi_{v \leftarrow r} \qquad (13)$$

where S is the absorbed dose per unit cumulated activity (rad/μCi-h). The unspecified sum in Equation 13 should be taken over all radiations emitted by the decay of each radionuclide. The dose-rate equation defined in Equation 12 can be rewritten making use of the S factor in the following manner:

$$\overline{R}_v = \sum_{r=a}^{v} A_r S_{v \leftarrow r} + A_{rem} S_{v \leftarrow rem} \qquad (14)$$

where

$$S_{v \leftarrow rem} = \frac{m_{tb}}{m_{rem}} (S_{v \leftarrow tb} - \sum_{r=a}^{v} \frac{m_r}{m_{tb}} S_{v \leftarrow r}) \qquad (15)$$

The first term in Equation 14 includes radiation exposing the target organ (r=v) including the nonpenetrating and all other separately identified organ-penetrating radiation exposing the target organ. The second term includes penetrating radiation from the remainder of the body to the target organ. Equation 15 defines the S factor for the remainder of the body which must be calculated since S factors for the remainder of the body are not included in ref. 17.

Representing the dose rate in the form of Equation 12 has two advantages. The first arises when the mean organ dose rate does not adequately represent the dose rate at the target site of interest and a more microscopic calculation is therefore desired. All emissions from a particular radionuclide which because of their short range need a microscopic analysis can be conveniently separated into the first term in Equation 12 and the dose rate contribution from them only calculated by a more microscopic approach. The dose-rate contribution from the long-range radiations can still be calculated by evaluation of the remaining terms in Equation 12. The second advantage of Equation 12 is appreciated when RBE data are available for each emission from, for instance, a theoretical model of RBE versus energy for various emissions, e.g., electrons, x-rays, gamma rays, and it is desired to correct each emission separately for RBE. This can be accomplished by introducing the RBE correction as an additional factor into each product of equilibrium dose constant and absorbed fraction before the sum over all emissions is carried out.

The total radiation dose delivered to a target tissue can be evaluated by integrating either Equation 12 or 14 over time. Since the activity A is the only time-dependent quantity in each term, substituting the cumulated activity $\tilde{A}$ at all places where A appears will accomplish this integration. Often the fraction of the administered activity retained, $F_r(t)$, can be expressed as a sum of exponential functions. In these cases Equation 9 can be rewritten in the form:

$$A_r(t) = A_o \, e^{-\lambda_{rj} t} \, \Sigma_j \, \alpha_{rj} \, e^{-\lambda t} \tag{16}$$

where A_o is the administered activity (μCi), λ is the physical decay constant (h^{-1}), α_{rj} are components of $F_r(t)$ having biologic parameters λ_{rj} (h^{-1}), and the summation over the index j is the number of exponentials which best represent the activity time distribution. The cumulated activity is obtained by integration of Equation 16:

$$\tilde{A}_r = A_o \, e^{-\lambda t} \, \Sigma \, \frac{\alpha_{rj}}{\lambda_{rj} + \lambda} \, (\mu\text{Ci-h}) \tag{17}$$

GENERAL RADIOTHERAPY PROTOCOL

In general, a radiotherapy protocol may consist of several separate and different parts the time-dose factors of which can be represented as TDF_a, TDF_b ... TDF_n. A general radiotherapy protocol may be designed equivalent to one where the TDF at full normal tissue tolerance, TDF_{tol}, is known by making use of the relationship:

$$TDF_{tol} = TDF_1 + TDF_2 + \ldots + TDF_n \tag{18}$$

where the TDFs on the right side of the equation are for the several separate and/or different parts, which are designated as separate parts by subscripts numbering from 1 to n and are not at any time being administered simultaneously. If any of the different parts of radiotherapy are being administered simultaneously, the total dose rate, R(t), from all parts should be added together linearly prior to performing the integration in Equation 8 for TDF evaluation. Equation 7 is used to evaluate correction factors for TDFs where rest periods have been interposed.

Table 2-1
Biologic Parameters for Single IV Administrations of 3 Radiolabeled Compounds

Radiolabeled Compound	Body Tissue	Fraction of Administered Activity/Organ			Biologic Disappearance Constants (hr^{-1})		
		α_1	α_2	α_3	λ_1	λ_2	λ_3
^{131}I-iodine	Total body	0.35	0.18	0.47	0.158	0.06	5.9×10^{-3}
	Marrow	9.6×10^{-2}	-6.5×10^{-3}	9.7×10^{-3}	0.313	0.027	0.0
^{32}P-EHDP	Trabecular bone	1.62×10^{-1}	4.37×10^{-2}	—	2.57×10^{-3}	0.0	—
	Cortical bone	2.17×10^{-1}	5.83×10^{-2}	—	2.57×10^{-3}	0.0	—
	Marrow	9.23×10^{-2}	2.15×10^{-2}	6.65×10^{-4}	1.61×10^{0}	3.39×10^{-1}	1.73×10^{-2}
^{35}S-sulfate	Marrow	1.22×10^{-2}	2.79×10^{-2}	2.8×10^{-5}	3.15×10^{-1}	4.81×10^{-3}	1.28×10^{-3}

Table 2-2

Time-Dose Factor (TDF) Estimate of Damage to Normal Red Marrow by Internally Deposited Radionuclides and Labeled Compounds

Radionuclide	Chemical Form	Administered Dose (mCi/kg body weight)	Radiation Dose to Marrow (rad)	TDF
[131]I	Sodium iodide	4.5	300	1.3
[125]I	Sodium iodide	8.0	630	1.3
[32]P	EHDP*	0.3	600	2.7
[33]P	EHDP*	2.6	670	2.7
[35]S	Sulfate	30.	750	4.4

*EHDP = Ethane-1-hydroxy-1, 1-diphosphonate.

THERAPY IN NUCLEAR MEDICINE APPLICATIONS

[131]I-Sodium Iodide Therapy for Metastatic Thyroid Cancer

Benua et al.[22] reported the experience of the Memorial Sloan-Kettering Cancer Center from 1946 to 1960 in treating patients with metastatic thyroid cancer. The majority of these patients had previously received a total surgical thyroidectomy. The administered dose of ^{131}I-sodium iodide was chosen for the majority of patients to result in a dose of 300 rads to the blood with the intent that this was the largest dose patients could tolerate in relative safety. Next to nausea, bone marrow depression was the most frequent complication of treatment.

Time and dose factor estimates for the effect on marrow from ^{131}I treatment were obtained using the blood and total-body retention data included in Table 2-1 and obtained from ref. 22, and assuming the isotope concentration of red marrow equal to blood. Nuclear and model dependent data were derived from the sources indicated earlier in this chapter. A TDF of 1.3 was found for this treatment procedure as indicated in Table 2-2.

[125]I-Sodium Iodide Therapy for Metastatic Thyroid Cancer

The administered dose and red marrow radiation dose for ^{125}I-sodium iodide treatment resulting in an equal TDF were calculated for two purposes. The first is to illustrate the possible predictive value of such estimates in evaluating the potential of substituting other radioactive isotopes of a given radionuclide for treatment or diagnosis. The second purpose is to point out that such estimates can not be relied on if the model assumed for the first isotope is not appropriate for the second isotope. Before this procedure could be expected to provide a reliable estimate of the effect of ^{125}I-sodium iodide therapy on red marrow, cellular level distribution studies should be carried out for red marrow. A more microscopic model may be needed for a reasonable estimate of the hazard associated with the use of ^{125}I due to the short-range nature of its emissions.

^{32}P-EHDP Treatment for Metastatic Osteogenic Sarcoma

The possibility of using ^{32}P-EHDP or ^{33}P-EHDP as an adjuvant in the prophylactic or palliative treatment of osteogenic sarcoma is under investigation.[23,24] Biologic data obtained from these patient investigations were used to derive the biologic parameters for ^{32}P-EHDP appearing in Table 2-1. An administered dose level of 0.3 mCi/kg body weight, derived from normal dog studies, was chosen because this level was reported[25] to result in depression of circulating lymphocytes and platelets with recovery at day 42 and with all other blood parameters essentially normal. Lower doses did not give a measurable effect. This dose would result in a TDF of 2.7 in humans as indicated in Table 2-2.

^{33}P-EHDP Treatment for Metastatic Osteogenic Sarcoma

This is another example of investigating the predictive value of radioactive isotope substitution (^{33}P for ^{32}P) by means of TDF estimations. This case differs from the iodine case in that distribution data are available showing that EHDP is taken up on bone surfaces. The present MIRD model assumes a uniform uptake within bone tissue (volume uptake). The relatively long range of the 1.7-MeV (maximum) beta particle emitted by ^{32}P relative to red marrow trabecular bone spacing[26] suggests that either a surface or volume uptake assumption would lead to essentially the same dose and TDF result for [32]P. The 0.25-MeV (maximum) beta particle emitted by ^{33}P has a much shorter range. Clearly, before the 2.7 TDF estimate derived from ^{32}P data can be used to predict the administered dose of ^{33}P required for equal effect, a more microscopic model calculation is needed.

[35]S-Sulfate Treatment

Distribution data needed to estimate the TDF for red marrow were derived from patient studies[27] (H. Q. Woodard, *personal communication*, 1977) and are included in Table 2-1. Two TDF estimates were obtained for ^{35}S-sulfate. The first assumes a single administration of 30 mCi/kg body weight, which results in a TDF of 4.4 and is included in Table 2-2 for comparison to the other TDF estimations. The second is according to a treatment plan carried out on one of the patients included in the ^{35}S study prepared by Dr. K. Mayer for this volume. Figure 2-2 illustrates graphically the increase of TDF with time, and Figure 2-3 the dose increase with time where multiple doses are administered at various times. The TDF and radiation dose for the treatment plan are 3.3 and 990 rads, respectively.

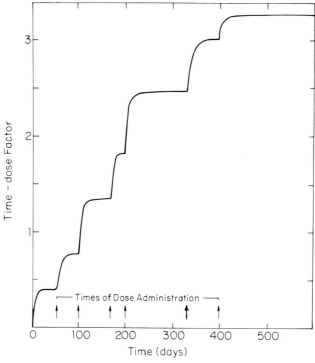

Fig. 2-2. Graph of TDF factor versus time for a ^{35}S-sodium sulfate patient treatment plan, where multiple administrations have been performed.

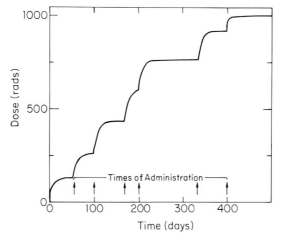

Fig. 2-3. Graph of the radiation dose versus time for a ^{35}S-sodium sulfate patient treatment plan, where multiple administrations have been performed.

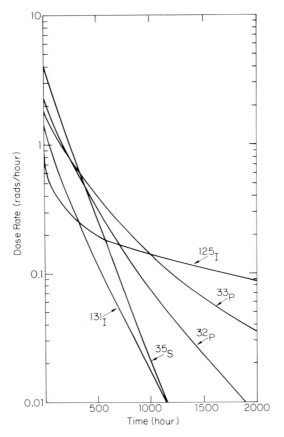

Fig.2-4. Graph of dose rate versus time for single administrations to humans of the radiolabeled compounds discussed
in the text.

This and other similar treatments resulted in sufficiently severe marrow toxicity to
contraindicate its use in patients according to Dr. Mayer's study.

DISCUSSION

The results of the time and dose-factor calculations in Table 2-2 and the
multiple administration protocol with ^{35}S suggest that any treatments resulting in a
TDF of no higher than about 2 to normal bone marrow are probably safe, whereas
treatments above 3 are likely to result in unacceptable results. However, at present considerable caution must be exercised in the use of any predictions of effects
on normal tissues derived from TDF calculations. The data used to establish the
TDF method for implant brachytherapy did not extend below 30 rads/hour, and no
empirical proof for the validity of the relationship for variable dose-rate procedures was given.[5] As is clear from Figure 2-4, the dose rates from which the TDF
calculations presented here were derived are well below 30 rads/minute at time of
administration and they decrease rapidly thereafter. The validity for the use of the

NSD concept in nuclear medicine procedures can and should be provided by a thorough analysis of currently existing treatment experience.

REFERENCES

1. Ellis, F.: Fractionation in radiotherapy. In: Modern Trends in Radiotherapy, Vol. I, Deeley, T. J., and Wood, C. A., (eds.). London, Butterworths, pp. 34–51, 1967.
2. Ellis, F.: Dose, time and fractionation: a clinical hypothesis. Clin. Radiol. 20:1–7, 1969.
3. Kirk, J., Gray, W. M., Watson, E. R.: Cumulative radiation effect. II: Continuous radiation therapy—long-lived sources. Clin. Radiol. 23:93–105, 1972.
4. Kirk, J., Gray, W. M., Watson, E. R.: Cumulative radiation effect. III: Continuous radiation therapy—short-lived sources. Clin. Radiol. 24:1–11, 1973.
5. Orton, C. G.: Time-dose factors (TDF's) in brachytherapy. Br. J. Radiol. 47:603–607, 1974.
6. Douglas, B. G., Fowler, J. F.: The effect of multiple small fractions of x-rays on skin reactions in the mouse. Radiat. Res. 66:401–426, 1976.
7. Bigler, R. E.: Dosimetry for evaluation of the biologic effects of radiation treatment using internally deposited radionuclides and labeled compounds. Proceedings of the Radiopharmaceutical Dosimetry Symposium, Oak Ridge, Tenn., April 26–29, 1976. Washington, D.C., HEW Publication (FDA) 76-8044.
8. Ellis, F.: NSD and TSD in 4π therapy. In: Second International Symposium on Radiation Therapy, New York, 1975, pp. 41–52. Afterloading: twenty years of experience, 1955–1975, B. S. Hilaris, (ed.). New York, Memorial Sloan-Kettering Cancer Center, 1975.
9. Orton, C. G.: Analysis and discussion of the time/dose/fractionation problem. AAPM Q. Bull. 6:173–175, 1971.
10. Orton, C. G., Ellis, F.: A simplification in the use of the NSD concept in practical radiotherapy. Br. J. Radiol. 46:529–537, 1973.
11. Winston, B. M., Ellis, F., Hall, E. J.: The Oxford NSD calculator for clinical use. Clin. Radiol. 20:8–11, 1969.
12. Ellis, F.: Radiation effect and tolerance. In: Handbook of Interstitial Brachytherapy, B. S. Hilaris (ed.). Acton, Mass., Publishing Sciences Group, Inc., pp. 45–52, 1975.
13. Loevinger, R., Berman, M.: A schema for absorbed dose calculations for biologically distributed radionuclides. MIRD Pamphlet No. 1. J. Nucl. Med. [Suppl. 1] 9:7–14, 1968.
14. Spencer, R. P.: Notations for tissue radionuclide distributions. J. Nucl. Med. 17:1110, 1976.
15. Woodard, H. Q., Bigler, R. E., Freed, B. R., Russ, G. A.: Expression of tissue isotope distribution. J. Nucl. Med. 16:958–959, 1975.
16. Woodard, H. Q., Bigler, R. E., Freed, B., Russ, G.: Reply to Notations for tissue radionuclide distributions. J. Nucl. Med. 17:1110–1111, 1976.
17. Snyder, W. S., Ford, M. R., Warner, G. G., Watson, S. B.: "S," absorbed dose per unit cumulated activity for selected radionuclides and organs. MIRD Pamphlet No. 11, p. 6. New York, Society of Nuclear Medicine, 1975.
18. Singh, B., Sharma, S. M., Patel, M. C., Raghavendran, K. V., Berman, M.: Kinetics of large therapy doses of ^{131}I in patients with thyroid cancer. J. Nucl. Med. 15:674–678, 1974.
19. Dillman, L. T., Von der Lage, F. C.: Radionuclide decay schemes and nuclear parameters for use in radiation-dose estimates. MIRD Pamphlet No. 10. New York, Society of Nuclear Medicine, 1975.

20. Snyder, W. S., Ford, M. R., Warner, G. G., Watson, S. B.: A tabulation of dose equivalent per microcurie-day for source and target organs of an adult for various radionuclides. Oak Ridge National Laboratory, ORNL-5000, Part 1 and 2, 1975.

21. Snyder, W. S., Ford, M. R., Warner, G. G.: Specific absorbed fractions for radiation sources uniformly distributed in various organs of a heterogeneous phantom. MIRD Pamphlet. New York, Society of Nuclear Medicine (*to be published*).

22. Benua, R. S., Cicale, N. R., Sonenberg, M., Rawson, R. W.: The relation of radioiodine dosimetry to results and complications in the treatment of metastatic thyroid cancer. Am. J. Roentgenol. 87:171–182, 1962.

23. Bigler, R. E., Rosen, G., Tofe, A. J., Russ, G. A., Francis, M. D., Benua, R. S., Woodard, H. Q.: Distribution of ^{32}P-diphosphonate in patients with osteogenic sarcoma. Proc. Am. Assoc. Cancer Res. 17:103, 1976.

24. Bigler, R. E., Rosen, G., Tofe, A. J., Russ, G. A., Francis, M. D., Benua, R. S., Woodard, H. Q., Kostick, J. A.: Comparative distribution of ^{32}P and ^{99m}Tc diphosphonates in patients with osteogenic sarcoma. J. Nucl. Med. 17:548, 1976.

25. Francis, M. D., Slough, C. L., Tofe, A. J.: Distribution and effect of P-32 EHDP in normal and bone tumor bearing dogs. J. Nucl. Med. 17:548, 1976.

26. Spiers, F. W.: Radionuclides and bone from ^{226}Ra to ^{90}Sr. Br. J. Radiol. 47:833–844, 1974.

27. Woodard, H. Q., Pentlow, K. S., Mayer, K., Laughlin, J. S., Marcove, R. C.: Distribution and retention of ^{35}S-sodium sulfate in man. J. Nucl. Med. 17:285–289, 1976.

Fazle Hosain and Parvathi Hosain

3
Selection of Radionuclides for Therapy

INTRODUCTION

The choice of radionuclide for nuclear medicine therapy depends on the physical characteristics of the radioisotope, chemical nature of the compound, and biological behavior of the radiopharmaceutical. In short, ideally one would like to have a suitable radionuclide in appropriate chemical form so that the biokinetics would facilitate selective uptake of radioactivity in the pathological site for internal radiation therapy. It is, therefore, most important to consider physical, chemical, and biological aspects together in selecting a radionuclide for therapy.

It is also desirable to examine similarities and differences between internal and external radiotherapy, and between therapeutic and diagnostic radiopharmaceuticals.

COMPARATIVE ASPECTS

The primary objective in radiation therapy is to control the disease and ultimately cure the patient. Salient features of external and internal radiation therapy are compared in Table 3-1. The fundamental difference lies in the source of radiation. For internal radiation therapy, we would be concerned with the radionuclides for the manufacture of appropriate radiopharmaceuticals. During recent years we have gained considerable experience in developing diagnostic radiopharmaceuticals. Comparative features of diagnostic and therapeutic radiopharmaceuticals are outlined in Table 3-2. The goal is to attain the highest radiation dose factor for the target site in comparison to the normal tissue. This could best be expressed by a figure of merit, a concept that has been used in radioactivity counting.[1] Wagner and Emmons[2] have dealt with the importance of

Supported by U.S. Public Health Service Grant CA-17802.

Table 3-1

Comparison of Salient Features of External and Internal Radiation Therapy

Feature	External	Internal
Objective	Delivery of an appropriate radiation dose to the target	Delivery of an appropriate radiation dose to the target
Precaution	Least exposure to the nontarget tissue	Least exposure to the nontarget tissue
Tool	Ionizing radiation from different machines	Ionizing radiations from radio-pharmaceuticals
Variables	Nature of beam, energy, and target geometry	Nature of nuclide, chemical, and metabolic status
Precondition	Precise localization of the target, and estimation of the size	Idea of location and function of the target, and estimation of the size

the figure of merit in designing radiopharmaceuticals for organ imaging. The figure of merit can be taken equal to $T/\sqrt{N}$, where T and N are specific activities in target and nontarget tissues. This could be easily adopted for radionuclide therapy with T and N representing radiation doses to target and nontarget tissues.

In the case of diagnostic radiopharmaceuticals , one is more concerned with sensitivity and specificity of the test with the least radiation dose. In therapy, the objective is to attain the highest differential radiation dose, and the figure of merit provides the most suitable criterion to compare different radiopharmaceuticals for a particular therapeutic application.

Table 3-2

Comparative Features of Diagnostic and Therapeutic Radiopharmaceuticals

Feature	Diagnostic	Therapeutic
Controlling factor	Depends on the status of kinetics and metabolism of the radiochemical under certain pathophysiological conditions	Depends on the status of kinetics and metabolism of the radiochemical under certain pathophysiological conditions
Radiation dose	In general, use of radionuclides with low equilibrium absorbed dose constant	In general, use of radionuclides with high equilibrium absorbed dose constant
Manufacturing process	Standardized chemical synthesis: less problem due to associated radiation	Standardized chemical synthesis: more problems due to associated radiation
Instrument requirement	Utilization of advanced nuclear instrumentation	Simple instrumentation, but accurate dosimetry
Primary objective	High specificity and sensitivity of the test for differential diagnosis	High figure of merit with respect to target and nontarget radiation doses

METABOLIC CONSIDERATIONS

A radionuclide is a radioisotope of an element. The chemical behavior and biological interactions are, thus, greatly defined by the elemental nature of the radionuclide. A variety of radioactive compounds can, however, be synthesized using a particular radioisotope. The biological behavior of the radioactive compound depends on several major factors: (1) pathophysiological condition of the patient, (2) chemical nature of the compound, and (3) route of the administration.

The importance of metabolic considerations in the choice of a radionuclide can be illustrated with a typical example of a radiopharmaceutical administered intravenously (Fig. 3-1). The biokinetics (active and passive transport) and the half-life of the radionuclide would control the time-dependent distribution of radioactivity in the body. It is desirable to have the highest accumulation of radioactivity in the target tissue (such as a malignant tumor). The radiation dose to the organ which is likely to produce the most harmful effect (critical organ) should be considered as the nontarget tissue to determine the figure of merit. The half-life of the associated radioisotope (especially when short) greatly alters the biokinetics of the radiopharmaceutical compared to the parent chemical compound (Fig. 3-2). Sometimes it might be possible to use a drug before, during, or after the administration of a radiopharmaceutical to alter the distribution pattern toward a higher figure of merit. Recently, Spencer[3] has emphasized a similar approach as a tissue displacement assay. Further, the radiation dose to the target from a therapeutic dose can also alter the distribution pattern of radioactivity as compared to that of a tracer dose.

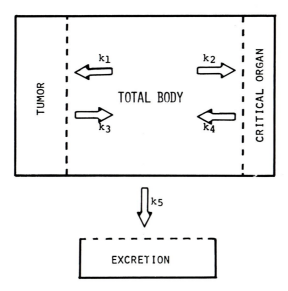

Fig. 3-1. Simplified model of biokinetics of the radiopharmaceutical following intravenous administration: k_1, k_2, k_3, k_4, and k_5 are the transfer rate constants between important pools.

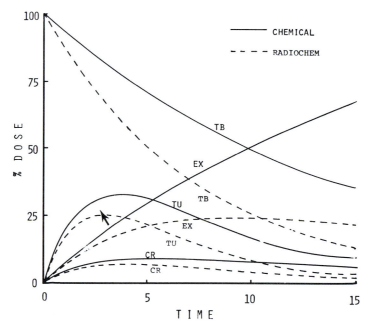

Fig. 3-2. Hypothetical clearance-distribution of a chemical compound (taking biological half-life for total body to be 10-units of time) and comparison with a radiochemical derivative (assuming radionuclide half-life of 10-unit time): TB, EX, TU, and CR representing total body, excretion, tumor, and critical organ, respectively. It is desirable to have a rapid higher accumulation of radioactivity in the target (TU) indicated by the arrow.

RADIOSENSITIVITY CONSIDERATIONS

The effectiveness of radiation therapy is based on the delivery of a radiation dose and the radiosensitivity of the target. The law of Bergonié and Tribondeau[4] outlines the general considerations that the radiosensitivity is directly proportional to the reproductive activity and inversely proportional to the degree of differentiation. Various organs differ in radiosensitivity, and various factors, such as oxygen tension,[5] can alter the radiosensitivity of the target.

A certain amount of total dose to the target is required for an effective therapeutic action. However, this dose must be distributed within a certain time to overcome the effectiveness of repair. The importance of dose rate is documented in Figure 3-3, which is based on an experimental work of Thomson and Tourtellotte.[6] Careful considerations are needed to accomplish the appropriate dose and dose rate from a radiopharmaceutical. The situation might lead beyond the tolerance limit of the critical organ. This would then mean administration of a higher total dose in several fractions. Dose fractionation is commonly encountered in external radiation therapy, and illustrated in Figure 3-4 (based on the work of Fowler[7] and Ellis[8]). Bigler[9] has recently attempted to formulate dose estimates for fractionated doses in terms of a time-dose-fractionation factor for radionuclide therapy. Further, special situations arise in case of internal dosimetry with respect to the exact location of the radionuclide at the cellular level. This has led to the

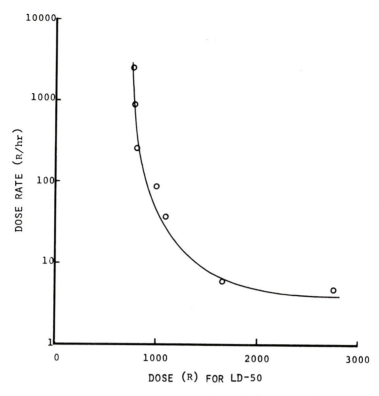

Fig. 3-3. Dose and dose rate in roentgens for LD$_{50}$ of mice exposed to gamma radiation. The total dose was independent of dose rate only at the higher range of the exposure rate.

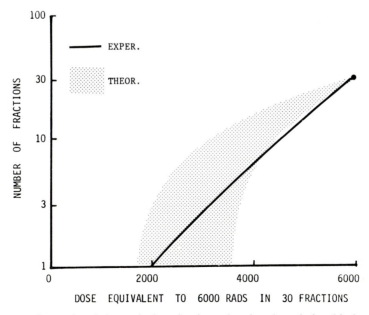

Fig. 3-4. Experimental and theoretical evaluations showing the relationship between the required dose and the fractionation number, equivalent to 6000 rads in 30 fractions.

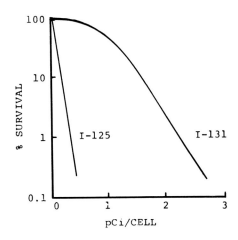

Fig. 3-5. The survival curves of V79 Chinese hamster cells in culture exposed to ^{125}I- and ^{131}I-labeled 5-iodo-2-deoxyuridine. ^{125}I appeared to be far more toxic compared to ^{131}I due to the incorporation of radioiodine into the cellular DNA.

considerations of microdosimetry.[10] Under this condition, absorption of low-energy radiation would induce far more effective therapeutic action as evident in Figure 3-5 (based on the work of Chan and coworkers[11]).

DOSIMETRY CONSIDERATIONS

The radiation dose to a target tissue depends mainly on two factors: (1) biological and (2) physical. The biological factor is related to the time concentration of radioactivity within the target (determined by the biokinetics of the radiopharmaceutical dose). The physical factor is associated with the type and the energy of the ionizing radiation arising from the radioactive decay. These ionizing radiations can be divided into three broad categories: (1) alpha particles; (2) electrons (negatrons, positrons, internally converted electrons and Auger electrons); and (3) photons (high-energy γ-rays and low-energy x-rays). Electrons are the most important component that have been used extensively in internal radiation therapy. Both low-energy and high-energy electrons have special value in radionuclide therapy. Generally, high-energy negatrons have been preferred for therapeutic purposes as they provide intrinsically higher radiation dose to any volume of tissue, except when the volume is too small. Low-energy electrons are specially useful for the irradiation of very small volumes (microdosimetry).

An understanding of the range-energy relation and specific ionization is important for radiation therapy. For internal radiation therapy, electrons of relatively low energy (beta particles of up to about 3 mev) are most important. The range (R), in terms of mg/cm^2, and the total specific ionization (S) as ion pairs per centimeter air corresponding to monoenergetic electrons of energy E (in mev) can be represented by the following equations:

$$R = 412E^{1.265-0.0954\ln E} \tag{1}$$

$$S = 33 + 63E^{-0.9} \tag{2}$$

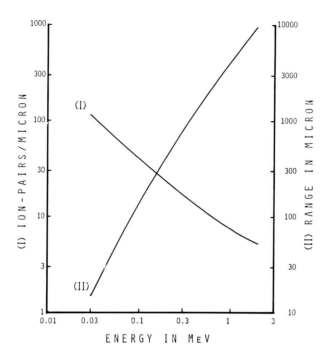

Fig. 3-6. The relationship between the electron energy in mev with (I) specific ionization (ion pairs/μm) and (II) the range (in μm) in a medium of unit density material (approximately the soft tissue).

Figure 3-6 shows such relationships graphically. High-energy electrons within an extended volume would produce higher ionization within the volume due to cross-ionization of long-range electrons from distributed radionuclides. In case of small volumes, the contribution of cross ionization of long-range electrons becomes minimal and the low-energy electrons with high specific ionization become more effective. Phosphorus 32 (with high-energy beta) and iodine 131 (with medium-energy betas) have been used in therapy more frequently. For lesions of over 1 cm diameter, the amount of ^{131}I needed for a certain radiation dose would be about 3.5 times more than that of [32]P. However, when the lesion becomes very small, the situation reverses and requires far greater amounts of specific concentration, specifically of ^{32}P, for the same radiation dose (Fig. 3-7).

The method of radiation dose calculation for internally distributed radionuclides has been greatly standardized and simplified for the general situation.[12] The radiation dose estimate for complete decay of radionuclide in a biological system can be represented by the following equation:

$$D\propto = \int C_t \, dt \times \Sigma \Delta_i \phi_i \qquad (3)$$

The factor $\int C_t \, dt$ represents the time concentration of radioactivity in the region of interest. This can be approximated by 1.44 $T_e C_o$ in simplified situations (T_e =

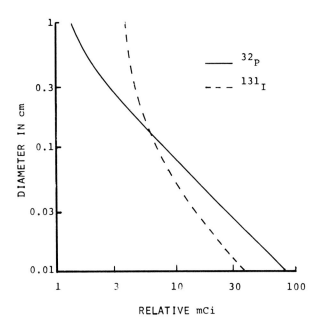

Fig. 3-7. Relative concentration in tissue (mCi/g) required for ^{32}P and ^{131}I for the same radiation dose level for target tissues of different sizes (0.01 to 1 cm in diameter).

effective half-life, and C_o = maximum specific concentration of radioactivity). The factor $\Sigma\Delta_i\phi_i$ is the equilibrium absorbed dose constant for the radionuclide within a specific geometric distribution. The value of Δ_i is given by $2.13 n_i \bar{E}_i$, where n_i is the fraction of disintegration corresponding to the ionizing radiation of average energy $\bar{E}_i$. The factor ϕ_i represents the absorbed fraction of the radiation within the given geometric configuration. The value of ϕ_i becomes very small for high-energy photons, especially for targets of smaller size. For low-energy photons and for all electrons, the value of ϕ_i can be taken equal to 1 unless the target size is very small.

An intrinsic radiation dose associated with a radionuclide can be represented by the equilibrium absorbed dose constant for a relatively small target (few grams). The inverse of this factor would indicate the relative amounts of radionuclide dose (A_j) needed for the same radiation dose level with different radiopharmaceuticals of identical biodistribution pattern (Fig. 3-8). It is evident that not only the pure beta emitters but also other radionuclides (especially positron emitters and radionuclide isomers with high internal conversion) could be used effectively in therapy. Astatine 211 (an alpha emitter) appears to be most promising with respect to both micro- and macrodosimetry. Further, it is important to consider relative tracer doses necessary for an optional result by selecting one of the several radiopharmaceuticals available for a similar diagnostic investigation.[13] Similarly, intercomparison of several radiopharmaceuticals for the same therapeutic application must be considered. Besides the cost, A_j provides one of the bases

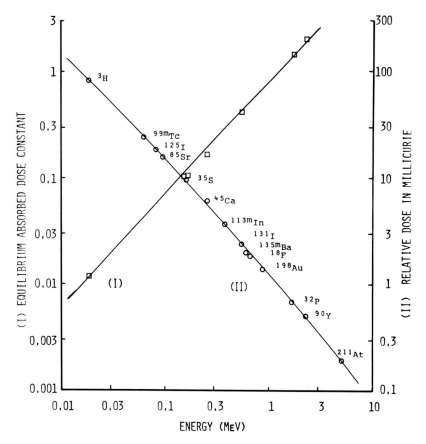

Fig. 3-8. The relationship between the energy (equivalent to E_{max} of beta particles) with (I) equilibrium absorbed dose constants of pure beta emitters, and (II) inverse plot of $\Sigma \Delta_i \phi_i$ for various radionuclides showing index of relative amounts in mCi (A_j).

for such comparison. The actual amount (Q_a) of radionuclide in a radiopharmaceutical for a particular radiation dose to the target (D_t) can be given by:

$$Q_a = D_t \, A_j \, F_c / t_c, \tag{4}$$

where t_c is the time-concentration fraction and F_c is the correction factor based on microdosimetry, tissue sensitivity, and dose fractionation.

DISCUSSION

Nuclear medicine is the application of radioactive materials to the diagnosis and treatment of patients and the study of human disease. The field can be symbolized by a triangle with radiopharmaceuticals, instruments, and biomedical problems at the three corners, and with the patient at the center.[14] Therapeutic nuclear medicine can be defined as the use of radioactive compounds for the treatment of disease. Here, in triangular concept, instruments can be replaced by dosimetry. The therapeutic nuclear medicine probably came into existence when radium chloride was used intravenously in patients with malignant lymphomas[15] (although the technique was discontinued later). Therapeutic uses of artificial radionuclides were reported in 1942.[16,17] Availability of various radionuclides and the potential uses of ionizing radiation in diverse ways opened up a new era. However, so far, ^{131}I is the most acceptable radionuclide in therapy. In 1967 Tabern[18] reviewed the uses of radioisotopes in therapy in a pamphlet published by Picker Nuclear. The major useful compounds appeared to be $Na^{131}I$, $Na_2H^{32}PO_4$, $Cr^{32}PO_4$, ^{198}Au-colloid and ^{90}Y-microspheres. During the past 35 years various radionuclides and radioactive compounds have been evaluated and suggested for therapy ranging from tritium[19] to astatine 211.[20] Indeed, any radionuclide can be used for therapy if an appropriate vehicle is available to obtain high concentration of radioactivity in the target tissue compared to the critical organ. The progress, so far, has been limited. The electrons of relatively short-lived radiopharmaceuticals, preferably obtained with the help of radionuclide generator systems, might be useful in delivering an appropriate radiation dose at a high dose rate with proper dose fractionation.

REFERENCES

1. Loevinger, R., Berman, M.: Efficiency criteria in radioactivity counting. Nucleonics 9(1):26–39, 1951.
2. Wagner, H. N., Jr., Emmons, H.: Characteristics of an ideal radiopharmaceutical. In: Radioactive Pharmaceuticals, G. A. Andrews, R. M. Kniseley, and H. N. Wagner, Jr., (eds.). Springfield, Virginia, Fed. Sci. Tech. Inf. (CONF-651171), U.S. Dept. Comm., pp. 1–32, 1966.
3. Spencer, R. P.: Tissue displacement assay (TDA): a theoretical tool for following radiopharmaceuticals. Med. Hypoth. 1:150–151, 1975.
4. Bergonié, J., Tribondeau, L.: Interpretation of some results of radiotherapy and an attempt at determining logical technique of treatment. Radiat. Res. 11:587–588, 1959. (Translation from C. R. Acad. Sci. [D] (Paris) 143:983–985, 1906.)
5. Gray, L. H.: Oxygenation in radiotherapy: I. Radiobiological considerations. Br. J. Radiol. 30:403–406, 1957.
6. Thomson, J. F., Tourtellotte, W. W.: The effect of dose rate on the LD 50 of mice exposed to gamma radiation from cobalt 60 sources. Am. J. Roentgenol. 69:826–829, 1953.
7. Fowler, J. F.: The estimation of total dose for different number of fractions in radiotherapy. Br. J. Radiol. 38:365–368, 1965.
8. Ellis, F.: Dose, time and fractionation: a clinical hypothesis. Clin. Radiol. 20:1–7, 1969.
9. Bigler, R. E.: Dosimetry for evaluation of the biologic effects of radiation treatment using internally deposited radionuclides and labeled compounds. In: Radiopharmaceutical Dosimetry Symposium, R. J. Cloutier, J. L. Coffey, W. S. Snyder, and E. E. Watson (eds.). Washington, D.C., HEW Publ. (FDA) 76-8044, pp. 221–229, 1976.
10. Reddy, A. R., Nagaratnam, A., Kaul, A., Haase, V.: Microdosimetry of internal emitters: a necessity? In: Radiopharmaceutical Dosimetry Symposium, R. J. Cloutier, J. L. Coffey, W. S. Snyder, and E. E. Watson (eds.). Washington, D.C., HEW Publ. (FDA) 76-8044, pp. 174–185, 1976.

11. Chan, P. C., Lisco, E., Lisco, H., Adelstein, S. J.: The radiotoxicity of iodine-125 in mammalian cells: II. A comparative study on cell survival and cytogenetic responses to ^{125}IUdR, ^{131}IUdR, and ^{3}HTdR. Radiat. Res. 67:332–343, 1976.
12. Loevinger, R., Berman, M.: A schema for absorbed-dose calculations for biologically-distributed radionuclides. J. Nucl. Med. [Suppl.] 1:9–14, 1968.
13. Hosain, P., Hosain, F.: A comprehensive approach for the evaluation of comparative dosimetry of internally administered radiopharmaceuticals. Proc. Int. Cong. Int. Rad. Prot. Assoc., Natl. Tech. Inf. Service (CONF-730907-P2). Springfield, Va., U.S. Dept. Comm., pp. 1175–1179, 1974.
14. Wagner, H. N., Jr.: Introduction. In: Principles of Nuclear Medicine, H. N. Wagner, Jr. (ed.). Philadelphia, W. B. Saunders Co., pp. 1–13, 1968.
15. Stevens, R. H.: The use of intravenous injections of radium chloride in some of the malignant lymphomas. Am. J. Roentgenol. 16:155–161, 1926.
16. Hertz, S., Roberts, A.: Applications of radioactive iodine in therapy of Graves' disease. J. Clin. Invest. 21:624, 1942.
17. Hamilton, J. G., Lawrence, H. H.: Recent clinical developments in the therapeutic application of radio-phosphorus and radio-iodine. J. Clin. Invest. 21:624, 1942.
18. Tabern, D. L.: The use of radioisotopes in therapy. Clin. Scintillator 11(2C):1–23, 1967.
19. Wood, P., Haruy, J., Davis, R., Wood, L.: Cancer radiochemotherapy with 7-tritiotetracycline: I. Rationale and preliminary animal results. In: Tritium, A. A. Moghissi and M. W. Carter (eds.). Las Vegas, Messenger Graphics Publ., pp. 710–723, 1973.
20. Zalutsky, M. R., Friedman, A. M.: Synthesis of a non-labile astatine-protein conjugate. *J. Label. Comp.* 13:181–182, 1977.

Niel Wald and Carol Rump Sherer

4
Chromosomal Alterations After Therapeutic Use of Radionuclides

Before discussing some areas of internal radionuclide therapy in which cytoge-netic changes have been informative, it might be useful to review briefly some pertinent effects of ionizing radiation on the genetic material of the cell. Three clinical areas will be considered in which such effects have been studied, and the information derived will be reviewed.

The effects of ionizing radiation on cell chromosomes were studied mainly on plants because of ease of preparation. Pioneering quantitative work was done by Sax (1938), Giles (1954), and others. A postulated mechanism of damage was developed by Lea (1946). Technical advancements in 1960 by Moorehead et al. led to a major cytogenetic improvement, the ability to analyze human peripheral blood lymphocyte chromosomes.

This revolutionary development immediately accelerated research in many areas, including the study of radiation effects. A number of reviews of the resul-tant new information have appeared, including those of Evans,[1] the United Na-tions Scientific Committee on the Effects of Atomic Radiation,[2] and Dolphin and Lloyd.[3]

It is not feasible to summarize all of the information concerning radiation cytogenetics in this chapter. Instead, the salient points pertinent to an understand-ing of chromosome damage arising from therapeutic uses of radionuclides will be considered briefly.

1. The test system utilized for most studies of cytogenetic radiation effects is the examination of the chromosomes of circulating human lymphocytes. The evaluation of lymphocyte chromosome damage is particularly appropriate when the radiation comes from radionuclides circulating in the blood. The information becomes more difficult to interpret when the radiation source is localized and concentrated in a particular organ or system.

2. The lymphocyte is an extremely radiosensitive cell. The inferences drawn by evaluating lymphocyte chromosome damage may be reasonably accepted as representative of some high turnover cell renewal systems such as the other blood cell precursors and the gastrointestinal lining. However, other tissues may be relatively less affected by the same radiation exposure.

3. The varying effect of the same radiation exposure administered at different dose rates is a highly important concept to recall when dealing with internal radiation emitters such as therapeutic radionuclides. Simple chromosome deletion, in which the end of the chromosome is broken off into a fragment separate from the original chromosome, is not related to the rate at which the radiation is delivered. This is because a single "hit" or radiation interaction is sufficient to produce a deletion and fragment. However, for the more complex chromosome aberrations such as the production of a "ring" or a dicentric chromosome, two "hits" or radiation interactions are required. Because of the transient "stickiness" which occurs at the breakage site as a result of alterations in the DNA-histone complex, the abnormal rejoinings, which are recognized as dicentric or ring chromosomes, must occur within a relatively short time. Also, the two breakage events have to occur in close physical proximity in order for the abnormal rejoining to take place. If the dose rate is low, the likelihood of the second event occurring close enough in time and space to produce the complex restructured chromosome is relatively low. At higher dose rates the same total dose is much more effective in producing these aberrations. The dose-response relationship curve is curvilinear, rising with a frequency which is close to the square of the dose rather than the linear dose-response relationship which is characteristic of the deletion and fragment phenomenon. Since therapeutic radionuclides are generally administered in a form to deliver a high dose within a short time, the dose rate characteristically falls off rapidly. This produces a rapidly and continually changing dose-response relationship over time which is difficult to interpret and use for the prediction of biological effect.

The interpretation of the dose-response data is made even more difficult when the radiation distribution in the body is nonuniform, allowing some of the circulating lymphocytes to receive a greater exposure and a higher dose rate than others. The difficulties involved in interpreting the cytogenetic effects of internal emitters, as compared to the greater simplicity in interpretation of external radiation exposure effects on the same test system, have limited the number of studies of therapeutic radionuclide effects on chromosomes.

Despite the foregoing considerations, the increasingly useful information derived from studies of external radiation exposure did stimulate a number of investigators to apply the technique to therapeutic radionuclide studies. The problems for which solutions have been sought using cytogenetic methods and the resultant studies and conclusions will be reviewed in the remainder of this chapter.

DO INTERNAL RADIATION EMITTERS ACT LIKE EXTERNAL IRRADIATION ON CHROMOSOMES?

Interest in the use of chromosomal techniques to establish a dose-response relationship was encouraged by an evaluation of the oncogenic effects of external radiation on patients with spondylitis.[4] In hopes of obtaining parallel information for internal radiation, Boyd, Buchanan, and Lennox[5] examined chromosomes from patients treated with radioiodine (^{131}I) for thyrotoxicosis or thyroid cancer. The percentage of normal cells declined and structural abnormalities appeared in circulating lymphocyte cultures from individuals treated with 100 to 150 mCi for thyroid cancer. Chromosome damage from a dose of 100 mCi of ^{131}I was found to be equivalent to damage produced in patients receiving a dose of 250 rads of x-rays to the spine, thus suggesting a relatively low risk of leukemogenesis.

Several investigators analyzed sequential chromosomal data to define the relationship between administration of ^{131}I and the cytogenetic effects present following such therapy. MacIntyre and Dobyns[6] noted an increase in the frequency of aneuploidy, breaks, fragments, and deletions as early as 20 minutes after administration of large doses of [131]I. The period of maximum exhibition of abnormalities was found to be 3 to 12 hours post-administration, which closely corresponded to the time at which the highest level of ^{131}I was detected in the blood. Some structural abnormalities were located in lymphocytes as many as 6 years after treatment, however, suggesting the importance of sublethal damage in the production of late effects.

Nofal and Beierwaltes[7] extended studies of magnitude and duration of increased aberration frequencies after radioiodine therapy. In patients with thyroid carcinoma treated with 150 to 250 mCi of ^{131}I, aberrations were found 30 minutes after treatment. The frequency and severity of numerical and structural aberrations were much greater following the large dosage used in the treatment for thyroid carcinoma than those found following the smaller dosage used in the treatment of hyperthyroidsm. Even in the latter, doses of about 10 mCi produced visible effects. Additional investigators, including Cantolino and colleagues[8] and Speight and coworkers[9] reported that chromosome damage following ^{131}I treatment for thyrotoxicosis persisted for at least several years after therapy.

CAN THE MEANINGFUL DOSE-RESPONSE RELATIONSHIP DERIVED FROM EXTERNALLY IRRADIATED PATIENTS BE USED IN THOSE RECEIVING ^{131}I THERAPY TO THE THYROID?

Utilizing more modern methods, such as 48-hour cultures to avoid a loss of aberrations through a second division of lymphocytes, Blackwell[10] attempted to relate dicentric chromosome occurrence to ^{131}I dose in order to compare with the dicentric chromosome frequencies previously related to external exposure doses. The dicentric frequency in patients treated with radioiodine did not follow the classic distribution expected from the random irradiation of cells. The investigators suggested that the dose of ^{131}I administered seemed to affect the lymphocytes not as if it had been evenly distributed throughout the entire body, but rather as if a portion of the lymphocytes received a much higher dose than the others.

By comparing the frequency of aberrations in lymphocytes of cancer patients treated with radioiodine to those from an in vitro calibration curve from a ^{60}Co source, Lloyd et al.[11] obtained estimates of the whole-body dosage equivalent. If the thyroid had been previously ablated for thyroid carcinoma, there was good agreement between the cytogenetic estimate of dose and the estimate based on thyroid uptake, plasma activity, and urinary activity. For individuals retaining partial or complete thyroid function, the cytogenetic estimation of dose was consistently higher than the calculated dose. In the latter cases, the investigators pointed out that there was always a concentration of ^{131}I found in the thyroid as well as in the liver, with resultant selective irradiation of some of the lymphocytes.

It is misleading, therefore, to assume that external radiation responses will be duplicated by internal irradiation when selective irradiation is a distinct possibility.

DO ALL IODINE ISOTOPES PRODUCE THE SAME
CYTOGENETIC DAMAGE?

Boyd and coworkers[12] investigated the possibility of utilizing ^{125}I rather than ^{131}I for therapy of thyroid disorders. It had been previously determined that ^{125}I causes more selective damage in the thyroid than ^{131}I due to its low-energy electron emissions. The therapeutic dose of ^{125}I, therefore, emits less radiation than the therapeutically equivalent dose of ^{131}I. Cytogenetic analysis demonstrated that ^{125}I is capable of inducing a level of chromosome damage in lymphocytes of treated patients at least as high as that found in patients treated with ^{131}I.

Further studies were instituted by Chan et al.[13] to compare the relative effects of ^{131}I, ^{125}I, and tritium in deoxyuridine compounds on hamster cells in tissue culture. Chromosomal studies indicated that ^{125}I had a 10-fold greater ability to produce chromosome damage as compared to ^{131}I in that particular test system, probably because of the intimate relation of the internal emitter to the DNA in the particular chemical form that was used.

IS LYMPHOCYTE CHROMOSOMAL DAMAGE
REPRESENTATIVE OF THAT OCCURRING IN OTHER CELLS
AND TISSUES?

The significance of damage found in mitotic lymphocytes as related to other organs such as the thyroid itself or the gonads has only rarely been investigated to determine if the lymphocyte is uniquely vulnerable to radiation injury. By studying the meiotic premetaphase and metaphase cells in the testes of male mice, Subramanyam et al.[14] demonstrated that ^{131}I induced translocations and polyploid cells, although these phenomena did not exhibit a clear dosage effect. The investigators suggested that only cells in radiosensitive stages of spermatogenesis (i.e., B and intermediate spermatogonia) will exhibit damage characteristic of irradiation. The dose of ^{131}I utilized relative to the size of the mouse was several-fold lower than the therapeutic doses administered to patients. It was therefore urged that caution be taken to prevent unnecessary ^{131}I irradiation that may be capable of inducing radiation damage in meiotic cells (although this has not been demonstrated directly in humans).

A different approach to estimating the gonadal effects of irradiation was utilized by Einhorn and colleagues,[15] who examined the children of parents treated with radioactive iodine. The investigators hoped to determine if children conceived after parental radioiodine therapy for hyperthyroidism or cancer of the thyroid demonstrated an increased frequency of aberrations which they would have inherited if the parental germ cell had been damaged. An increase in the frequency of abnormal cells in the children of parents given ^{131}I therapy was noted. The extent of such damage was related generally to the magnitude of the exposure of the parent, indicating that a causal relationship may exist. One child had been exposed in utero when his mother had been treated with 1.5 mCi 5 months before delivery. The child exhibited the highest frequency of breaks among the children studied, although the parent received the lowest treatment dose among the parents treated.

Finally, Moore and Colvin[16] looked directly at thyroid cells in Chinese hamsters which had received 0.01 to 1 μ Ci ^{131}I at 7 to 10 days of age. At 30 days after treatment there was a high aberration frequency which dropped markedly by 1 year post-exposure. Some damaged cells persisted for life, however.

WHAT IS THE RELATIVE CYTOGENETIC EFFECT OF A PURE β EMITTER (^{32}P) COMPARED TO THAT OF ^{131}I?

The problems involved in cytogenetic analysis of blood cells from patients receiving ^{32}P for polycythemia vera or related blood disorders are considerably more complex than those of hematologic normals. Macdiarmid[17] reported that even before treatment an elevated frequency of abnormal bone marrow cells was present in many of the cases, including the major chromosome lesions seen after irradiation. Fourteen of the patients showed a significant increase in the frequency of aberrations following treatment, which was above the somewhat increased pretreatment level. There was a subsequent fall in aberration frequency. Repeated doses resulted in a continuous high level of abnormalities. In this particular system, therefore, radiation damage adds to an already hematologically unstable situation. The usual dose-response relationship cannot be utilized because the target cells are initially defective.

Investigators attempted to discern whether radiation or the natural course of polycythemia vera was producing the abnormalities. To distinguish between disease and treatment abnormalities, Barnes, Holmes, and Ilbery[18] studied chromosomes of patients following administration of ^{32}P or venesection. The frequency of major chromosomal lesions increased markedly in patients who received ^{32}P. However, some aberrations appear to be imposed by the disease state. In a similar study the diseased cells responded well to radiation treatment, but Schwartz and Ehrlich[19] felt that irradiation might be involved in the leukemic transformations of some polycythemia patients. This concept was supported by epidemiologic studies of Modan and Lillienfeld[20] and may reflect an unusually high sensitivity to irradiation in this disease.

CAN CYTOGENETIC STUDY DETECT AN UNEXPECTED INTERNAL DISTRIBUTION OF A THERAPEUTIC RADIONUCLIDE AND ITS CAUSE?

Radiocolloids ^{198}Au and ^{90}Y are utilized in the treatment of joint diseases by injection into the joint, primarily the knee, to relieve pain and effusion and increase joint mobility. The beneficial effects of injections of ^{198}Au were first realized by Ansell and coworkers[21] and Makin and colleagues.[22] The use of similar agents including ^{90}Y quickly followed.

Lymphocytes of treated individuals were analyzed by Stevenson et al.,[23] who found that in a number of cases there was a marked increase in the frequency of dicentric chromosomes. Unfortunately, the dose-response relationship remained unclear because the total dose administered did not correlate well with the frequency of dicentrics. Patients receiving low doses often presented high levels of chromosomal damage, whereas several patients with low damage levels received high doses.

Within the same year, Oka et al.[24] reported that as much as 10 percent of the ^{90}Y injected into patients' joints could be located in the inguinal lymph nodes. The group discovered that leakage from the joint to the lymph nodes could be reduced by complete bed rest for 3 days. Two years after the initial discovery of cytogenetic aberrations following treatment by radiocolloids, Stevenson and a large cooperative study group[25] were able to demonstrate that the frequency of dicentrics versus the amount of radioactivity found in the area of the nodes did indeed show a meaningful dose-response relationship. It is clear that leakage was occurring from the joint and the response was due to the concentration of radiation in the lymph nodes through which the lymphocytes were circulating. This was borne out in Stevenson's review[26] of the frequency of abnormal chromosomes found following administration of several radioisotopes in five sets of clinical data from radioisotope therapy patients. There was a relatively similar effect from the ^{198}Au and the ^{90}Y treatment except in one series where there was much less of an effect. It was noted that in this series the patients were restricted to bed rest for 48 hours on the hypothesis that immobilization of the joint results in much less leakage. This was supported by the cytogenetic evidence.

It is interesting to note that a melanoma patient who was treated with ^{32}P-lipiodol injected into the lymphatic system demonstrated a much higher frequency of dicentrics per millicurie than was found in the other isotope treatments. This finding substantiates the concept that the concentration of radiation in localized areas produces the damage in lymphocytes circulating in and out of the lymphoid tissue.

Further studies of intraarticular therapy led to the use of different compounds which had a decreased leakage from the joint and which showed less chromosomal effects.[27]

SUMMARY

In summary, several benefits can be derived from the assessment of radiobiologic damage from therapeutic radionuclides through chromosomal analysis. Such studies provide a technique by which risk can be given quantitative values rather than estimated values obtained through a risk equation. Through cytogenetics, investigators can compare the relative hazard of two different materials where nonuniform distribution makes either measurement or calculation questionable. Cytogenetic analysis opens the door to microdosimetry at the cellular and intracellular level that can allow such comparisons as that between ^{125}I and ^{131}I in a biologically meaningful way. Special hazards, such as the joint leakage phenomenon in intraarticular therapy, can be identified and the effectiveness of efforts to reduce these special hazards can be evaluated. Cytogenetic analysis can also be a possible tool for determination of the relative radiosensitivity of the target organ in order to predict the likelihood of related late effects, as in the ^{32}P therapy for polycythemia vera.

Most studies under controlled conditions to evaluate the biological effects require the analysis of a large number of cells. It is a slow and tedious task to carry out cytogenetic analysis for radiation effects in which the investigator must score hundreds of cells. Our laboratory[28] and various others in different parts of the world are attempting to automate the technique of radiation-induced aberration scoring. If we succeed, we will have an even more practical tool for facilitating and improving nuclear medicine therapy.

REFERENCES

1. Evans, H. J.: Actions of radiations on chromosomes. In: The Scientific Bases of Medicine. London, Athalone Press, pp. 321–339, 1967.
2. United Nations Scientific Committee on the Effects of Atomic Radiation: 24th Session, Supplement 13 (A/7613), Annex C, Radiation-induced chromosome aberrations in human cells. New York, United Nations, pp. 98–155, 1969.
3. Dolphin, G. W., Lloyd, D. C.: The significance of radiation induced chromosome aberrations in radiological protection. J. Med. Genet. 11:181–189, 1974.
4. Tough, I. M., Buckton, K. E., Baikie, A. G., et al.: X-ray induced chromosome damage in man. Lancet 2:849–851, 1960.
5. Boyd, E., Buchanan, W. W., Lennox, B.: Damage to chromosomes by therapeutic doses of radioiodine. Lancet 1:977–978, 1961.
6. MacIntyre, M. N., Dobyns, B. M.: Anomalies in chromosomes of the circulating leukocytes in man following large doses of radioactive iodine. J. Clin. Endocrinol. Metab. 22:1171–1181, 1962.
7. Nofal, M. M., Beierwaltes, W. H.: Persistent chromosomal aberrations following radioiodine therapy. J. Nucl. Med. 5:840–850, 1964.
8. Cantolino, S. J., Schmickel, R. D., Ball, M., et al.: Persistent chromosomal aberrations following radioiodine therapy for thyrotoxicosis. N. Engl. J. Med. 275:739–744, 1966.
9. Speight, J. W., Smith, E., Baba, W. I., et al.: Lymphocyte chromosomes in untreated and ^{131}I treated thyrotoxic patients. J. Endocrinol. 42:277–282, 1968.
10. Blackwell, N.: Chromosomal findings in patients treated with small doses of iodine 131. Mutat. Res. 26(3):397–402, 1974.
11. Lloyd, D. C., Purrott, R. J., Dolphin, G. W., et al.: A comparison of physical and cytogenetic estimates of radiation dose in patients treated with iodine 131 for thyroid carcinoma. Int. J. Radiat. Biol. 30(5):473–485, 1976.
12. Boyd, E., Ferguson-Smith, M. A., McDougall, I. R., et al.: Chromosome breakage in human peripheral lymphocytes after radioactive iodine ^{125}I treatment. Radiat. Res. 57:482–487, 1974.
13. Chan, P. C., Lisco, E., Lisco, H., et al.: The radiotoxicity of iodine-125 in mammalian cells. II. A comparative study on cell survival and cytogenetic responses to ^{125}IUdR, ^{131}IUdR, and ^{3}HTdR. Radiat. Res. 67(2):332–343, 1976.
14. Subramanyam, S., Murthy, D., Reddi, O. S.: Cytological investigations on the effects of ^{131}I in male mice. Indian J. Med. Res. 63(12):1680–1687, 1975.
15. Einhorn, J., Hulten, M., Lindsten, J., et al.: Clinical and cytogenetic investigation in children of parents treated with radioiodine. Acta. Radiol. [Ther.] (Stockh.) 11:193–207, 1972.

16. Moore, W., Colvin, M.: Persistence of chromosomal aberrations in Chinese hamster thyroid following administration of iodine 131. J. Nucl. Med. 9(4):165–167, 1968.
17. Macdiarmid, W. D.: Chromosome changes following treatment of polycythemia with radioactive phosphorus. Q. J. Med. 34:133–143, 1965.
18. Barnes, C. A., Holmes, H. L., Ilbery, P. T. L.: Chromosomal aberration following phosphorus treatment of polycythemia. Aust. Radiol. 13:396–417, 1969.
19. Schwartz, S. O., Ehrlich, L.: The relationship of polycythemia vera to leukemia; a critical review. Acta. Haematol. (Basel) 4:129–147, 1950.
20. Modan, B., Lillienfeld, A. M.: Polycythemia vera and leukemia—the role of radiation treatment. Medicine (Baltimore) 44:305–344, 1965.
21. Ansell, B. M., Crook, A., Mallard, J. R., et al.: Evaluation of intraarticular colloidal gold [198]Au in the treatment of persistent knee effusions. Ann. Rheum. Dis. 22:435, 1963.
22. Makin, M., Robin, G. C., Stein, J. A.: Radioactive gold in the treatment of persistent synovial effusion. Isr. Med. J. 22:107–111, 1963.
23. Stevenson, A. C., Bedford, J., Hill, A., et al.: Chromosome damage in patients who have had intraarticular injections of radioactive gold. Lancet 1:837–839, 1971.
24. Oka, M., Rekonen, A., Ruotsi, A., et al.: Intra-articular injection of Y-90 resin colloid in the treatment of rheumatoid knee joint effusions. Acta. Rheum. Scand. 17:148–160, 1971.
25. Stevenson, A. C., Bedford, J., Dolphin, G. W., et al.: A cytogenetic and scanning study of patients receiving intra-articular injection of gold-198 and yttrium-90. Ann. Rheum. Dis. 32:112–123, 1973.
26. Stevenson, A. C.: Chromosomal damage in human lymphocytes from radioisotope therapy. Ann. Rheum. Dis. [Suppl.] 32:19–22, 1973.
27. Gumpel, J. M., Beer, T. C., Crawley, J. C. W., et al.: Yttrium 90 in persistent synovitis of the knee—a single centre comparison. The retention and extra articular spread of ^{90}Y radiocolloids. B. J. Radiol. 48:377–381, 1975.
28. Wald, N., Li, C. C., Herron, J. M., et al.: Automated analysis of chromosome damage. In Automation of Cytogenetics. CONF-751158, Livermore, Calif. Lawrence Livermore Laboratory, pp. 39–50, 1976.

Mohamed A. Antar and Richard P. Spencer

5
Effects of Therapy on Major Organ Function and Imaging

The task of nuclear medicine is not only to aid in establishing a diagnosis, but also to assist in the planning of treatment, often in delivering therapy, in evaluating the results of treatment, and in detecting recurrence. In other words, nuclear medicine has a role in the *overall management* of many patients (Table 5-1). In the present discussion we will focus on one aspect—what effect does therapy have on tissues as reflected in organ function and imaging studies? A broad perspective is that although diseases can cause changes in organ structure and function, so can therapy. Separating out the individual effects of the initial disorder and those of the treatment may be difficult, but it can often be essential to patient management. By therapy we mean the full range of surgical intervention, radiation therapy, and the use of chemotherapeutic agents (Table 5-2). Although we can not dwell on the role of nuclear medicine in treatment planning, several authors have pointed out particular applications in delineating location of specific structures such as esophagus, stomach, kidneys, bladder, and spleen for radiation therapy.[1,2] In the present discussion, the emphasis is focused on one major aspect—what effects does therapy have on tissues as reflected in organ functions and imaging studies?

In order to gauge the effects of therapy, we must have information about the natural history of a disorder. Figure 5-1 provides a pertinent example of this. The upper portion is a liver scan performed on a 36-year-old man. Both hepatomegaly and splenomegaly are apparent, as well as uneven distribution of radiocolloid, suggesting space-occupying lesions. The patient had a past history of ethanol intake and at least one episode of pancreatitis. Both the alkaline phosphatase and 5'-nucleotidase were elevated. This was an example of hepatitis. It did not represent an intrahepatic malignancy. On conservative therapy, the patient improved. A repeat study, 26 months later, showed a decrease in size of both the liver and spleen and a more normal pattern of radionuclide distribution. Conversely, a patient with a known malignancy can still be subject to other medical and surgical

---

Supported by U.S. Public Health Service Grant CA 17802 from the National Cancer Institute.

Table 5-1
Role of Nuclear Medicine in
Overall Management of Patients

---

1. Establish diagnosis
    a. What is wrong and how extensive
    b. Defining natural history of the disorder
2. Assist in treatment planning
    a. Outline organs or masses
    b. Aid in guiding biopsies
3. Occasionally aid in delivering therapy
4. Evaluating the results of treatment
5. Detecting recurrence or complications

---

problems. Studies with radiopharmaceuticals can be of use in defining the natural history of a disorder.

Radiation-induced lesions result in highly variable clinical manifestations in different anatomic sites. These include such diverse findings as pulmonary fibrosis, gastric ulceration, intestinal obstruction, nephritis and hypertension, cessation of bone growth, bone necrosis, decrease in salivation, liver failure, cardiomyopathy, neurologic disorders, functional spinal cord transection, and cataract.

Furthermore, radiation injury may be mistaken for recurrent cancer. Additional irradiation or aggressive chemotherapy of a radiation-associated lesion, mistaken for a recurrent neoplasm, can be detrimental.

BRAIN

The initial clinical response of the central nervous system to irradiation may be increased intracranial pressure due to radiation edema; this may be difficult to analyze, since cerebral edema may exist before radiation treatment for brain tumors. In the subacute phase, severe manifestations of infarction and gliosis may show themselves as brain necrosis. In the chronic phase, after total brain irradiation in children, poor cerebration and mental retardation may manifest them-

Table 5-2
Nuclear Medicine Role in Assessing the Effects of Therapy on Major Organs

---

The effects may be caused by different modalities, e.g.,
1. External radiation (e.g., radiotherapy of cancer and bomb survival in Japan); "Chicago endemic due to radiation to neck"
2. Internally administered radioisotopic therapy, consequences of fallout
3. Chemotherapy for cancer and other medications
4. Surgical procedures
5. Any combination of the above

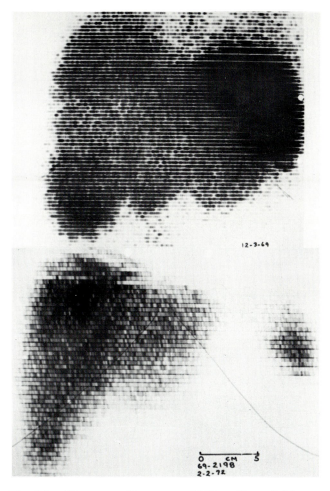

Fig. 5-1. The top rectilinear scan (^{99m}Tc-sulfur colloid) was performed on a 36-year-old man. The bottom scan, on the same patient, was obtained 26 months later.

selves.[3] However, preexisting hydrocephalus due to a posterior fossa tumor may also cause cerebral atrophy and poor mentation, independent of the radiation effect.[4,5] The peak latent period between irradiation and onset of necrosis ranges between 1 and 3 years.[5]

The mechanism of delayed damage of the brain is not yet clearly established. Although some authors consider that direct damage to the neurons plays a part, this is likely to be of importance only in those rare cases with acute demyelination. Most of the evidence indicates that impairment of the fine vasculature of the brain is the dominant mechanism in radiation damage.[5] In general, the vasculoastrocytic unit is considered the most radiovulnerable component of the CNS. The white matter suffers damage more easily than the gray matter, presumably because the blood supply to the gray matter is more abundant.

Clinically, radiation damage appears as a mass lesion in the brain, the symptoms depending on the site of the lesion. The differential diagnosis lies between recurrence of intracranial tumor, brain abscess, and brain necrosis. Postirradiation necrosis can also present as a glioma[6]; occlusion or hypoplasia of the internal carotid artery and its primary branches following radiation therapy for intracranial tumor in children has also been reported.[7] Postradiation cortical atrophy with or without ventricular dilation may occur.[5,8]

It has been difficult to obtain objective evidence of the role to be played by the procedures in nuclear medicine in evaluating the response of intracranial lesions to therapy.

1. If intracranial surgery has been employed, then the bone flap may cause increased accumulation of radionuclides for weeks to months afterward.
2. Often it is possible to document decrease in apparent intracranial lesion size, or avidity of accumulation of radiotracer, after radiation therapy or chemotherapy (Fig. 5-2). However, there is still much uncertainty as to whether this indicates an absolute change in lesion size or simply reflects altered permeability or binding of radiotracer. The role to be played by cerebral dynamic studies and brain scans in the evaluation of brain tumor response to therapy,[9] as well as the role of computerized tomography in such cases,[10] must still be defined.

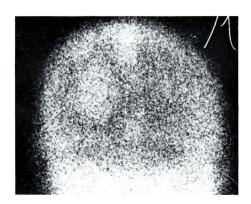

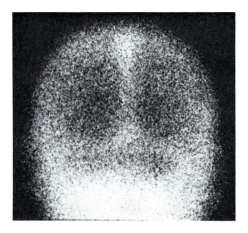

Fig. 5-2. Posterior scintiphotos in a 39-year-old woman with metastatic adenocarcinoma of the lung. After the top study was obtained, the patient was given an estimated 3800 R whole brain irradiation by external radiation as well as chemotherapy and irradiation of the chest lesion. Bottom: The brain scan was repeated 11 months after the initial study. The lesion is not visualized (^{99m}Tc-pertechnetate, after oral perchlorate in both studies).

Nordman and Rekonen[9] obtained ^{99m}Tc-pertechnetate scintigraphy on 31 patients with cerebral tumors, both before and after radiotherapy. The radiation total dose varied from 3500 to 6000 rads. Immediately after irradiation, pertechnetate accumulation in brain tumors remained the same in 22 percent of the cases. It increased in a large proportion of the cases (58 percent). Three months after the irradiation, the uptake remained increased in 50 percent of the patients studied, and decreased in the remaining patients.

The increased accumulation of ^{99m}Tc-pertechnetate may be caused by increased capillary permeability in the irradiated area. Irradiation of cerebral lymphoma in mice showed an increase of 200 percent in the capillary permeability of the tumor region.[11] On the other hand, Nordman and Rekonen[9] reported that accumulation of ^{75}Se-sodium selenite diminished in the majority of the irradiated cases (76 percent), and in no case did this uptake increase.

In a recent study of several patients who received radiation therapy for brain metastasis, the ^{99m}Tc-pertechnetate scintigraphy showed that the lesions had decreased uptake post-irradiation, and such decreased uptake was associated with improvement of the clinical condition of the patients.[12] On the other hand, in another patient, such decreased uptake in the lesion after radiation therapy was not associated with an improvement in signs and symptoms. Three weeks after the last postirradiation scan the patient died. On autopsy, there was still a large metastatic lesion in the area originally seen in the pretreatment scan. The decrease of ^{99m}Tc uptake in this case may be related to gliosis as well as to changes in the fine vasculature of the tumor and the adjacent brain tissue. These cases point out again the difficulty in the interpretation of ^{99m}Tc-pertechnetate brain scans after irradiation.

The administration of corticosteroids is frequently beneficial in the treatment of cerebral neoplasms associated with cerebral edema. Fletcher et al.[13] and the authors[12] have shown that dexamethasone administration resulted in a decrease in the apparent size of the original lesions on ^{99m}Tc-pertechnetate scan. They attributed the change in apparent size of the original lesion to a decrease in peritumor edema.

PITUITARY GLAND

The pituitary gland has been considered to be radiation resistant and to manifest minimal or no acute damage following therapeutic dose levels. A recent report,[14] however, pointed out that chronic damage following external irradiation of the normal pituitary, delivered incidentally during radiotherapy of neoplasms of the head and neck, may be more common than has been appreciated in the past. There were decreases in the levels of human gonadotropins, and of the ^{131}I uptake by the thyroid, as well as other evidence of hypopituitarism.

The availability of synthetic hypothalamic hormones for clinical investigations and the radioimmunoassay of hormones have both been useful to document hypopituitarism after external radiotherapy for nasopharyngeal cancer.[15] Samaan et al.[15] reported that such hypopituitarism is of both hypothalamic and pituitary origin.

One of the complications of radiation therapy for pituitary tumor is the development of an "empty sella," i.e., intrasellar extension of the subarachnoid space.[5] The mechanism of the empty sella syndrome under these conditions is as yet poorly understood. Fibrosis and contraction presumably take place. Pushing or pulling of the optic chiasm into the empty sella that was originally occupied by the tumor prior to the therapy may occur and thus give rise to the visual disturbance and headaches so frequent in the syndrome.[5]

THYROID

The thyroid gland was among the first organs to be studied by radionuclides. We must consider radiation and the thyroid from several aspects:

1. Results of atomic bomb exposure or fallout.
2. Prior childhood external irradiation of head or neck for benign lesions (moderate radiation doses).
3. External irradiation to the neck and head for cancer therapy.
4. Results of radioiodide therapy for hyperthyroidism and cancer of the thyroid.

In some animal species, the thyroid has been shown to be sensitive to radiation-induced tumors (Parker and coworkers[16] give reference to the literature).

Results of Atomic Bomb Exposure of Fallout

In a human population, the citizens of Hiroshima and Nagasaki, thyroid carcinoma was more common in women and in those exposed to a whole-body dose of 50 rads (or greater) of atomic radiation 13 to 26 years previously. No radiosensitive period was demonstrated. That is, even persons aged 50 at the time of exposure to the radiation were not exempt from developing thyroid carcinoma. There is a continuing higher risk in women up to 26 years after exposure, in contrast to the incidence of leukemia, which peaked at 6 years after exposure. Euthyroidism was the general rule, suggesting cellular mutation rather than atrophy with subsequent loss of function. Of the tumors found, 76 percent were papillary or papillary sclerosing, and 24 percent were follicular (of 74 total cases).[16] It should be pointed out that in these cases there was a radiation dose not only to the thyroid, but also to the whole body (which ranged from 69 to 175 rads). Fallout radiation has been associated with thyroid disorders in 31 percent of the cases in the Marshall Islands.[17] The findings included hypothyroidism, benign adenomatous nodules, and malignant lesions. Although the radioactive debris in that incident was largely composed of radioiodide, other radionuclides were also involved. The preponderance of lesions occurred in children exposed at less than 10 years of age who had received greater thyroid exposures (500 to 1400 rads) and a whole-body dose of 175 rads. Fortunately, there have been no comparable major fallout events in North America. Rallison and coworkers[18] studied the incidence of thyroid disease in children who might have been exposed to fallout in Utah and Nevada from U.S. bomb tests in the 1950s. Although there was only a short follow-up, no significant increase of thyroid carcinoma or nodular goiter was found in the children.

In the above instances of atomic bomb- or fallout-associated cases of thyroid neoplasia, the lesions are almost always "cold" in terms of lack of uptake of radioiodide, and palpable nodules were present. Given a high-risk group, should they be screened by means of radionuclide scans? This question assumes urgency because of the high incidence of thyroid carcinoma associated with prior external radiation of the neck. What was once termed "a Chicago endemic"[19] is now recognized as a national problem.

Prior Childhood External Radiation of Head or Neck
for Benign Lesions: Low and Moderate Doses

The association of thymic or tonsillar radiation in children with subsequent thyroid neoplasia was first detected by Duffy and Fitzgerald in 1950.[20] From half to three-quarters of all children with thyroid neoplasia were found to have a history of prior radiation to the neck, typically 300 to 600 rads delivered during the first 5 years of life.[21] The thyroid neoplasms were detected approximately 10 years after the radiation exposure.[22] In another series of patients, however, DeGroot and Paloyan[19] found that these patients developed tumors an average of 20 years after x-ray exposure. Clinical findings were similar to those of the "nonir-radiated" carcinoma patients, but the tumors were less invasive and never undif-ferentiated.

Individuals with radiation of the head or neck as a child should be carefully examined. Those with thyroid nodules, and probably those with scan-demonstrated thyroid defects, should likely be subject to operation. Although this is not definitively proven, it appears that the distribution of types of thyroid cancers found in the irradiated population, as well as the biological behavior of the tumors, does not differ from thyroid cancer found in the general population (al-though the incidence is of course much higher in those with prior irradiation). There are those who might argue that suppressive therapy (by means of exogen-ous thyroid hormone) might be indicated. Another question focuses on which radiotracer should be utilized in screening these irradiation-associated patients. Most centers employ ^{99m}Tc-pertechnetate for thyroid scans. However, the dispa-rate handling of ^{99m}Tc-pertechnetate and radioiodide in occasional cases raises doubts.[139,140] There is, thus, some rationale for employing ^{123}I if it is of high radionuclidic purity and available.

Arnold et al.[23] evaluated 1452 persons who had x-ray therapy to the neck region for benign conditions 18 to 35 years previously. The usual radiation dose was 300 to 600 rads. Thyroid abnormalities were found in 21 percent. The inci-dence of nodules as detected by palpation was 9.3 percent in men and 15.5 percent in women. This is much higher than in the Framingham survey of 5127 persons aged 30 to 59 years (there were palpable nodules in 1.5 percent of men and 6.4 percent of women[24]). Furthermore, the incidence of nodules detected by thyroid ^{99m}Tc-pertechnetate scintigram was considerably higher (17.8 percent for men and 22.6 percent for women) than the already high incidence detected by palpation alone. The authors have not detected any positive scan findings in areas where the thyroid gland was normal by subsequent surgical pathology, suggesting that the nuclear image was not "too sensitive." Thyroid scintigram detected 96 percent of the thyroid abnormalities. It, however, did not appear to help differentiate benign from malignant abnormalities.

In 193, patients with abnormal studies who were explored surgically, the incidence of malignant lesions was 29 percent.[24] In these patients the incidence of malignancy in thyroids with a solitary cold area by nuclear imaging (25.4 percent) was not greater than that in glands with multiple cold areas (35.4 percent). Their findings are not in agreement with the widely accepted belief that malignancy is more likely to be found in a thyroid containing a solitary cold nodule than in a multinodular gland.[25]

A retrospective study of 11,000 children irradiated for ringworm of the scalp and two matched groups was reported by Modan and Mart.[26] The radiation dose was approximately estimated to be 140 rads to the brain and 6.5 rads to the thyroid. Twelve patients developed thyroid cancer during follow-up of 12 to 23 years after x-ray exposure. The irradiated group had a significantly higher risk of malignancy. The increased rate of thyroid carcinoma in these cases is puzzling since the dose absorbed by the thyroid was only 6.5 rads. The authors mentioned some alternative explanations: carelessness during irradiation (retrospective study), extreme sensitivity of the thyroid gland to irradiation, or tumor production through a hypophyseal/thyroid axis after a relatively high radiation dose absorbed by the hypophysis.

External Irradiation to the Neck and Head for Cancer Therapy: Large Dose

Among the problems of the earlier studies on the effect of external irradiation on the thyroid gland were the lack of the more sophisticated thyroid function tests (e.g., RIA) currently available, and the short follow-up period of assessment for hypothyroidism which did not allow meaningful conclusions. The study with a long follow-up of patients was that reported by Einhorn and Wikholm.[27] In 41 patients followed for a mean period of 18 years after treatment for carcinoma of the larynx and hypopharynx, the incidence of established hypothyroidism was 7.3 percent. However, the 24-hour ^{131}I uptake following TSH stimulation was decreased in all 41 patients, indicating thyroid dysfunction. Recently, Fuks et al.[14] studied thyroid functions in a series of patients (363) who received a large dose of external irradiation to the neck. All patients had been treated with external radiation therapy for Hodgkin's disease, non-Hodgkin's lymphoma, or carcinoma of the head and neck (52). The radiation dose for the first two groups ranged from 4000 to 5000 rads and that for carcinoma was between 5000 and 6000 rads. The interval between irradiation and thyroid function tests ranged from 6 months to 14 years.

All patients with Hodgkin's disease and other lymphomas had a lower-limb lymphogram prior to treatment, whereas none of the patients with carcinoma of the head and neck had lymphograms. The incidence of thyroidal dysfunction (overt and compensated hypothyroidism) was significantly increased (58 to 64 percent) compared to that in patients with carcinoma of the head and neck (38 percent). Such increase occurred even though the former group received less

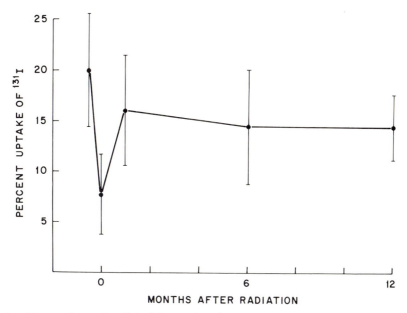

Fig. 5-3. Mean values of radioiodide uptake after external radiation of the thyroid in 18 adults. The mean dose was 6258 rads (range 3750 to 7000 rads). This radiation was delivered over a period of 6 to 7 weeks. The zero point is set at the time irradiation was completed. This figure constructed from mean values in ref. 30.

irradiation to the neck. This apparent paradox may be related to the lymphogram performed prior to irradiation in the lymphoma patients. A large iodide load may be an important cofactor contributing to radiation-induced thyroid disease. However, such an iodide load is not essential for the development of thyroid dysfunction after irradiation alone since the incidence was 38 percent in patients with carcinoma of the head and neck who did not receive a lymphogram.[14]

The effects of external radiation (500 to 1500 rads) on thyroidal radioiodide uptake have been documented in guinea pigs.[28,29] In human subjects there has been an extensive experience with thyroid function after external radiation for Hodgkin's disease, other lymphomas, and tumors of the head and neck. Lanaro and associates[30] reported data from which Figure 5-3 is constructed. Thyroid radioiodide uptake fell from 20 percent to 8 percent at the end of therapy (mean dose of 6258 rads over 6 to 7 weeks). By 1 year later it had climbed to 14 percent. Other series have commented on the development of both primary and secondary hypothyroidism after head and neck irradiation, the long time lapse involved, and the frequent finding of circulating thyroid antibodies.[14,27,31,32]

Radioiodide Therapy for Hyperthyroidism and Thyroid Cancer

What of thyroid malignancy occurring after radioiodide therapy for hyperthyroidism?

1. There are only rare case reports of thyroid carcinoma following radioiodide therapy for the overactive thyroid.[33] The impaired reproductive capacity of the

thyroid is thought to be behind the low occurrence of subsequent thyroid neo-plasms.[34] Some have argued for thyroid ablation, so that no radition-damaged thyroid cells would remain. Of particular interest would be the long-term followup of patients who had thyroid ablation with radioiodide for ophthalmopathy in Graves' disease. Such patients may have relief of the ocular symptoms.[35] It has not been demonstrated that the output of long-acting thyroid stimulators (LATS) in such individuals leads to thyroid neoplasia. The suggestion that certain medica-tions, such as propylthiouracil, render the thyroid radioresistant[36] has to be con-firmed by other workers.

2. Radioiodide therapy, of course, also delivers whole-body irradiation. Al-though it has been stated that the therapeutic doses used in treating the overactive thyroid may increase the incidence of leukemia, at least one detailed analysis does not confirm this finding (when the incidence was compared with those treated by surgery.[37] However, when large doses of radioiodide (50 to 100 mCi) are used, as in the treatment of thyroid carcinoma, there appears to be a definite increase in the incidence of leukemia.[38]

The limitations in treating thyroid carcinoma by means of radioiodide are recognized.[39] But what of the use of external radiation, in conjunction with surgery, in locally invasive papillary thyroid carcinoma? The results are not en-tirely encouraging,[40] and further approaches are needed.

Bone marrow damage is the most frequent serious complication resulting from the use of ^{131}I for thyroid cancer. Severe marrow depression is usually related to a retention of more than 120 mCi of ^{131}I. Acute myeloblastic leukemia has been seen following radioiodide therapy for thyroid cancer. In Pochin's se-ries[41] of 215 patients treated with ^{131}I for metastatic thyroid cancer, 4 died of acute leukemia, and 4 developed cancer of the breast. The incidence of leukemia is significant, but it does not seem high enough to contraindicate therapy.[42]

Radiation pneumonitis and pulmonary fibrosis complicating ^{131}I treatment of diffuse pulmonary metastasis has been reported by Rall and coworkers.[43] Since such changes were seen only in patients who retained 100 mCi or more in the lung, doses now are limited so that such areas contain no more than 80 mCi at 48 hours, as determined from the urinary excretion of a prior tracer. Other less serious side effects after ^{131}I therapy for cancer include nausea, vomiting, decreased sper-matogenesis, amenorrhea, and parotitis.

Data concerning the occurrence of malignant and benign thyroid neoplasms in patients treated for hyperthyroidism were collected at 26 medical centers in the Cooperative Thyrotoxicosis Therapy Follow-up Study, and have been reviewed.[44] The analysis was based on 34,684 patients treated for hyperthyroidism between 1946 and 1968 by ^{131}I, thyroidectomy, antithyroid drugs, x-irradiation, or various combinations of these therapeutic measures. Table 5-3, reconstructed from these data, summarizes the incidence of malignant tumor and benign adenoma after the four modalities of treatment. The authors concluded that if the occurrence of 19 malignant lesions found 1 year or more after ^{131}I is viewed from the standpoint of the incidental malignant lesions found in patients treated primarily by thyroidec-tomy, the risk from ^{131}I is not significant. The occurrence of thyroid adenomas is higher when ^{131}I therapy is used for treatment in the first two decades of life than when used in older individuals.[41] The significant difference in the incidence of malignancy after external irradiation versus that after radiation by administration

Table 5-3
Cooperative Thyrotoxicosis Therapy (1946–1968)*

Modality	All Patients			Grave's Without Nodules Only		
	No. of Patients	No. of Malignancies		No. of Patients	Malignancy ($>$ 1 yr)	Benign ($>$ 1 yr)
		within 1 yr	$>$ 1 yr			
^{131}I therapy	21,714	9	19†	16,042	9	20
Thyroidectomy	11,732	50	4	8,860	3	5
Antithyroid drugs	1,238	0	4	998	3‡	13‡
Irradiation	448	—	2	—	—	—

*From ref. 44.

†In view of the incidental malignant lesions in patients treated by thyroidectomy, the risk from ^{131}I is not significant.

‡Significantly higher.

of ^{131}I is not yet clear. However, most of the doses of ^{131}I in the past have been relatively high, and delivered approximately 8000 to 16,000 rads to the thyroid gland. It appears that such single large doses eventually lead to death of the cells rather than to mutation and carcinogenesis. In view of the high incidence of hypothyroidism in patients treated with ^{131}I, some investigators recently advocate using much smaller and multiple doses of ^{131}I so as to deliver 2000 rads. One should raise the question, Will these low doses of ^{131}I have a higher risk for tumor development? Further research is needed to answer such an important question. Other investigators suggested using ^{125}I instead of ^{131}I. In another chapter in this volume, Dr. Atkins discusses that aspect in detail. Also, the incidence of hypothyroidism after ^{131}I therapy for hyperthyroidism is discussed elsewhere.

^{131}I-THERAPY AND SUBSEQUENT REPRODUCTIVE HISTORY

Hyperthyroidism in children.   Safa et al.[45] evaluated the long-term results of ^{131}I therapy in 87 children with Graves' disease. The mean dose of ^{131}I per patient was 9.75 ± 6.5 mCi, and the mean follow-up period was 12.3 ± 3.5 years. The fertility rate of patients, the number of spontaneous abortions, and the health status of the progeny of ^{131}I-treated patients were not different from those of the general population. Since the number of the patients is small, no statistically valid conclusion can be drawn from these data. But no deaths and no cases of cancer or leukemia were observed in these patients or their offsprings. Hypothyroidism developed in 46 percent of the patients.

Thyroid cancer in children.   Sarkar and coworkers[46] studied 33 children who were treated with ^{131}I after surgery for papillary-follicular thyroid carcinoma. The mean age at the time of the first ^{131}I therapeutic dose was 14.6 years, and the mean follow-up period was 18.7 years. The mean total dose of ^{131}I was 196 mCi (range 80 to 691). Estimated cumulative radiation doses ranged from 20 to 166 rads to the whole body, and from 8 to 69 rads to the gonads. They reported that the inci-

Table 5-4

Effect of ^{131}I Therapy, in Children, on Fertility and
Anomalies in Their Offspring

	Therapy for Hyperthyroidism*	Therapy for Thyroid Cancer†
No. of patients	87	40
No. of live offspring	86	71
Age at therapy (years)	3–18	6–20
Dose (mCi)	9.8 (3–31)	196 (80–691)
Follow-up period (years)	12.3 (5–24)	18.7 (14–25)
Hypothyroidism incidence	46%	100%
Infertility	4/43 (9%)	3/33 (12%)
Spontaneous absorption and mole per pregnancies	7/93 (8%)	1/72 (1.4%)
Anomalies in offspring	3/86 (3.5%)	1/71 (1.4%)
Cancer	0	—
Leukemia	0	—

*From ref. 45.
†From ref. 46.

dences of infertility (12 percent), miscarriage (1.4 percent), prematurity (8 percent), and major congenital anomalies (1.4 percent) found in this series were not significantly different from those in the general population. Again, the number of the patients in this sample is too small for valid statistical analysis. Table 5-4 compares the two studies.

Does the diagnostic use of radioiodide in children increase the incidence of thyroid neoplasms? Despite an isolated report,[47] there is no conclusive evidence at present. The thyroid gland is small in the first year of life Thus, there is considerable radiation for each unit of radioactivity accumulated. Because of the need to reduce the radiation dose in young children, there is little indication for radioiodide uptake studies. Scans, however, might be indicated for evaluation of neck masses, or to determine if thyroid tissue is located ectopically or is present at all (thyroid agenesis).

RESPIRATORY SYSTEM

Pulmonary neoplasms had provided a nearly unique opportunity to study the rate of growth of tumors (indeed, prior to radionuclide scans, the only other tumors subject to such analysis were bone neoplasms). By means of carefully controlled chest radiographs, it was possible to graph tumor size as a function of time. These studies were largely pioneered by Spratt and Spratt.[48] Since the tumors could be followed only over a limited part of their life cycle, it was often difficult to identify "best fit" growth curves. Therefore, a readily measured parameter, *linear radial growth rate* (mm/day), was utilized. Survival was inversely proportional to the growth rate (the faster the growth, the shorter the survival). We will utilize the concept of linear growth rate in a later section when discussing hepatic lesions.

Imaging studies have been used in an effort to stage pulmonary lesions.

1. Perfusion lung scans may reveal a defect in the area of a bronchogenic carcinoma. These tumors, of course, have a blood supply from the bronchial circulation, and not from the pulmonary. In addition, tumor involvement of mediastinal nodes may compromise blood supply, further accentuating the defect. Some authors have used perfusion lung scans in staging pulmonary tumors, but this has not proved to be entirely reliable.
2. Gallium citrate (^{67}Ga) has been used to study lung tumors.[49,50] The radionuclide does not distinguish between malignant and benign pulmonary lesions (such as tuberculosis, sarcoidosis, pneumonia, abscesses). However, positive uptake can direct attention to otherwise inapparent areas of spread or secondary involvement.

Several studies have indicated that there was a probable increase of lung cancer in atom bomb survivors in Hiroshima and Nagasaki.[51] Cihak et al.[51] found lung cancer in 204 of 3778 autopsies on radiation-exposed survivors and controls. Small cell anaplastic carcinomas were definitely increased in irradiated persons compared to controls (relative risk 3.9). Epidermoid and bronchogenic adenocarcinoma also showed increased risk, but this was not statistically significant.

Irradiation to the whole thorax with additional radiotherapy to the mediastinum may cause severe acute radiation pneumonitis. Littman et al.[52] reported two fatalities in children.

A significant portion of intrapulmonary tumors are treated by external irradiation. The response of human lung to therapeutic levels of ionizing radiation is well established pathologically.[53] In the acute state there is hyperemia, bronchial epithelitis, and depletion of lymphoid elements. Later there is a degenerative stage of parenchymal cellular damage or death. This stage is marked by fibrinopurulent pleuritis, swelling and sloughing of alveolar lining cells, and the appearance of fibrinoid material within alveoli. The latter may form a continuous hyaline membrane. The final, regenerative stage is characterized by metaplasia of bronchial epithelium and alveolar lining cells, connective tissue proliferation, and obliterative pulmonary arteriolitis. Grossly, the lung exhibits loss of elasticity and volume. Studies with light and electron microscopy have shown striking changes in the pulmonary capillaries following large radiation doses.[54] There is an early increase in capillary permeability, followed by sloughing of capillary endothelium and obliteration of the endovascular space by cells and acellular debris. Arterioles exhibit intimal thickening and proliferation of adventitial fibrous tissue. This is accompanied by interstitial parenchymal fibrosis.

The clinical counterparts of these events may emerge in the variable syndrome of so-called radiation pneumonitis and radiation fibrosis of the lung. Postirradiation pulmonary fibrosis has been observed radiographically in 70 percent of long-term survivors with carcinoma of breast; usually asymptomatic, it may be associated with disabling pulmonary insufficiency.[55]

Using serial pulmonary perfusion scans, Johnson et al.[56] have shown that pulmonary blood flow is reduced regionally in the irradiated segment of the lung in patients who have undergone radiation therapy. These patients also exhibit pulmonary fibrosis, pleural thickening, or both; these radiographic findings are less extensive than the corresponding deficit in pulmonary flow.

Teates and Cooper[57] studied long-term effects up to 40 months after thoracic irradiation (3100 to 4100 rads tissue dose in 24 to 40 days) using roentgenographic examination and physiologic studies (vital capacity, maximum breathing capacity, and arterial oxygen percentage saturation). The adverse changes were evident within 6 months and showed little progression after 12 months. They concluded that the physiologic tests they employed were not as sensitive as roentgenographic examination in detecting radiation damage in the lung.

Recent studies with serial perfusion scans and [133]Xenon ventillation studies are even more sensitive.[56,58,59] The effects of thoracic irradiation are incompletely reflected by x-ray changes, i.e., the area of radiation-induced ischemia noted on the radioisotopic perfusion scan was larger than the fibrotic changes seen on the roentgenogram.[58] In a recent report,[59] Bateman and Croft reported that 11 of 12 scans revealed perfusion defects on the irradiated side, with ventilation-perfusion mismatches (normal ventilation, impaired perfusion). Radiotherapy of the thorax may cause breathlessness and nonspecific chest pains in the presence of a normal chest radiograph, thus clinically mimicking pulmonary embolism. In these circumstances, the diagnosis will depend heavily on the lung perfusion and ventilation scans. Since radiotherapy may produce ventilation-perfusion mismatch similar to that of pulmonary embolism, special care should be exercised in the interpretation of lung scans in patients who have received radiation therapy to the thorax.

Using serial regional measurements of pulmonary blood flow and ventilation in 25 patients irradiated for breast cancer, Prato et al.[60] concluded that blood flow showed the earliest and greatest decrease. They noted that changes in blood flow at 60 days are predictive of the changes at 300 days and recommended earlier studies during irradiation for predicting long-term effects.

Subclinical radiation injury has been reported to become overt after rapid withdrawal of high-dose corticosteroids in patients with Hodgkin's disease after "mantle" radiation therapy.[61] The importance of recognizing this condition, which responds to high doses of corticosteroids tapered during many months, is emphasized.[61]

GASTROINTESTINAL TRACT

During radiotherapy for cancer, the gastrointestinal viscera are at especially high risk because of their relatively limited tolerance to ionizing radiation. Organic damage and serious impairment of digestive function may interfere greatly with the enjoyment of life and are sometimes lethal.[62] For the therapeutic radiologist, the margin for error is small while the penalty to the patient may be great. For a comprehensive review of the pathophysiology of radiation effects on the gastrointestinal tract, reference should be made to the treatise of Rubin and Casarett.[63]

Many cancer patients receive combined chemotherapy and radiation. A range of cancer chemotherapeutic agents may cause a significant augmentation of radia-

Table 5-5

Nuclear Medicine Procedures for Detection of Radiation Effects in the
Gastrointestinal Tract

1. Imaging, e.g., ^{99m}Tc scan of esophagus[65]
2. Gastric emptying study using Na $^{51}CrO_4$ or ^{99m}Tc-S-colloid[66]
3. $^{14}CO_2$ breath test with ^{14}C-glycocholic acid, e.g., majority of patients with prior abdominal radiotherapy showed abnormal results[67,68]
4. $^{14}CO_2$ breath test using ^{14}C-fatty acids and esters for malabsorption due to radiation or chemotherapy[68,69]
5. ^{51}Cr-albumin for gastrointestinal loss
6. ^{51}Cr-labeled RBC for bleeding ulcers

tion injury in the gastrointestinal tract.[64] Table 5-5 presents examples of nuclear
medicine procedures which may be employed in studying the function of the
gastrointestinal tract after radiation therapy.

Two groups of investigators from England[67] and Switzerland[68] have utilized the
breath $^{14}CO_2$-cholic acid test to study the effect of radiotherapy for abdominal malignancy on the intestine. The majority of the patients showed abnormal tests.
Late radiation damage may cause permanent alteration of bowel habit and an
interruption of the enterohepatic circulation. It has been suggested that both of
these phenomena originate in the small bowel. Chronic large bowel injury was
lacking in one series,[67] since only 1 of 13 patients had an inflamed rectal mucosa,
and none had blood in the stools. Inflammation of the colon or rectum causes
neither alteration of the enterohepatic circulation nor abnormal small intestinal
x-rays.

Stagnant loops and/or ileal damage might have caused the abnormal breath
tests. It should be pointed out that $^{14}CO_2$ breath tests, after ^{14}C-bile salts, do not
distinguish between these two entities.

Several investigators[67-72] have confirmed the clinical usefulness of this test,
and it is gaining widespread acceptance in many medical centers. Lutölf et al.[68]
also reported that pulmonary excretion of $^{14}CO_2$, after administration of glycine-
1-^{14}C, was increased in patients with Crohn's disease and in patients receiving
radiotherapy to the abdomen for malignancy as opposed to pretherapy excretion
values.

LIVER AND SPLEEN

The spleen and liver are considered together here since they share drainage
via the same venous system, and also are repositories of reticuloendothelial cells.

Until recently, the normal liver had been considered an organ resistant to
ionizing radiation when given in the usual therapeutic range for neoplasms.[73] Few
changes have been noted on the commonly used liver function tests after local
irradiation. These tests, however, are insensitive parameters of hepatic radiation
response in the intact organism, particularly to irradiation of 50 percent or less of
the liver.[74] This is due in part to their dependence on the functional state of the
liver as a whole.

Recent observations based on the study of liver scans of patients receiving therapeutic doses of irradiation suggest hepatic radiation injury.[75–81] On scans performed after administration of [198]Au or ^{131}I-Rose Bengal, there have been areas of decreased activity which seem to correspond to the regions exposed to x-irradiation. Studies of hepatic reticuloendothelial cells (with radiolabeled colloid) and hepatic parenchymatous cells (with ^{131}I-Rose Bengal) have been shown to give a more sensitive index of function and relative location than other available means (such as biochemical estimation of certain enzymes).[80] Thus, the photoscanning procedure can be used to obtain a functional as well as an anatomical evaluation prior to initiation of radiation. Further, the studies can potentially be used serially during radiation and in the recovery period.

The mechanism of the radiation-induced defect on photoscans is not clear. The decreased uptake of radionuclide within the irradiated portion of the liver may be due to a direct radiation effect on the hepatic cells or due to alteration in the local blood flow. Ingold et al.[75] characterized the acute radiation effect on the liver as "centrolobular hemorrhage and sinusoidal congestion with adjacent minimal hepatic cellular atrophy."

Several statements can be made about the response of the liver to radiation.

1. If tumors compressing the liver are successfully treated with external radiation, normal hepatic tissue can grow back into the area.[82]
2. When there is tumor obstruction to portal venous outflow, hepatic irradiation may partly relieve the obstruction.[83]
3. The left lobe of the liver is often included in the radiation portal when paraaortic nodes or the pancreas is treated by irradiation. The typical finding (if the radiation dose is above 2000 rads) is decreased reticuloendothelial function in the affected area.
4. When the right hepatic lobe undergoes radiation, radiocolloid can be seen to be shifted to the left lobe and spleen.[84]
5. If the radiation dose to the affected area of the liver is below about 2500 rads, there may be a return of function. There is a different radiation sensitivity of parenchymal and reticuloendothelial (RE) cells.[80,81] Nebesar and coworkers[85] have discussed the combined use of radionuclide scans and angiography in radiation "hepatitis."

Radionuclide scans can be used to quantify and depict the rate of growth of intrahepatic tumors,[86] and of their response to radiation or chemotherapy.[87] That is, the linear growth rate (and rate of regression) can be estimated. Even when the liver is diffusely involved by tumor, scans can be used to estimate the rate of response to treatment.

The RE cells of the nonleukemic spleen appear to be relatively more resistant to external local radiation than has been previously appreciated. On the other hand, the white pulp of the spleen, the area of lymphocyte production, is rapidly depleted of lymphocytes after a moderate whole-body radiation exposure.

Samuels[89] reported that serial ^{99m}Tc-sulfur liver and spleen colloid scans of 10 children whose spleens were previously normal in size revealed enlargement of the spleen following megavoltage radiotherapy for Wilms's tumor or adrenal neuroblastoma. The increase in splenic size was transient; perhaps reversible outflow obstruction was occurring.

URINARY SYSTEM

Because of the danger of radiation nephritis, the kidneys are usually shielded during abdominal radiation. However, in the course of splenic irradiation or wide-field treatment for metastases, the kidneys may be irradiated leading to various complications.[90] A dose of 2300 rads or more to the kidneys in 5 weeks may result in a serious or fatal radiation nephritis.[91] Radiation effect on the kidneys has been categorized as follows.[90−92]

1. Acute radiation nephritis: occurring within 6 to 13 months in adults and within a shorter period in children, and can be assessed by radioisotopic renogram.
2. Chronic radiation nephritis: resembles chronic glomerulonephritis. It may arise de novo or as an aftermath of the acute stage.
3. Hypertension—benign and malignant: probably due to endothelial damage which may initiate the release of renin and angiotensin.
4. Proteinuria: may be asymptomatic.

The ureters are fairly radioresistant; they rarely exhibit fibrosis and obstruction after radiation. The radiation injuries to the urinary bladder may result in cystitis, ulcers, obstruction of the bladder neck, and urethral stricture.

Cohen and Robinson[93] have reported on the radioisotope renogram (^{131}I-hippuran) in three cases of acute radiation nephritis. More extensive studies, by means of radiopharmaceuticals which are excreted in the glomerular filtrate, are needed. There can also be radiation damage to the lower urinary tract from therapeutic external radiation or from internally implanted sources.[94] A typical finding is obstruction of a ureter in its lowermost portion. The differential diagnosis must include involvement by tumor or the results of radiation-induced stricture.

BONE AND BONE MARROW

The deleterious effects of radiation on growing bones have been recognized for many years.[95] Shortly after the turn of the century, Perthes et al. demonstrated that exposure to x-rays caused retardation in the growth of bones in animals.[141] In 1924 Blum reported "radium poisoning" and described "radium jaw" in radium dial workers.[142] In recent years, more workers have reported on the side effects of radiation therapy in children and adults.[96−104] The abnormality produced depends primarily on the radiation dose, the age of the patient at the time of irradiation, and the area irradiated and its blood supply. The effects of radiation on bone have been summarized as follows:[104]

1. Epiphyseal irradiation: results in an arrest of chondrogenesis.
2. Metaphyseal irradiation: results in a failure of the absorptive processes of calcified cartilage and bone.
3. Diaphyseal irradiation: produces alterations in periosteal activity, which, in turn, gives modeling abnormalities.
4. Bone irradiation: results in hypoplasia, as seen in the ilium and ribs: or radiation necrosis, as seen in the femoral neck and in the mandible.
5. Late radiation effects: include benign exostosis or sarcoma (infrequent).

The threshold of radiation roentgenographic changes in bone is estimated to be 3000 rads, and cell death occurs with 5000 rads.[97] However, in children, lower doses can cause certain damage to the bone, e.g., 1000 to 2000 rads for subcortical lucent zones and 2000 to 3000 rads for scalloping of the vertebrae.

The bone changes commonly reported include scoliosis, structural alterations in the vertebral bodies, exostosis, epiphyseal destruction, shortening or bowing of the extremities, radiation-induced sarcoma, and hypoplasia of the ilium, rib cage, and orbit. Fortunately, radiation-induced sarcoma is an uncommon sequela of bone irradiation in children. Among radiation-induced sarcomas, the osteogenic type is the most common form, followed by fibrosarcoma and chondrosarcoma. The latent period between radiation therapy and the diagnosis of radiation-induced neoplasm ranged from 3 to 30 years, with an average of about 10 years.[101]

The use of ^{99m}Tc-polyphosphate complexes for skeletal scintigraphy has led to improved detection of metastatic disease, particularly in the early stages when there has not yet been sufficient bone erosion to render the lesions visible to x-ray examination. Recently Castronovo, Potsaid, and Pendergrass[102] have suggested that these radiopharmaceuticals might be useful in monitoring the effect of irradiation therapy on such lesions. They report reduced uptake of ^{99m}Tc-diphosphonate in bone lesions following an 18-day irradiation therapy treatment involving an exposure of 3000 rads. Other investigators[103,105] have also reported such decreased accumulation of ^{99m}Tc-phosphates in the areas of bones which have been previously irradiated. Cox[103] suggests that the reduced uptake observed in lesions after irradiation therapy is related to: (1) reduced blood flow caused by degenerative changes in the blood vessels; and (2) reduced phagocytosis in bone marrow and inflamed areas. The regions bordering the irradiated area may show increased activity or a ''flare-up'' resulting in a false-positive effect. This may be related to increased cell wall permeability, destruction of tumor cells, removal of necrotic products, and the beginning of reparative events. A ''flare'' can also occur on the scan of malignant lesions in bone during chemotherapy.[143,133] This might indicate a favorable response, rather than a progression of the malignant process.

Bone Marrow

In the course of treatment of localized Hodgkin's disease and lymphoma, some radiotherapists have advocated extending the radiation fields to cover most lymph node-bearing areas to prevent spread of the lymphoma to uninvolved regions.[106] Fields for ''total nodal irradiation'' expose from one-half to three-fourths of the hemopoietic tissue in adult patients to more than 3500 rads. Studies by Sykes et al.[107] in women receiving radiotherapy for breast cancer and by other investigators using morphologic and scanning techniques[108] suggest that repopulation of the marrow fails to persist after doses exceeding 2500 to 3500 rads delivered in 2 to 4 weeks. Moreover, several recent studies have demonstrated decreased bone marrow reserve[109] and increased sensitivity to chemotherapy[110] in patients who have had extensive radiotherapy.

Using radionuclide scanning, Rubin et al.[111] concluded that following radiation doses ranging from 4000 to 5000 rads in 4 to 6 weeks, recovery of marrow function continued for more than 2 years after treatment. Sykes et al.[112] found no evidence of recovery of sternal marrow for up to 14 years after treatment with exposure of 4500 rads in 3 to 3.5 weeks. Recovery might be related to the specific marrow site irradiated, although no studies pertinent to this question have been recorded.

Many associations between the medical use of ionizing radiations and leukemia have been presented in the literature.[101] Stewart et al.[113] estimated that therapeutic uses of x-rays accounted for 3.6 percent of adult leukemia. An excess incidence of leukemia has been reported in those previously irradiated during childhood for enlargement of the thymus.[101] In a recent survey of 10,000 patients with Hodgkin's disease treated with radiation, Crosby[114] reported a 10-fold increase over that expected. On the other hand, no increased incidence of leukemia was reported with radioactive iodine therapy for thyrotoxicosis,[37] or after heavy irradiation of the pelvis in the treatment of cancer of the cervix.[115]

The spontaneous occurrence of leukemia in patients with various lymphomas makes correlation of any slightly increased incidence with treatment very difficult, particularly as such treatment prolongs life and consequently the risk for these patients.

In their review of late effects of therapeutic irradiation of bone marrow, Parker and Berry[101] conclude that leukemia rarely develops in therapeutically

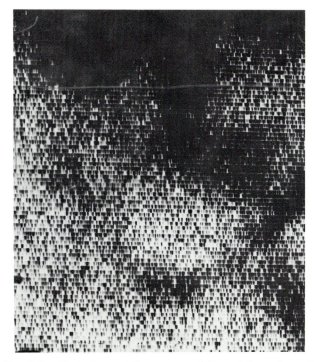

Fig. 5-4. Posterior rectilinear scan of the pelvis performed after intravenous administration of ^{99m}Tc-sulfur colloid. The patient, a 75-year-old woman, had a known carcinoma of the breast. The bone marrow scan revealed decreased activity in the left pelvis and femoral head. A biopsy revealed metastatic carcinoma.

irradiated bone marrow, and that most evidence which documents a causative relationship is based on treatments no longer used.

The bone marrow accumulates iron (and radioiron) as part of the erythropoietic pathway. Hence, radioiron could be used to obtain images of erythrocyte precursors (erythrons) in bone marrow. Unfortunately, ^{52}Fe (T½ = 8 hours) is difficult to obtain, and ^{59}Fe has a high-energy gamma ray as well as a long physical half-life. DeGowin and coworkers[106] have used a special collimator on a rectilinear scanner in order to obtain a rough idea of the distribution of intravenously administered ^{59}Fe. The technique showed that irradiation, usually employed in treating lymphomas, might prevent local regrowth of bone marrow for 1 to 3 years. Other workers have used the iron analogue ^{111}In for bone marrow scanning. If the assumption is made that erythrons usually have the same distribution as reticuloendothelial cells in bone marrow, then radiocolloids can be employed to evaluate the bone marrow.[81] Here, we are looking for *decreased* activity in the locale in which bone marrow has been replaced by tumor (Fig. 5-4) or rendered ineffectual by irradiation. Recall that this finding of decreased activity at the site of tumor in bone marrow is just the opposite of the increased uptake of radiotracer (bone matrix scan) observed in metastatic tumor in the mineral-rich phase of bone.

OTHER ORGANS AND OBSERVATIONS

The eye is usually included in the field of irradiation for treatment of malignant tumors of the orbit, nasal cavity, or paranasal sinuses.[116] Cataract formation has been found at doses in excess of 1200 rads. However, eyesight has been preserved even with higher doses (up to 6000 rads in 30 fractions in 6 weeks). When 5-fluorouracil (5-FU) was used in conjunction with high-dose radiotherapy, loss of vision was much more frequent. All patients treated with combined therapy had either visual loss or major clinical difficulties. Brizel et al.[117] used ^{99m}Tc-pertechnetate dacryoscintigraphy to evaluate the effects of radiotherapy on the nasolacrimal system. They reported that the technique yielded useful information about flow mechanisms and tear transit times.

The often nonspecific entry of radiotracers into tumors has been well documented. Less well-explored is the subject of radiopharmaceutical uptake in irradiated areas. Thus, the observation that ^{67}Ga citrate accumulates in salivary glands of patients after radiation therapy[118] stands as an interesting observation that has still to be incorporated into an overall view of how to monitor radiation effects in man. Such increased uptake in the salivary gland occurred, although experiments in animals showed that whole-body radiation resulted in decreased whole-body Ga-67 retention.[119,120] There was decreased activity in the liver, spleen, and blood, but increased tracer in the bone.

Ionizing irradiation may damage the heart and produce changes in pericardium, myocardium, and endocardium. The epicardium is the area most severely damaged by irradiation. McReynolds et al.[121] reported two cases of severe coronary heart disease in patients several years after mediastinal irradiation for Hodgkin's disease (mantle type, 4000 to 5000 rads). Autopsy studies indicated thickening of the epicardium and mural endocardium. The coronary arteries showed severe thickening of the walls by both intimal and adventitial fibrous proliferation. The coronary artery sclerosis found in these cases was different from that seen in the usual coronary heart disease.

Levinson et al.[122] also reported cerebrovascular insufficiency caused by atypical atherosclerotic lesions in cervical arteries which developed in three patients who had received external cervical irradiation more than 25 years previously. Also, chronic damage to medium and large arteries following therapeutic irradiation was documented.[123]

Other important radiation effects are radiation-induced lymphocyte-immune deficiency[124-126] and possible genetic consequences of irradiation of tumors in children.[127,128] The association between systemically administered radioisotopes for therapy and subsequent malignant disease has been recently reviewed.[129]

Adrenal cortical scanning with [131]I-19-iodocholesterol delivers to the glands up to 30 rads/mCi.[130] Such a dose has been investigated by Beierwaltes' group in Michigan as a means to control metapyralone-induced adrenal cortical hyperplasia in dogs.[130]

EFFECTS OF CHEMOTHERAPY ON NUCLEAR MEDICINE FINDINGS

The drugs used in cancer chemotherapy possess a potential for affecting normal tissues and developing organs, with manifestations appearing many years later. Although emphasis has usually been placed on immediate and early toxicity, there is justifiable concern about chronic or delayed effects.[131] Combining chemotherapy and irradiation modifies the damage in the tissues. The antibiotic cancer chemotherapeutic agents are the most likely to enhance radiation injury. The second most common type of injury appears to occur with drugs causing injury to the normal tissue on their own, such as adriamycin in the heart and methotrexate in the central nervous system.[64] Table 5-6 presents several examples of the effects of chemotherapy on nuclear medicine findings as measured by scans or radioisotopic functional studies.

Table 5-6
Effects of Chemotherapy on Nuclear Medicine Findings (Examples)

1. *Brain scan:* Corticosteroid may mask a small metastatic lesion.[12,13]
2. *Bone scan:* Chemotherapy for breast metastases → initial "flare," increased activity.[133]
3. *[67]Ga kinetics:* Vincristine and mustargen in animals → Decreased ^{67}Ga retention.[119]
4. *Lung pneumonitis:* Acute withdrawal of corticosteroids → worsening of condition.[61]
5. *RE function:* Chemotherapy → decreased function as seen in scans.[110,134]
6. *Intestinal malabsorption:* Chemotherapy → decreased absorption of fat as measured by breath $^{14}CO_2$.[67,68]
7. *Eye:* 5-Fluorouracil and radiotherapy for tumors of nasal cavity → loss of vision was more frequent than after radiotherapy alone.[116]
8. *Tumors:* Actinomycin-D after radiation → decreased risk for developing a second tumor (by a factor of 7).[135]

Table 5-7

Role of Radioimmunoassay in Detection of Radiation Effects (Examples)

---

1. Pituatary irradiation: Growth hormone, insulin, cortisol, TSH, etc.
2. Thyroid dysfunction: TSH, T4, T3, etc.
3. Kidney: In radiation hypertension; renin-angiotensin
4. Adrenals: Corticosteroids (cortisol)
5. Gonads: Several hormone assays
6. Tumors: Carcinoembryonic antigen, [137]DNA (using ^{125}I-iodide oxyuridine-labeled DNA as an antigen), [138]alpha-fetoprotein[136]

ROLE OF RADIOIMMUNOASSAY PROCEDURES

Use of radioimmunoassays has been one of the fastest growing areas of nuclear medicine in recent years. Table 5-7 gives some examples of the procedures which may be used to study the function of different organs exposed to therapeutic radiation or chemotherapy. The use of blood levels of such markers as alpha-fetoprotein[136] and carcinoembryonic antigen[137] (determined by radioimmunoassay) may be of value, in conjunction with dynamic and static images, in determining the response of tumors to treatment.

SUMMARY

1. Different modalities of therapy, especially radiation, can have profound effects on organ morphology and function.
2. The latent period may extend to several years or decades.
3. The range of nuclear medicine procedures, encompassing static imaging, dynamic evaluation, and radioimmunoassay, plays an important role in detecting such changes. In certain instances these procedures are superior to traditional methods.
4. The physician should be alert to the effect of therapy on nuclear medicine images and tests, for proper interpretation of the results and management of the patient.

REFERENCES

1. Feldman, M. I., Anderson, B. G., Shetty, S. K.: Some applications of scintiscanning to radiation therapy. Radiology 112:740–741, 1974.
2. Spencer, R. P., Knowlton, A.: Radiocolloid scans in evaluating splenic response to external radiation. J. Nucl. Med. 16:123–126, 1975.
3. Bamford, F. N., Jones, P. M., Pearson, D., et al.: Residual disabilities in children treated for intracranial space-occupying lesions. Cancer 37:1149–1151, 1976.
4. Rubin, P.: The radiographic expression of radiotherapeutic injury: an overview. Semin. Roentgenol. 9:5–13, 1974.
5. Kramer, S., Lee, K. F.: Complications of radiation therapy: the central nervous system. Semin. Roentgenol. 9:75–83, 1974.

6. Diengdoh, J. V., Booth, A. E.: Postirradiation necrosis of the temporal lobe presenting as a glioma. J. Neurosurg. 44:732–734, 1976.

7. Wright, T. L., Bresnan, M. J.: Radiation-induced cerebrovascular disease in children. Neurology (Minneap.) 26:540–543, 1976.

8. Wilson, G. H., Byfield, J., Hanafee, W. N.: Atrophy following radiation therapy for central nervous system neoplasms. Acta Radiol. 2:361–368, 1972.

9. Nordman, E., Rekonen, A.: Interpretation of ^{99m}Tc-pertechnetate scintigraphy after irradiation of brain tumors. Int. J. Nucl. Med. Biol. 2:25–29, 1975.

10. Carella, R. J., Pay, N., Newall, J. et al.: Computerized (axial) tomography in the serial study of cerebral tumors treated by radiation: a preliminary report. Cancer 37:2719–2728, 1976.

11. Potchen, E. J., Kinzie, J., Curtis, C., et al.: Effect of irradiation on tumor microvascular permeability to macromolecules. Cancer 30:639–642, 1972.

12. Antar, M. A.: The effect of irradiation therapy on serial brain scans; correlation with autopsy findings. *In preparation.*

13. Fletcher, J. W., George, E. A., Henry, R. E., et al.: Brain scan, dexamethasone therapy, and brain tumors. J.A.M.A. 232:1261–1263, 1975.

14. Fuks, Z., Glatstein, E., Marsa, G. W., et al.: Long term effects of external radiation on the pituitary and thyroid glands. Cancer 37:1152–1161, 1976.

15. Samaan, N., Bakdash, M. M., Caderao, J. B., et al.: Hypopituitarism after external irradiation: Evidence for both hypothalamic and pituitary origin. Ann Intern. Med. 83:771–777, 1975.

16. Parker, L. N., Belsky, J. L., Yamamoto, T., et al.: Thyroid carcinoma after exposure to atomic radiation: a continuing survey of a fixed population, Hiroshima and Nagasaki, 1958–1971. Ann. Intern. Med. 80:600–604, 1974.

17. Conard, R. A., Dobyns, B. M., Sutow, W. W.: Thyroid neoplasia as late effect of exposure to radioactive iodine in fallout. J.A.M.A. 214:316–324, 1970.

18. Rallison, M. L., Dobyns, B. M., Keating, F. R., et al.: Thyroid disease in children: a survey of subjects potentially exposed to fallout radiation. Am. J. Med. 56:457–463, 1974.

19. DeGroot, L. Paloyan, E.: Thyroid carcinoma and radiation: a Chicago endemic. J.A.M.A. 225:487–491, 1973.

20. Duffy, B. J., Fitzgerald, P. J.: Cancer of the thyroid in children: a report of 28 cases. J. Clin. Endocrinol. Metab. 10:1296–1308, 1950.

21. Hempelmann, L. H.: Risk of thyroid neoplasms after irradiation in childhood. Science 160:159–163, 1968.

22. Wilson, S. M., Platz, C., Block, G. M.: Thyroid carcinoma after irradiation. Arch. Surg. 100:330–337, 1970.

23. Arnold, J., Pinsky, S., Ryo, U. Y., et al.: ^{99m}Tc-pertechnetate thyroid scintigraphy in patients predisposed to thyroid neoplasms by prior radiotherapy to the head and neck. Radiology 115:653–657, 1975.

24. Vander, J. B., Gaston, E. A., Dawber, T. R.: The significance of nontoxic thyroid nodules. Final report of a 15-year study of the incidence of thyroid malignancy. Ann. Intern. Med. 69:537–540, 1968.

25. Wright, H. K., Burrow, G. N., Spaulding, S., et al.: Current therapy of thyroid nodules. Surg. Clin. North Am. 54:277–288, 1974.

26. Modan, B., Mart, H.: Radiation-induced head and neck tumours. Lancet 1:277–279, 1974.

27. Einhorn, J., Wikholm, G.: Hypothyroidism after external irradiation to the thyroid region. Radiology 88:326–328, 1976.

28. Lach, H., Dymarczyk, B.: Influence of X-rays on the rate of accumulation of ^{131}I in the

thyroid of guinea pigs in the initial stage of radiation disease. Acta Biol. Acad. Sci. Hung. 27:1–7, 1976.

29. Lach, H., Dymarczyk, B.: Influence of X-rays on diurnal variation in ^{131}I uptake by guinea pig thyroid. Acta Biol. Acad. Sci. Hung. 27:9–13, 1976.

30. Lanaro, A. F., Bosch, A., Frais, Z.: Effect of irradiation on the normal thyroid gland ^{131}I uptake. Am. J. Roentgènol. 114:600–605, 1972.

31. Adler, R., Corrigan, D. F., Wartofsky, L.: Hypothyroidism after X irradiation to the neck: three case reports and a brief review of the literature. Johns Hopkins Med. J. 138:180–184, 1976.

32. Rosenthal, M. B., Goldfine, I. D.: Primary and secondary hypothyroidism in nasopharyngeal carcinoma. J.A.M.A. 236:1591–1593, 1976.

33. McDougall, I. R.: Thyroid cancer after iodine-131 therapy. J.A.M.A. 227:438, 1974.

34. Ashkar, F. S., Maile, A., Smoak, W. M., III, et al.: The role of surgery and ^{131}I therapy for hyperthyroidism in the etiology of thyroid carcinoma. South. Med. J. 66:1014–1016, 1973.

35. Fawell, W. N., Catz, B.: Attempt at thyroid ablation with radioactive iodine for the treatment of ophthalmopathy in Graves' disease. Am. J. Med. Sci. 265:467–472, 1973.

35. Krassas, G., Jacobs, H. S., McHardy-Young, S.: The comparative effect of propylthiouracil and carbimazole on the therapeutic response to radioiodine therapy. J. Endocrinol. 71:38P, 1976.

37. Saenger, E. L., Tomkins, E., Thoma, G. E.: Radiation and leukemia rates. Science 171:1096–1097, 1971.

38. Brincker, H., Hansen, H. S., Andersen, A. P.: Induction of leukaemia by ^{131}I treatment of thyroid carcinoma. Br. J. Cancer 28:232–237, 1973.

39. Leeper, R. D.: The effect of ^{131}I therapy on survival of patients with metastatic papillary or follicular thyroid carcinoma. J. Clin. Endocrinol. Metab. 36:1143–1152, 1973.

40. Lenio, P. T.: External irradiation in treatment of papillary carcinoma of the thyroid. Am. J. Surg. 131:281–283, 1976.

41. Pochin, E. E.: Long term hazards of radioiodine treatment of thyroid carcinoma. Thyroid Cancer, U.I.C.C. Monograph series, Springer-Verlag, Berlin, 12:293–304, 1969.

42. Pochin, E. E.: The occurrence of leukaemia following radioiodine therapy. In: Advances in Thyroid Research, Transactions of the Fourth International Goiter Conference, R. Pitt-Rivers (ed.). London, Pergamon Press, p. 392, 1961.

43. Rall, J. E., Alpers, J. B., Lewallen, J. B., et al.: Radiation pneumonitis and fibrosis, a complication of radioiodine treatment of pulmonary metastases from cancer of the thyroid. J. Clin. Endocrinol. Metab. 17:1263, 1957.

44. Dobyns, B. M., Sheline, G. E., Workman, J. B., et al.: Malignant and benign neoplasms of the thyroid in patients treated for hyperthyroidism: a report of the cooperative thyrotoxicosis therapy, followup study. J. Clin. Endocrinol. Metab. 38:976–998, 1974.

45. Safa, A. M., Schumacher, O. P., Rodriguez-Antunez, A.: Long-term follow-up results in children and adolescents treated with radioactive iodine (^{131}I) for hyperthyroidism. N. Engl. J. Med. 292:167–171, 1975.

46. Sarkar, S. D., Beierwaltes, W. H., Gill, S. P., et al.: Subsequent fertility and birth histories of children and adolescents treated with ^{131}I for thyroid cancer. J. Nucl. Med. 17:460–464, 1976.

47. Pilch, B. Z., Kahn, R., Ketcham, A. S., et al.: Thyroid cancer after radioactive iodine diagnostic procedures in childhood. Pediatrics 51:898–902, 1973.

48. Spratt, J. S., Jr., Spratt, T. L.: Rates of growth of pulmonary metastases and host survival. Ann. Surg. 159:161–171, 1964.

49. Cellerino, A., Filippi, P. G., Chiantaretto, A., et al.: Operative and pathologic survey of 50 cases of peripheral lung tumors scanned with 67 gallium. Chest 64:700–705, 1973.

50. Van Der Schoot, J. B., Groen, A. S., DeJong, J.: Gallium-67 scintigraphy in lung diseases. Thorax 27:543–546, 1972.

51. Cihak, R. W., Ishimaru, T., Steer, A., et al.: Lung cancer at autopsy in A-bomb survivors and controls, Hiroshima and Nagasaki, 1961–1970: I. Autopsy findings and relation to radiation. Cancer 33:1580–1588, 1974.

52. Littman, P., Davis, L. W., Nash, J., et al.: The hazard of acute radiation pneumonitis in children receiving mediastinal radiation. Cancer 33:1520–1525, 1974.

53. Warren, S., Spencer, J.: Radiation reaction in the lung. Am. J. Roentgenol. 43:682–701, 1940.

54. Von Babler, R., Buchwald, W.: Experimentelle entzündung. und fibrose des lungengerüstes durch ionisierend Strahlen. Fortschr. Röntgenstr. 104:192–206, 1966.

55. Bates, D., Guttman, R. J.: Changes in lung and pleura following 2 mev therapy for carcinoma of the breast. Radiology 69:372–383, 1957.

56. Johnson, P. M., Sagerman, R. H., Jacox, H. W.: Changes in pulmonary arterial perfusion due to intrathoracic neoplasia and irradiation of the lung. Am. J. Roentgenol. 102:637–644, 1968.

57. Teates, D., Cooper, G., Jr.: Some consequences of pulmonary irradiation: a second long term report. Am. J. Roentgenol. 96:612–619, 1966.

58. Goldman, S. M., Freeman, L. M., Nemetallah, A., et al.: Effects of thoracic irradiation on pulmonary arterial perfusion in man. Radiology 93:289–296, 1969.

59. Bateman, N. T., Croft, D. N.: False-positive lung scans and radiotherapy. Br. Med. J. 1:807–808, 1976.

60. Prato, F. S., Kurdyak, R., Saibil, E. A., et al.: Physiological and radiographic assessment during the development of pulmonary radiation fibrosis. Radiology 122:389–397, 1977.

61. Castellino, R. A., Glatstein, E.: Latent radiation injury of lungs or heart activated by steroid withdrawal. Ann. Intern. Med. 80:593–599, 1974.

62. Roswit, B.: Complications of radiation therapy: the alimentary tract. Semin. Roentgenol. 9:51–63, 1974.

63. Rubin, P., Casarett, G. W.: A direction for clinical radiation pathology. The tolerance dose. In: Frontiers of Radiation Therapy and Oncology, Vol. 6, J. M. Vaeth (ed.). Baltimore, University Park Press, pp. 1–16, 1972.

64. Phillips, T. L., Fu, K. K.: Quantification of combined radiation therapy and chemotherapy effects on critical normal tissues. Cancer 37:1186–1200, 1976.

65. Feldman, M. I., Anderson, B. G., Shetty, S. K.: Some applications of scintiscanning to radiation therapy. Radiology 112:740–741, 1974.

66. Frankendal, B.: Gastric emptying and small intestinal propulsion in mice following irradiation of the abdomen. Acta Radiol. 12:529–540, 1973.

67. Newman, A., Blendis, L. M., Katsaris, J., et al.: Small-intestinal injury in women who have had pelvic radiotherapy. Lancet 2:147–1473, 1973.

68. Lütolf, U. M., Glanzmann, C., Renk, I. W., et al.: Exhalationsdiagnostik mit ^{14}C-markierten verbindungen, methode und resultate. Schweiz. Med. Wochenschr. 104:729–736, 1975.

69. Antar, M. A., Spencer, R. P., Binder, H. J.: A simple test for measurement of fat absorption using breath $^{14}CO_2$ patterns after ingestion of ^{14}C-labeled fat. Am. J. Clin. Nutr. 25:450, 1972.

70. Fromm, H., Thomas, P. J., Hofmann, A. F.: Sensitivity and specificity in tests of distal ileal function: prospective comparison of bile acid and vitamin B_{12} absorption in ileal resection patients. Gastroenterology 64:1077–1090, 1973.

71. James, O. F. W., Agnew, J. E., Bouchier, I. A. D.: Assessment of the ^{14}C-glycocholic acid breath test. Br. Med. J. 3:191–195, 1973.

72. Sasaki, Y., Someya, K., Matsumoto, N., et al.: Deconjugation of bile salts by intestinal bacteria in cirrhotic patients. J. Nucl. Med. 15:530, 1974.

73. Ellinger, F.: Response of liver to irradiation. Radiology 44:241–251, 1945.

74. Kurohara, S. S., Swensson, N. L., Usselman, J. A. et al.: Response and recovery of liver to radiation as demonstrated by photoscans. Radiology 89:129–135, 1967.

75. Ingold, J. A., Reed, G. B., Kaplan, H. S., et al.: Radiation hepatitis. Am. J. Roentgenol. 93:200–208, 1965.

76. Johnson, P. M.: Radiation induced hepatic injury and its detection by scintillation scanning. Am. J. Roentgenol. 99:453–462, 1967.

77. Usselman, J. A.: Liver scanning in the assessment of liver damage from therapeutic external irradiation. J. Nucl. Med. 7:761–772, 1966.

78. Concannon, J. P., Eldermann, A., Frich, J. C., Jr. et al.: Localized "radiation hepatitis" as demonstrated by scans. Radiology 89:136–139, 1967.

79. Fellows, K. E., Jr., Vawter, G. F., Tefft, M.: Hepatic effects following abdominal irradiation in children: detection by ^{198}Au scan and confirmation by histologic examination. Am. J. Roentgenol. 103:422–431, 1968.

80. Antar, M. A., Spencer, R. P., Lang, R. C., et al.: Radionuclide studies on effects of different doses of focal radiation on the function of the liver. J. Nucl. Med. 11:297, 1970.

81. Antar, M. A., Spencer, R. P.: Effects of radiation therapy on major organ scans. Invest. Radiol. 9:321–322, 1974.

82. Spencer, R. P., Kligerman, M. M.: Scan evidence of hepatic "refunction" after tumor irradiation. J. Nucl. Med. 11:140–141, 1970.

83. Spencer, R. P., Antar, M. A., Toulookian, R. J., et al.: Relief of massive splenomegaly after irradiation of liver involved by Wilm's tumor. J. Nucl. Med. 14:939–940, 1973.

84. Spencer, R. P., Knowlton, A. H.: Redistribution of radiocolloid uptake after focal hepatic irradiation. Oncology 32:266–268, 1975.

85. Nebesar, R. A., Tefft, M., Vawter, G. F., et al.: Angiography in radiation "hepatitis." Br. J. Radiol. 471:588–593, 1974.

86. Spencer, R. P., Witek, J. T.: Radionuclide studies on the growth of intrahepatic tumors and of the infiltrated liver. Cancer 32:838–842, 1973.

87. Witek, J. T., Spencer, R. P.: Scan evidence of decrease in size of intrahepatic tumors after chemotherapy. Gastroenterology 67:516–518, 1974.

88. Spencer, R. P., Turner, J. W., Syed, J. B.: Regression of hepatic metastases from oat cell carcinoma after chemotherapy. Clin. Nucl. Med. 1:82–83, 1976.

89. Samuels, L. D.: Paradoxical splenic enlargement following radiation therapy. Radiology 104:389–391, 1972.

90. Aron, B. S., Schlesinger, A.: Complications of radiation therapy: the genitourinary tract. Semin. Roentgenol. 9:65–74, 1974.

91. Luxton, R. W.: Radiation nephritis: a long-term study of 54 patients. Lancet 2:1221–1224, 1961.

92. Madrazo, A., Schwarz, G., Churg, J.: Radiation nephritis: a review. J. Urol. 114:822–827, 1975.

93. Cohen, Y., Robinson, E.: The role of the radioisotope renogram in the diagnosis and evaluation of radiation nephritis. J. Urol. 112:268–271, 1974.

94. Ignatoff, J. M., Graham, J. B.: Bilateral ureterovaginal fistula: complication of radiation therapy. Urology 4:585–589, 1974.

95. Rutherford, H., Dodd, G. D.: Complications of radiation therapy: growing bone. Semin. Roentgenol. 9:15–27, 1974.

96. Loutit, J. F.: Malignancy from radium. Br. J. Cancer 24:195–207, 1970.

97. Dalinka, M. K., Edeiken, J., Finkelstein, J. B.: Complications of radium therapy: adult bone. Semin. Roentgenol. 9:29–40, 1974.

98. Probert, J. C., Parker, B. R.: The effects of radiation therapy on bone growth. Radiology 114:155–162, 1975.

99. De Smet, A. A., Kuhns, L. R., et al.: Effects of radiation therapy on growing long bones. Am. J. Roentgenol. 127:935–939, 1976.

100. Gates, G. F., Goris, M. L.: Maxillary-facial abnormalities assessed by bone imaging. Radiology 121:677–682, 1976.

101. Parker, R. G., Berry, H. C.: Late effects of the therapeutic irradiation on the skeleton and bone marrow. Cancer 37:1162–1171, 1976.

102. Castronovo, F. P., Potsaid, M. S., Pendergrass, H. P.: Effects of radiation therapy on bone lesions as measured by ^{99m}Tc-diphosphonate. J. Nucl. Med. 14:604–605, 1973.

103. Cox, P. H.: Abnormalities in skeletal uptake of ^{99m}Tc-polyphosphate complexes in areas of bone associated with tissues which have been subjected to radiation therapy. Br. J. Radiol. 47:851–856, 1974.

104. Rubin, R., Andrews, J. R., Swaim, R., et al.: Radiation-induced dysplasia of bone. Am. J. Roentgenol. 82:206–216, 1959.

105. Osmond, J. D., III, Pendergrass, H. P., Potsaid, M. N.: Accuracy of ^{99m}Tc-diphosphonate bone scans and roentgenograms in the detection of prostate, breast, and lung carcinoma metastases. Am. J. Roentgenol. 125:972–977, 1975.

106. DeGowin, R. L., Chaudhuri, T. K., Christie, J. H., et al.: Marrow scanning in evaluation of hemopoiesis after radiotherapy. Arch. Intern. Med. 134:297–303, 1974.

107. Sykes, M. P., Chu, F. C., Savel, H., et al.: The effects of varying dosage of irradiation upon sternal-marrow regeneration. Radiology 83:1083–1088, 1964.

108. Bell, E. G., McAfee, J. G., Constable, W. C.: Local radiation damage to bone and marrow demonstrated by radioisotopic imaging. Radiology 92:1083–1088, 1969.

109. Vogel, J. M., Kimball, H. R., Foley, H. T., et al.: Effect of extensive radiotherapy on the marrow granulocyte reserves of patients with Hodgkin's disease. Cancer 21:798–804, 1968.

110. Hoogstratten, B., Holland, J. F., Kramer, S., et al.: Combination chemotherapy-radiotherapy for stage III Hodgkin's disease: an acute leukemia group B study. Arch. Intern. Med. 131:424–428, 1973.

111. Rubin, P., Landman, S., Mayer, E., et al.: Bone marrow regeneration and extension after extended field irradiation in Hodgkin's disease. Cancer 32:699–711, 1973.

112. Sykes, M. P., Chu, F., Gee, T. S., et al.: Followup on the long term effects of therapeutic irradiation on bone marrow. Radiology 113:179–180, 1974.

113. Stewart, A., Pennybacker, W., Barber, R.: Adult leukaemias and diagnostic x-rays. Br. Med. J. 5309:882–890, 1962.

114. Crosby, W. H.: Acute granulocytic leukemia, a complication of therapy in Hodgkin's disease? Clin. Res. 17:463, 1969.

115. Hutchison, G. B.: Leukemia in patients with cancer of the cervix uteri treated with radiation—A report covering the first 5 years of an international study. J. Natl. Cancer Inst. 40:951–982, 1968.

116. Chan, R. C., Shukovsky, L. J.: Effects of irradiation on the eye. Radiology 120:673–675, 1976.

117. Brizel, H. E., Shells, W. C., Brown, M.: The effects of radiotherapy on the nasolacrimal system as evaluated by dacryoscintigraphy. Radiology 116:373–381, 1975.

118. Bekerman, C., Hoffer, P. B.: Salivary gland uptake of ^{67}Ga-citrate following radiation therapy. J. Nucl. Med. 17:685–687, 1976.

119. Fletcher, J. W., Herbig, F. K., Donati, R. M.: [67]Ga citrate distribution following whole-body irradiation or chemotherapy. Radiology 117:709–712, 1975.

120. Swartzendruber, D. C., Hübner, K. F.: Effect of external whole-body X-irradiation on gallium-67 retention in mouse tissues. Radiat. Res. 55:457–468, 1973.

121. McReynolds, R. A., Gold, G. L., Roberts, W. C.: Coronary heart disease after mediastinal irradiation for Hodgkin's disease. Am. J. Med. 60:39–45, 1976.

122. Levinson, S. A., Close, M. B., Ehrenfeld, W. K., et al.: Carotid artery occlusive disease following external cervical irradiation. Arch. Surg. 107:395–397, 1973.

123. St. Louis, E. L., McLoughlin, M. J., Wortzman, G.: Chronic damage to medium and large arteries following irradiation. J. Can. Assoc. Radiol. 25:94–104, 1974.

124. Meyer, K. K.: Radiation-induced lymphocyte-immune deficiency: a factor in the increased visceral metastases and decreased hormonal responsiveness of breast cancer. Arch. Surg. 101:114–121, 1970.

125. Stewart, C. C., Perez, C. A.: Effect of irradiation on immune responses. Radiology 118:201–210, 1976.

126. Order, S. E.: The effects of therapeutic irradiation on lymphocytes and immunity. Cancer 39:737–743, 1977.

127. Lewis, E. B.: Possible genetic consequences of irradiation of tumors in childhood. Radiology 114:147–153, 1975.

128. Lushbaugh, C. C., Casarett, G. W.: The effects of gonadal irradiation in clinical radiation therapy: a review. Cancer 37:1111–1120, 1976.

129. Berlin, N. I., Wasserman, L. R.: The association between systemically administered radioisotopes and subsequent malignant disease. Cancer 37:1097–1101, 1976.

130. Anderson, B. G., Beierwaltes, W. H., Nishiyama, R. H., et al.: Effect of large doses of [131]I-19-iodocholesterol on metapyralone-induced adrenal cortical hyperplasia in dogs. J. Nucl. Med. 16:928–932, 1975.

131. Jaffe, N.: Non-oncogenic sequelae of cancer chemotherapy. Radiology 114:167–173, 1975.

132. Phillips, T. L.: Chemical modification of radiation effects. Cancer 39:987–999, 1977.

133. Gillespie, P. J., Alexander, J. L., Edelstyn, G. A.: Changes in [87m]Sr concentrations in skeletal metastases in patients responding to cyclical combination chemotherapy for advanced breast cancer. J. Nucl. Med. 16:191–193, 1975.

134. Henry, R. E., Solaric-George, E., Donati, R. M.: Effect of granulocytopenia, marrow suppressive drugs, and infection on marrow reticuloendothelial (RE) patterns. J. Nucl. Med. 14:407–408, 1973.

135. D'Angio, G. J., Meadows, A., Mike, V., et al.: Decreased risk of radiation-associated second malignant neoplasms in actinomycin-D-treated patients. Cancer 37:1177–1185, 1976.

136. Bourgeaux, C., Martel, N., Sizaret, P., et al.: Prognostic value of alpha-fetoprotein radioimmunoassay in surgically treated patients with embryonal cell carcinoma of the testis. Cancer 38:1658–1660, 1976.

137. Sugarbaker, P. H., Bloomer, W. D., Corbett, E. D., et al.: Carcinoembryonic antigen (CEA) monitoring of radiation therapy for colorectal cancer. Am. J. Roentgenol. 127:641–644, 1976.

138. Leon, S. A., Shapiro, B., Sklaroff, D. M.: DNA in the serum of cancer patients and the effect of therapy. J. Nucl. Med. 17:550, 1976.

139. Shambaigh, G. E., Quinn, J. L., Oyzsu, R., et al.: Disparate thyroid imaging: combined studies with sodium pertechnetate and radioactive iodine. J.A.M.A. 228:866–869, 1074.

140. Turner, J. W., Spencer, R. P.: Thyroid carcinoma presenting as a pertechnetate "hot" nodule, but without I-131 uptake. J. Nucl. Med. 17:22–23, 1976.

141. Perthes, G.: Ueber den Einfluss der Rontgenostrahlen auf epitheliale Gewebe, insbesoudere auf des Carcinom. Arch. f. Klin. Chir. 71:955, 1903.
142. Blum, T.: Osteomyelitis of the mandible and maxilla. J. Am. Dental Assoc. 11:802, 1924.
143. Alexander, J. L., Gillespie, P. J., Edelstyn, G. A.: Serial bone scanning using technetium 99m diphosphonate in patients undergoing cyclical combination chemotherapy for advanced breast cancer. Clin. Nucl. Med. 1:13–17, 1976.

SECTION II

Thyroid

Harold L. Atkins

6
Treatment of Hyperthyroidism:
Use of ^{131}I and ^{125}I

The late occurrence of myxedema as a consequence of ^{131}I therapy for hyperthyroidism is the major concern in the present-day management of this condition. It is now over 30 years since the initiation of widespread use of radioiodine in therapy for hyperthyroidism. The rapid onset of myxedema in a significant number of patients following treatment was recognized at an early date.[1] The report of Beling and Einhorn[2] in 1961 drew attention to the cumulative incidence of myxedema each year at a rate of 3 percent per year after the first year. Since then many others have confirmed this finding with incidence rates ranging from 2 to 6.3 percent per year for longer than 15 years.[3-8]

A review of post-thyroidectomy patients has revealed a cumulative incidence of late-onset myxedema in these patients as well, although at somewhat lower rates.[4,7,9-11] Chemotherapy for hyperthyroidism probably results in no increase in myxedema as a late outcome, but there is a high recurrence rate in addition to problems encountered with side reactions.[12]

Radioiodine therapy remains the treatment of choice for most patients suffering from hyperthyroidism. Various strategies are being undertaken by investigators to overcome the problem of late-onset hypothyroidism. This is of particular importance since ^{131}I is now used in the treatment of younger individuals with the former restrictions on use in patients under 40 years of age no longer applied. It is the purpose of this review to discuss the factors which may be important in the etiology of this complication and to indicate the approaches that have been used or proposed to overcome this problem.

FACTORS RELATED TO POST-THERAPY HYPOTHYROIDISM

Investigators who have reviewed their long-term experience have indicated a number of factors which appear to be important in relation to the development of

Supported by U.S. Energy Research and Development Administration.

hypothyroidism. Consideration of these factors may yield clues to the etiology of post-therapy myxedema and lead to the development of methods to reduce its incidence.

Size of gland. In all series reviewed in which this factor was taken into account, the incidence of post-treatment hypothyroidism was significantly greater in patients who had small glands, either nonpalpable or of normal size.[2–4,6,7] The administered level of ^{131}I has been adjusted downward from the usual calculated amount in some series in consideration of this factor.[7,13]

In the review of their surgical series, Nofal et al.[7] also described this feature, but normal sized glands were rarely operated on.[7] This may be a point of bias in favor of surgery when attempting to compare ^{131}I with surgery in relation to resultant hypothyroidism.[14]

Presence of nodules. The multinodular gland appears to be more resistant to treatment, whether it be radioiodine or surgery. It usually requires multiple doses of ^{131}I more frequently and has a much lower incidence of post-therapeutic hypothyroidism.[2,5–7] Surprisingly, in patients with a single functioning nodule the incidence of subsequent hypothyroidism is greater.[3,7] In these patients it would ordinarily appear appropriate to give large doses since the nonnodular tissue would be relatively spared. However, the same results are found following surgery.[7] Therefore, the incidence of hypothyroidism must be related to something other than just the distribution of radioactivity in the gland following a therapeutic dose of [131]I.

Age of patient. There is a suggestion that the thyroid of younger individuals is more sensitive to radiation than that of older individuals and in some institutions the dose is reduced somewhat for the younger patient. The study of Segal et al.[3] showed a slightly higher incidence of myxedema in the younger patients. In some series the ^{131}I-treated younger patients tended to have larger glands,[4] whereas in other series these patients tended to be treated surgically. This factor can certainly bias results. Nofal et al.[7] demonstrated a slightly higher incidence of post-therapy hypothyroidism in the younger age group with ^{131}I treatment, whereas the highest incidence following surgery was in the patients who were between 40 and 49 years when treated.

Size of dose. The size of the initial dose does appear to have an effect on subsequent development of hypothyroidism and has been the basis for several series using lower doses to control the disease.[13,15–19] This may possibly slow the rate of the late cumulative incidence, but it certainly reduces the incidence of hypothyroidism in the first year. It does result in an increased requirement for multiple doses.

Number of doses. There is an inverse relationship between number of doses (and total doses) and the development of late-onset hypothyroidism in most studies.[2,3,7,14] Usually patients requiring multiple doses had multinodular glands. In addition, response to the first dose selected out those patients whose glands were more radiosensitive.

Race. In two series race is taken into account. Apparently blacks are more resistant to therapy, requiring multiple doses more often than whites.[8] In addition, there is less spontaneous, idiopathic, and post-therapeutic (^{131}I and surgery) myxedema in black patients.[14]

Previous surgery. In all series the use of ^{131}I following a partial thyroidectomy resulted in a greatly increased incidence of hypothyroidism.[2-4]

Size of postsurgical remnant. The size of the postsurgical remnant has no correlation with the incidence of subsequent hypothyroidism.[11,20]

Immune status. The incidence of post-therapy hypothyroidism has been considered in relationship to a number of immune factors.

In the surgical series of Green and Wilson,[4] there appeared to be a higher incidence of hypothyroidism in patients whose surgical specimens showed evidence of focal thyroiditis. A slight correlation existed between focal thyroiditis and the titer in the tanned red cell agglutination and complement fixation tests. No consistent effect of operation on the titers was found. Others have also noted the association of thyroiditis in the surgical specimens with postsurgical hypothyroidism.[4,10,21]

On the other hand, in ^{131}I-treated patients, there was no correlation between the results of serologic tests and the clinical state following treatment. In addition, the ^{131}I therapy had no effect on titer levels in patients in whom this was tested prior to and 2 to 3 years after treatment.[4]

The results of other studies are not clear. Burke and Silverstein[22] demonstrated a relationship between increased levels of circulating antithyroid antibodies and ^{131}I-induced hypothroidism in the first year. Others have also found transitory increases in thyroid autoantibodies in the first year following radioiodine therapy for hyperthyroidism, greater in those becoming hypothyroid in the first year, but probably not significant for the occurrence of late hypothyroidism.[23,24]

A lack of significant relationship of humoral antibodies to development of post-therapeutic hypothyroidism following ^{131}I has been found by others.[7,25,26] There does appear to be a higher incidence of postsurgical hypothyroidism in patients who have high titers of antithyroid antibodies.[25,26]

Relationship to prior nondestructive therapy. Segal et al.[3] found the lowest incidence of post-^{131}I hypothyroidism in patients who had received iodine or antithyroid drugs and iodine prior to [131]I. The incidence in this group was 4.1 percent compared to 9.4 percent in those having no prior treatment and 23.6 percent in those who had prior drugs and destructive therapy such as x-ray and/or surgery.

ETIOLOGY OF POST-THERAPEUTIC HYPOTHYROIDISM

The reason for the high incidence of post-therapeutic hypothyroidism following ^{131}I is still unknown, but a number of hypotheses have been proposed. Although radiation effects may be a major cause, it does not explain why a similar situation, albeit somewhat more mild, exists relative to surgical treatment. A means to reduce post-therapeutic hypothyroidism may be found when there exists a better understanding of the etiology of this complication.

A thesis for the effects of ^{131}I has been proposed by Greig.[27] The reproductive capacity of thyroid cells is more radiosensitive than the functional capacity. However, damage to the reproductive capacity is not manifest until the cell attempts to undergo mitosis, which may not occur for some years following [131]I. Some cells may die immediately. With time there is an increasing stress on the remaining cells with shortening of life span and inhibition of DNA synthesis under the influence of thyroid stimulating hormone.[28] These cells then attempt to divide but die in the process, eventually resulting in hypothyroidism.

Another possibility is related to the well-known late effects of radiation on blood vessels. The delayed development of endarteritis obliterans can result in the deprivation of an adequate blood supply to the gland. This, in turn, would lead to reduced function and/or cell death.

Early hypothyroidism occurs when all the thyroid cells have received a lethal dose of radiation. Usually, however, the dose distribution is uneven throughout the gland resulting in a frequency distribution of radiation injury. The most marked irregularity in distribution of radioiodine occurs in nodular glands accounting for the relative radioresistance of these glands and the low incidence of postradiation hypothyroidism.

Hypothyroidism developing late after partial thyroidectomy remains unexplained in the light of the above thesis. It is possible that the remnant of gland is put under severe stress to maintain a normal level of function and eventually is "exhausted." Another factor may be increased scarring and consequent reduction in blood flow to the gland. These possibilities are generally unsatisfactory explanations when considered along with the accumulated experience in this field.

There is now important evidence that hyperthyroidism, like Hashimoto's thyroiditis, is a disease related to a defect in the autoimmune surveillance mechanism.[29-31] Although it is thought to be primarily a disease involving cell-mediated immune processes, humoral factors may also play a role.[32,33] Except for some mildly positive evidence in those patients developing postsurgical hypothyoidism, as stated above, the role of autoimmunity in post-therapeutic hypothyroidism is unclear. However, it has been suggested that with both surgery and radiation, partial destruction of the gland releases more thyroidal antigens, in turn leading to eventual complete destruction of the gland.[14]

It is difficult to determine the natural course of hyperthyroidism in the untreated individual in the modern era. Spontaneous remissions occur but the disease can readily have a fatal outcome. It is estimated that only about 1 percent of such cases would end up as hypothyroid.[3] Therefore, the high incidence of late hypothyroidism cannot be attributed to the natural history of the disease or considered a fortuitous occurrence. Most likely it is related to the underlying etiology of the disease as well as to the treatment of it.

THERAPEUTIC STRATEGIES

Attempts to deal with the high incidence of postradioiodine hypothyroidism were energetically pursued by many investigators once this major complication was recognized. Several strategies have evolved but long-term follow-up over 15 to 20 years is required in order to be sure that any apparent improvement in the first few years is maintained. In addition, it must be ascertained that no selection bias, related to the several factors discussed above, will affect the results.

Reduction of Initial Dose

Estimation of the radiation dose delivered to the thyroid is difficult due to errors in estimating size of the gland by palpation, irregular distribution of radioiodine in the gland, and variations in biological half-life. In early series the activity delivered to the gland tended to be high (150 to 300 μCi/g) resulting in radiation doses in excess of 10,000 rads. The result was a high incidence of hypothyroidism.

Goolden and Fraser[13] devised a treatment schedule which varied the radioiodine concentration per gram of thyroid depending on the overall size of the thyroid. With this method smaller glands received a lower radiation dose ($\sim$3500 rads at 60 μCi/g) than larger glands. Their previous schedule called for a uniform dose of 150 μCi ^{131}I per gram except for glands estimated to be greater than 70 grams, which were dosed to a level of 300 μCi/g. Unfortunately, only 1-year results were reported. These showed a hypothyroidism rate of 5 percent compared to their previous experience of 17 percent at 1 year. However, at 1 year 38.5 percent of the group were still toxic and required antithyroid drug therapy.

Two other groups have demonstrated a reduced incidence of hypothyroidism at 5 or more years following initial ^{131}I treatment but at the price of prolonging the hyperthyroid status of some patients. Smith and Wilson[16] reduced the rate of hypothyroidism from 29.0 percent to 7.4 percent at 5 years by reducing the estimated radiation dose delivered to the thyroid from 7000 rads to 3500 rads. Further treatment with antithyroid drugs for persistent hyperthyroidism was necessitated in 43 percent of the high-dose group and 64 percent of the low-dose group. Apparently, additional ^{131}I treatment was not administered for persistent disease.

In the series of Cevallos et al.,[19] patients receiving ^{131}I at 160 μCi/g had a 5.6 year incidence of hypothyroidism of 45.7 percent while 22.9 percent required further [131]I. In their lower dose group (80 μCi/g) the hypothyroidism incidence at 5.5 years was 23.5 percent, and 26.5 percent required additional treatment.

In both the series of Smith and Wilson and that of Cevallos et al. there was a continuing rise in the cumulative incidence of hypothyroidism, but the rate of increase was slowed in comparison with the high-dose group in the Smith and Wilson study. In the series of Cevallos et al. the initial incidence at 1 year showed a marked reduction in the low-dose group, but the rate of increase thereafter was higher than in the high-dose group indicating that at some time in the future the two groups would converge.[19]

Another group receiving 50 μCi/g ^{131}I was reported by Rapoport et al.[17] These patients also had a low incidence of hypothyroidism but there was a high retreatment rate. Since that report a dosage scheme was devised similar to that of Goolden and Fraser taking into account the increased radiosensitivity of the smaller glands.[34] Results of this plan are not yet available.

A rather successful long-term result has been obtained by Jackson[18] with the delivering of 3500 rads ($\sim$40 μCi/g) to a large series of patients. Approximately 38

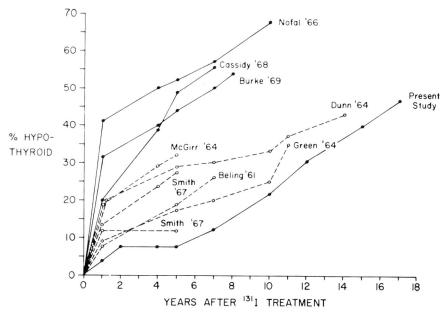

Fig. 6-1. Cumulative incidence of hypothyroidism in study of Glennon et al. (present study) compared with previously reported data. Solid lines indicate data originally reported using the life table method; broken lines indicate data recalculated from the reported data using the life table method. Reproduced with permission from Glennon J.A. et al., Ann. Int. Med. 76:721–723, 1972.

percent required more than one dose. The 10-year incidence of hypothyroidism was an acceptable 18 percent.[35]

Less satisfactory were the results of Glennon et al.[36] who observed the results of a single dose of 3 mCi or less for up to 17 years. Although the incidence of hypothyroidism was low at 1 year (3.7 percent) and at 5 years (7.5 percent), there was an annual increase of 3.4 percent thereafter, equalling the rates for higher dose series (Fig. 6-1). This illustrates the necessity for long-term follow-up and suggests that the eventual cumulated incidence of hypothyroidism cannot be reduced by low dose [131]I.

There seems to be no doubt that the incidence of hypothyroidism at 1 and 5 years can be substantially reduced by lowering the administered dose of ^{131}I, but probably at the price of increasing the need for retreatment and prolonging the duration of hyperthyroidism for many patients. The longer term results at 10 to 15 years or more are not yet available in many of these series, and there is the suggestion in the data of Cevallos et al. that the differences due to the different dose regimens may be less marked at that time.[19] The data of Glennon et al. indicate that the long-term follow-up does show a high rate of hypothyroidism even after low doses.[16]

Multiple Small Doses

The advantage of using multiple small doses (less than 50 μCi/g) is that it permits observation of the response prior to retreatment and permits individualization of the treatment regimen for each patient. Again, it prolongs the time for most patients to become euthyroid, but the results in one such trial appear promising with only 3 percent hypothyroidism at 7 to 16 years following initiation of therapy in 334 patients.[37]

High-Dose Radioiodine Followed by Replacement Therapy

Since it is felt by some that every patient treated with ^{131}I will eventually become hypothyroid, and since the onset may be very gradual and unnoticed by the patient until the process is advanced, an opposite approach has been taken. Using an initial dose which is rather high (160 to 200 μCi/g) causes rapid reversal of the hyperthyroid state with 90 percent of the patients controlled within 3 months.[38] Thyroid replacement therapy was instituted in the controlled patients, to be continued for the remainder of each patient's life. Although this approach appears to be practical in that it brings the hypothyroid state under rapid control and reduces the possibility of an advanced stage of unrecognized hypothyroidism, it is intellectually not satisfactory. This is especially true at this time when patients under the age of 40 years receive [131]I. In selected patients with cardiac disease and in the older age group this method is certainly a valid one. A continued search for a way to achieve a euthyroid state in each patient with hyperthyroidism is indicated.

Use of External Beam Irradiation

The hyperthyroid gland is more sensitive than the normal gland to ionizing radiation. Radiation doses which do not affect normal rat thyroid cell function (1000 rads, x-ray, or 5000 rads, ^{131}I) can have a marked effect on human thyrotoxic thyroid cells.[39]

External beam therapy was used in the treatment of hyperthyroidism prior to the availability of antithyroid drugs and radioiodine.[40-43] The older literature is difficult to evaluate precisely because of problems with specification of dose and in the diagnosis of thyroid status. However, it is apparent that the success rate in curing hyperthyroidism was good (80 to 90 percent) with doses probably under 2000 rads to the thyroid. Post-therapeutic hypothyroidism appears to have been low, both short term and long term, but the adequacy of follow-up and ability to detect developing hypothyroidism are in question.

It is of interest, in view of recent theories of the etiology of hyperthyroidism, that Groover et al.[40] also irradiated the thymus in addition to the thyroid.

On the other hand, much higher doses of radiation delivered to the thyroid in the course of treatment of malignancies in the pharynx and larynx produce only minor suppression of radioiodine uptake without long-term effects. A biphasic suppression is noted at 3 to 4 weeks and again at 3 to 4 months with slightly higher uptakes in the intervening period.[44,45] Einhorn and Wikholm[46] found only 3 cases of hypothyroidism 10 or more years following high-dose irradiation to 43 patients. However, they did demonstrate diminished reserve as evidenced by lack of response to TSH stimulation in the clinically euthyroid patients.

A more recent attempt to treat thyrotoxicosis with external beam therapy has been described by Philp et al.[47] Cobalt 60 irradiation in doses of 115 to 900 rads in

28 patients failed to control the hyperthyroid state in 25. It is interesting that 3 patients did become euthyroid with doses of 400, 600, and 800 rads. The trial was then abandoned.

The advantage of external beam irradiation is the rather precise control of radiation dose. This permits the depletion of a specified fraction of thyroid cells, a situation not possible with an internally deposited radionuclide.

Trotter and Willoughby[48] have demonstrated a biphasic effect of radiation on thyroidal radioiodine uptake following a dose of 400 to 800 rads of ^{60}Co gamma rays on a portion of the thyroid. There is an initial 30 to 50 percent reduction in uptake, demonstrated on scans, which occurs at an interval of 24 hours between irradiation and administration of the dose. A slight compensatory increase in uptake is then noted for 2 weeks followed by a second decrease in uptake at 3 weeks lasting for about 2 weeks.

Fifty patients were treated with radioiodine following irradiation of a portion of the gland with 800 rads in the hope that the portion of the gland temporarily suppressed by ^{60}Co would take up less of a therapeutic dose of ^{131}I and thus be spared destruction. However, no difference in the rate of hypothyroidism was noted in the early results at less than 1 year. Further details have not been published.

With the development of accurate methods for localizing charged particle beams, there is the possibility of using the Bragg peak for precise delineation of a target area within the thyroid while sparing normal tissue. With such a beam of heavy ions it would be possible to selectively irradiate a portion of the thyroid while sparing the remainder, as well as adjacent normal tissues. This approach has not yet been undertaken.

Use of ^{125}I

The highly energetic beta emission combined with the gamma photons of ^{131}I results in a rather uniform distribution of the radiation dose in the individual thyroid cell. Since, as stated above, the reproductive capacity of thyroid cells is more radiosensitive than the functional aspect, it seems very unlikely that reduction of the functional integrity can occur following ^{131}I without subsequent cell death and eventual hypothyroidism.

With ^{125}I the situation is theoretically quite different. Most of the radiation effect is probably due to the very low energy conversion and Auger electrons.[49-51] The lower energy Auger electrons (0.8–2.9 kev) are particularly abundant (Table 6-1). The range of these electrons in tissue is very small (from < 0.4 to 20 μm). Since the radioiodine is primarily in the colloid, the radiation dose distribution is markedly nonhomogeneous, affecting the cellular cytoplasm at the apex of the cell to a much greater extent than the nucleus (Fig. 6-2).

Dose estimates for whole-gland distribution can be in serious error relative to the microscopic distribution. Difficulties in calculation are evident because of the marked variation in follicle size and cell size in the normal and hyperthyroid gland. Several authors have made such calculations,[49-54] and these have shown ratios of about 3-4 to 1 for the colloid-cell interface dose to the dose at the nucleus (Table 6-2).

Theoretically this concentration of dose at the colloid-cell interface should

Table 6-1
Decay Characteristics of ^{125}I*

	Radiation	Energy (kev)	N/100 Disintegrations
Photons	Gamma	35.4	6.66
	$K_{\alpha 1}$ x-ray	27.4	76.15
	$K_{\alpha 2}$ x-ray	27.2	39.06
	$K_{\beta 1}$ x-ray	30.9	20.56
	$K_{\beta 2}$ x-ray	31.8	4.26
	L x-rays	3.7	22.26
Electrons	K int. conv.	3.6	80.0 ⎫
	L int. conv.	30.9	11.42 ⎬ $\Delta_i = 0.0151$
	M int. conv.	34.6	1.9 ⎭
	KLL Auger	22.6	14.16 ⎫
	KLX Auger	26.4	5.97 ⎬ $\Delta_i = 0.0107$
	KXY Auger	30.1	0.96 ⎭
	LMN Auger	2.9	154.42 ⎫ $\Delta_i = 0.0159$
	MXY Auger	0.8	364.61 ⎭

*Half-life: 60.2 days.

result in more marked effects on the site of hormonogenesis than on the replicative capacity. Studies comparing the effects of ^{131}I and ^{125}I in animal systems have demonstrated recovery of function after initial suppression by ^{125}I. A more marked effect was seen on iodine-concentrating mechanisms than on goitrogenesis,[56–59] and histopathological studies have confirmed the localization of dose.[59]

The cell survival studies of Greig et al.[57] are confirmatory. Only the work of Jongejan and Van Putten[60] indicates an opposite conclusion. They found no difference in the ^{125}I/^{131}I ratio for administered levels of activity to produce identical effects on hormonal function and on cell killing.

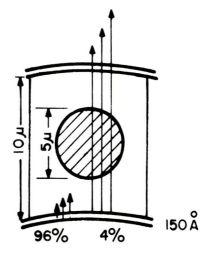

Fig. 6-2. Schematic representation of percentage distribution of electron radiation dose inside thyroid cell. The radiations emanate from ^{125}I in the follicular colloid. (Reproduced with permission from Lewitus Z. et al., Seminars in Nucl. Med. *1*:411–421, 1972.)

Table 6-2
Calculated Radiation Dose to the Thyroid From ^{125}I (1 mCi in a 20-g Gland)

	Initial Dose Rate (rads/day)			Total Dose (rads)*		
Author	Whole Gland	Colloid-Cell Interface	Nucleus	Whole Gland	Colloid-Cell Interface	Nucleus
Harper et al.[52]	36.8			795		
Gillespie et al.[49]	75	170	46	1620	3672	994
Reddy et al.[50]		457	112		9871	2419
Gavron and Feige[51]	78	63.6	32.4	1685	1374	700
Lewitus et al.[53]	88.8	151.2	37.2	1918	3266	804
Ben-Porath et al.[54]		77.8	25.9		1680	559
MIRD†	72			1555		

*Assumes T½ eff. of 115 days.
†Author's calculation using MIRD tables for absorbed dose per unit cumulated activity.[55]

Several clinical trials of ^{125}I for hyperthyroidism were initiated in the hope that late hypothyroidism could be substantially reduced (Table 6-3). These have varied in the dose of ^{125}I used relative to the conventional ^{131}I dose and the results have been mixed. At least two groups have discontinued their study because of lack of improvement in results.

In Glasgow the initial trial used a dose in millicuries of ^{125}I four times the usual dose of ^{131}I. This resulted in a rapid reversal of the hyperthyroid state but with a substantial percentage of ensuing hypothyroidism. With reduction in the amount of ^{125}I administered the incidence of hypothyroidism decreased, but with an increase in persistent hyperthyroidism.[62–64]

On the other hand, Israeli investigators have used fewer millicuries of ^{125}I than of ^{131}I, assuming a quality factor of 3 for the rad dose in the apical region of the cell from the low-energy Auger electrons.[65] The relapse rate was high leading to the use of increased doses and finally to a combination of ^{125}I and ^{131}I in equal millicurie amounts.[66] With this combined therapy it was felt that a rapid response by affecting hormonogenesis was initiated by ^{125}I and that long-term effects were maintained by the cell killing action of ^{131}I. This combination led to the lowest incidence of recurrence but without much effect on the incidence of hypothyroidism.

A series of patients treated by Siemsen et al.[67] initially showed a low rate of hypothyroidism but with a high rate of persistent hyperthyroidism. No further patients are being added to this study because of the conclusion that the results were no better than with ^{131}I. The series of Werner et al.[68] and that of Weidinger et al.[69] continue, and a recent study by Glanzmann and Horst[70] shows promising results.

In this last study there was no hypothyroidism at 18 to 24 months and 18 percent persistent hyperthyroidism. Of those patients with persistent or relapse of thyrotoxicosis, more than 30 percent had T_3 thyrotoxicosis.

Another small series of patients was treated with ^{125}I by Gimlette and Hoschl.[71] The dose of ^{125}I was identical to the dose of ^{131}I used in a control group.

Table 6-3
Results of ^{125}I Therapy for Thyrotoxicosis

Author	Radioactivity Level (N)		Euthyroid (%)	Hyperthyroid (%)	Hypothyroid (%)	Follow-up (years)
Bremner et al.[63]	1000 μCi/g	(18)	64	0	36	3.3 (ave.)
	600 μCi/g	(86)	42	24	34	3 (ave.)
	300 μCi/g	(193)	64	18	18	2.3 (ave.)
Lewitus et al.[66]	12–72 μCi/g	(45)	44.4	48.9	6.7	0.5–2
	87–94 μCi/g	(11)	54.5	36.4	9.1	
	24–107 μCi/g^{125}I +					
	35–100 μCi/g^{131}I	(43)	90.7	2.3	7.0	
Weidinger et al.[69]	4–9.5 mCi	(30)	73.3	20	6.7	0.3–4
	10–19.5 mCi	(21)	42.9	38.1	19	
	20–36 mCi	(12)	50	41.7	8.3	
	Total	(63)	58.7	30.2	11.1	
Siemsen et al.[67]	200 μCi/g	(60)	71	24	5	1–2
	100 μCi/g	(40)	43	53	4	0.75–2
Glanzmann and Horst[70]	~50 μCi/g	(99)	82	18	0	1.5–2
Gimlette and Hoschl[71]	3–6 mCi	(31)	32.3	58	9.7	1.9–3

The study was discontinued after 36 months follow-up because of the high rate of persistent hyperthyroidism (58 percent) along with an incidence of 9.7 percent hypothyroidism. This compares with 32 percent hyperthyroidism and 10.7 percent hypothyroidism following [131]I.

For full evaluation of ^{125}I more time must pass and the late results at 15 to 20 years be apparent. Hypothyroidism following ^{125}I may be more transient than after [131]I. Assessment of ^{125}I at this time does not appear to be particularly encouraging with regard to its ability to restore the euthyroid state without excessive hypothyroidism.

CONCLUSIONS

Hypothyroidism occurring within the first year of radioiodine therapy can be reduced by lowering the amount of administered [131]I. The incidence appears to be directly related to the dose in $\mu Ci/g$.[72] This probably reflects direct killing of thyroid cells or a mechanism related to interphase death.

Late-onset hypothyroidism does not appear to be directly related to the administered dose of radioiodine. It is probably a result of cell death during mitosis and may be related to biological factors affecting the rate of cell replication.

This late-onset hypothyroidism remains a problem. The various methods that have been applied to reduce the incidence have had unimpressive results. The wide variation in results from one locality to another suggests that environmental and dietary factors may also be important.

The differences between surgical and radioiodine therapy results may be due largely to a bias in selection of patients. If so, improved results with less post-therapeutic hypothyroidism must await a better understanding of the etiology of thyrotoxicosis, and treatment must be directed toward that etiology.

REFERENCES

1. Chapman, E. M., Maloof, F.: The use of radioactive iodine in the diagnosis and treatment of hyperthyroidism: ten years' experience. Medicine (Baltimore) 34:261–321, 1955.
2. Beling, V., Einhorn, J.: Incidence of hypothyroidism and recurrence following ^{131}I treatment of hyperthyroidism. Acta Radiol. 56:275–288, 1961.
3. Segal, R. L., Silver, S., Yohalem, S. B., et al.: Myxedema following radioactive iodine therapy of hyperthyroidism. Am. J. Med. 31:354–364, 1961.
4. Green, M., Wilson, G. M.: Thyrotoxicosis treated by surgery or iodine-131. With special reference to development of hypothyroidism. Br. Med. J. 1:1005–1010, 1964.
5. McGirr, E. M., Thomson, J. A., Murray, I. P. C.: Radioiodine therapy in thyrotoxicosis. A review of 908 cases. Scot. Med. J. 9:505–513, 1964.
6. Dunn, J. T., Chapman, E. M.: Rising incidence of hypothyroidism after radioactive-iodine therapy in thyrotoxicosis. N. Engl. J. Med. 271:1037–1042, 1964.
7. Nofal, M. M., Beierwaltes, W. H., Patno, M. E.: Treatment of hyperthyroidism with sodium iodide I 131. A 16 year experience. J.A.M.A. 197:605–610, 1966.
8. Blahd, W. H., Hays, M. T.: Graves' disease in the male. A review of 241 cases treated with an individually calculated dose of sodium iodide I 131. Arch. Int. Med. 129:33–40, 1972.

9. VanderLaan, W. P., Swenson, O.: The results of surgical treatment in Graves' disease. N. Engl. J. Med. 236:236–238, 1947.

10. Beahrs, O. H., Sakulsky, S. B.: Surgical thyroidectomy in the management of exophthalmic goiter. Arch. Surg. 96:512–516, 1968.

11. Hedley, A. J., Flemming, C. J., Chesters, M. I., et al.: Surgical treatment of thyrotoxicosis. Br. Med. J. 1:519–523, 1970.

12. Hershman, J. M.: The treatment of hyperthyroidism. Ann. Intern. Med. 64:1306–1314, 1966.

13. Goolden, A. W. G., Fraser, T. R.: Treatment of thyrotoxicosis with low doses of radioactive iodine. Br. Med. J. 2:442–443, 1969.

14. Bronsky, D., Kiamko, R. T., Waldstein, S. S.: Posttherapeutic myxedema. Relative occurrence after treatment of hyperthyroidism by radioactive iodine (^{131}I) or subtotal thyroidectomy. Arch. Intern. Med. 121:113–117, 1968.

15. Hagen, G. A., Ouelette, R. P., Chapman, E. M.: Comparison of high and low dosage levels of ^{131}I in the treatment of thyrotoxicosis. N. Engl. J. Med. 277:559–562, 1967.

16. Smith, R. N., Wilson, G. M.: Clinical trial of different doses of ^{131}I in treatment of thyrotoxicosis. Br. Med. J. 1:129–132, 1967.

17. Rapoport, B., Caplan, R., DeGroot, L. J.: Low-dose sodium iodide I 131 therapy in Graves' disease. J.A.M.A. 224:1610–1613, 1973.

18. Jackson, G. L.: Calculated low dose radioiodine therapy of thyrotoxicosis. Int. J. Nucl. Med. Biol. 2:80–81, 1975.

19. Cevallos, J. L., Hagen, G. A., Maloof, F., et al.: Low-dosage ^{131}I therapy of thyrotoxicosis (diffuse goiters). N. Engl. J. Med. 290:141–143, 1974.

20. Taylor, G. W., Painter, N. S.: Size of the thyroid remnant in partial thyroidectomy for toxic goitre. Lancet 1:287–289, 1962.

21. Whitsell, F. M., Black, B. M.: A statistical study of the clinical significance of lymphocytic and fibrocytic replacements in the hyperplastic thyroid gland. J. Clin. Endocrinol. Metabl. 9:1202–1215, 1949.

22. Burke, G., Silverstein, G. E.: Hypothyroidism after treatment with sodium iodide I 131. J.A.M.A. 210:1051–1058, 1969.

23. Einhorn, J., Einhorn, N., Fagraeus, A., et al.: Hypothyroidism and humoral antibodies after radioactive treatment of hyperthyroidism. In: Thyrotoxicosis, Proceedings of an International Symposium, W. James Irvine (ed.). Baltimore, Williams & Wilkins Co., pp. 123–134, 1967.

24. Blagg, C. R.: Antibodies to thyroglobulin in patients with thyrotoxicosis treated with radioactive iodine. Lancet 2:1364–1365, 1960.

25. Buchanan, W. W., Koutras, D. A., Crooks, J., et al.: The clinical significance of the complement-fixation test in thyrotoxicosis. J. Endocrinol. 24:115–125, 1962.

26. Irvine, W. J., Macgregor, A. G., Stuart, A. E.: The prognostic significance of thyroid antibodies in the management of thyrotoxicosis. Lancet 2:843–847, 1962.

27. Greig, W. R.: Radiation, thyroid cells and ^{131}I therapy—a hypothesis. J. Clin. Endocrinol. Metab. 25:1411–1417, 1965.

28. Al-Hindawi, A. Y., Wilson, G. M.: The effect of irradiation on the function and survival of rat thyroid cells. Clin. Sci. 28:555–571, 1965.

29. Volpé, R.: The immunologic basis of Graves's disease. N. Engl. J. Med. 287:463–464, 1972.

30. Farid, N. R., Munro, R. E., Row, V. V., et al.: Peripheral thymus-dependent (T) lymphocytes in Graves's disease and Hashimoto's thyroiditis. N. Engl. J. Med. 288:1313–1317, 1973.

31. Lamki, L., Row, V. V., Volpé, R.: Cell-mediated immunity in Graves' disease and in Hashimoto's thyroiditis as shown by the demonstration of migration inhibition factor (MIF). J. Clin. Endocrinol. Metab. 36:358–364, 1973.

32. Werner, S. C., Wegelius, O., Fierer, J. A., et al.: Immunoglobulins (E, M, G,) and complement in the connective tissues of the thyroid in Graves's disease. N. Engl. J. Med. 287:421–425, 1972.

33. Werner, S. C., Fierer, J. A.: Cell-mediated immunity in Graves' disease? N. Engl. J. Med. 287:1215, 1972.

34. DeGroot, L. J.: Graves Disease: Diagnosis and Treatment In: The Thyroid and Its Diseases, 4th Ed., Leslie J. DeGroot and John B. Stanbury (eds.). New York, Wiley Biomedical Division, pp. 314–367, 1975.

35. Jackson, G. L.: Personal communication, 1977.

36. Glennon, J. A., Gordon, E. S., Sawin, C. T.: Hypothyroidism after low-dose ^{131}I treatment of hyperthyroidism. Ann. Intern. Med. 76:721–723, 1972.

37. Reinwein, D., Schaps, D., Berger, H., et al.: Hypothyreoserisijiko nach fraktionierter Radiojodtherapie. Dtsch. Med. Wochenschr. 98:1789–1795, 1973.

38. Safa, A. M., Skillern, P. G.: Treatment of hyperthyroidism with a large initial dose of sodium iodide I 131. Arch. Intern. Med. 135:673–675, 1975.

39. Greig, W. R., Crooks, J., Macgregor, A. G.: Clinical and radiobiological consequences of therapeutic thyroid irradiation. Proc. R. Soc. Med. (Lond.) 59:599–602, 1966.

40. Groover, T. A., Christie, A. C., Merrit, E. A., et al.: Roentgen irradiation in the treatment of hyperthyroidism. A statistical evaluation based on three hundred and five cases. J.A.M.A. 32:1730–1734, 1929.

41. Harris, J. H.: Radiation treatment of hyperthyroidism: Report of results at the Hospital of the University of Pennsylvania during the seven and one-half years ending July 1, 1934. Am. J. Roentgenol. Rad. Ther. 38:129–144, 1937.

42. Pfahler, G. E.: Roentgen-ray treatment of hyperthyroidism. Radiology 34:43–52, 1940.

43. Soley, M. H., Stone, R. S.: Roentgen ray treatment of hyperthyroidism. Arch. Intern. Med. 70:1002–1016, 1942.

44. Lanaro, A. E., Bosch, A., Frias, Z.: Effects of irradiation on the normal thyroid gland uptake. Am. J. Roentgenol. Rad. Ther. 114:600–609, 1972.

45. Greig, W. R., Boyle, J. A., Buchanan, W. W., et al.: Clinical and radiobiological observations on latent effects of irradiation on the thyroid gland. J. Clin. Endocrinol. Metab. 25:1009–1014, 1965.

46. Einhorn, J., Wikholm, G.: Hypothyroidism after external radiation to thyroid region. Radiology 88:326–328, 1967.

47. Philp, J. R., Harrison, M. T., Ridley, E. F., et al.: Treatment of thyrotoxicosis with ionizing radiation. Lancet 2:1307–1310, 1968.

48. Trotter, W. R., Willoughby, P.: The effect of external irradiation on ^{131}I uptake by the thyrotoxic thyroid. In: Thyrotoxicosis, Proceedings of an International Symposium, Edinburgh, May, 1967, W. J. Irvine (ed.). Baltimore, Williams & Wilkins Co., pp. 147–154, 1967.

49. Gillespie, F. C., Orr, J. S., Greig, W. R.: Microscopic dose distribution from ^{125}I in the toxic thyroid gland and its relation to therapy. Br. J. Radiol. 43:40–47, 1970.

50. Reddy, A. R., Sastre, K. G. K., Gupta, M. H., et al.: Microdosimetry of ^{125}I in hyperthyroidism. In: Basic Mechanisms in Radiation Biology and Medicine, Bombay, Bhabbs Atomic Research Center, pp. 711–719, 1971.

51. Gavron, A., Feige, Y.: Dose distribution and maximum permissible burden of ^{125}I in the thyroid gland. Health Phys. 23:491–499, 1972.

52. Harper, P. V., Siemans, W. D., Lathrop, K. A., et al.: Production and use of iodine-125. J. Nucl. Med. 4:277–289, 1963.

53. Lewitus, Z., Ben-Porath, M., Feige, Y., et al.: Differences in the radiobiological action of 125I and 131I in the thyroid cell. In Biophysical Aspects of Radiation Quality. IAEA, Vienna, pp. 405–417, 1971.

54. Ben-Porath, M., Feige, Y., Lubin, E., et al.: Microdosimetry of I-125 in the thyroid follicle. J. Nucl. Med. 11:300–301, 1970 (Abst.).

55. Snyder, W. S., Ford, M. R., Warner, G. G., et al.: "S" absorbed dose per unit cumulated activity for selected radionuclides and organs. MIRD Pamphlet No. 11, Society of Nuclear Medicine, 1975.

56. Gross, J., Ben-Porath, M., Rosin, A., et al.: A comparison of radiobiologic effects of ^{131}I and ^{125}I respectively on the rat thyroid. In: Thyroid Neoplasia, S. Young and D. R. Inman (eds.). London and New York, Academic Press, pp. 291–306, 1968.

57. Greig, W. R., Smith, J. F. B., Orr, J. S., et al.: Comparative survivals of rat thyroid cells *in vivo* after ^{131}I, ^{125}I and X irradiations. Br. J. Radiol. 43:542–548, 1970.

58. Vickery, A. L., Jr., Williams, E. D.: Comparative biological effects of ^{125}I and ^{131}I on the rat thyroid. Acta Endocrinol. (Kbh.) 66:201–212, 1971.

59. Lewitus, Z., Rechnic, J.: Electron-microscopic and isotopic evidence for a difference between the radiobiological effects of iodine-131 and iodine-125. In: Radioactive Isotope in Klinik und Forschung, Band II, Gasteiner Internationales Symposion 1974, R. Hofer (ed.). Vienna, Urban & Schwarzenberg, pp. 44–51, 1975.

60. Jongejan, W. J., Van Putten, L. M.: The effects of ^{131}I and ^{125}I on mouse and rat thyroid. Int. J. Radiat. Biol. 22:489–499, 1972.

61. Greig, W. R., Smith, J. F. B., Gillespie, F. C., et al.: Iodine-125 treatment for thyrotoxicosis. Lancet 1:755–757, 1969.

62. McDougall, I. R., Greig, W. R., Gillespie, F. C.: Radioactive iodine (^{125}I) therapy for thyrotoxicosis. N. Engl. J. Med. 285:1099–1104, 1971.

63. Bremner, W. F., McDougall, I. R., Greig, W. R.: Results of treating 297 thyrotoxic patients with [125]I. Lancet 2:218–282, 1973.

64. McDougall, I. R., Greig, W. R.: [125]I therapy in Graves's disease. Ann. Intern. Med. 85:720–723, 1976.

65. Lewitus, Z.: Iodine-125 treatment for thyrotoxicosis. Lancet 2:1368, 1969.

66. Lewitus, Z., Lubin, E., Rechnic, J., et al.: Treatment of thyrotoxicosis with ^{125}I and [131]I. Semin. Nucl. Med. 1:411–421, 1971.

67. Siemsen, J., Wallack, M. S., Martin, R. B., et al.: Early results of ^{125}I therapy of thyrotoxic Graves' disease. J. Nucl. Med. 15:257–260, 1974.

68. Werner, S. C., Johnson, P. M., Goodwin, P. N., et al.: Long term results with iodine-125 treatment for toxic diffuse goiter. Lancet 2:681–685, 1970.

69. Weidinger, P., Johnson, P. M., Werner, S. C.: Five years' experience with iodine-125 therapy of Graves's disease. Lancet 2:74–77, 1974.

70. Glanzmann, C., Horst, W.: Ergebnisse der Therapie der Hyperthyreose mit 125- Jod. Nucl. Med. 14:207–218, 1975.

71. Gimlette, T. M. D., Hoschl, R.: Treatment of thyrotoxicosis with iodine-125 in moderately low dosage. Clin. Radiol. 24:263–266, 1973.

72. Malone, J. F., Cullen, M. J.: Two mechanisms for hypothyroidism after ^{131}I therapy. Lancet 2:73–75, 1976.

William H. Beierwaltes

7

Radioiodide in the Therapy
for Thyroid Carcinoma

[131]I TREATMENT OF WELL-DIFFERENTIATED THYROID
CARCINOMA: A WELL-EVALUATED THERAPEUTIC MODEL

One of the least traumatic, least invasive, and most effective methods of treating any cancer metastatic to lymph nodes and lungs today is the use of ^{131}I to treat metastatic well-differentiated thyroid carcinoma after surgery.[1–9]

This treatment differs most obviously from conventional teletherapy (and pi meson therapy) in that:

1. The source of radiation therapy is swallowed in a few milliliters of water through a paper straw.
2. In some instances, only one dose need be given.
3. The *therapeutic* amount of radiation is given in a *tracer* amount of chemical.
4. Even small thyroid cancer metastases not detected externally will concentrate the ^{131}I selectively in a high target-to-nontarget ratio.
5. The ^{131}I in the metastasis irradiates the metastasis from the inside out relatively selectively.
6. The ionization produced by the 609-kev beta rays (10 rads/μCi/g) is greater than from conventional x-ray therapy and is confined to a smaller area because the beta radiation penetrates only a few millimeters in tissue.[10]

   Assuming a half-life b of 4 days, 0.1 percent of the therapy dose of ^{131}I per gram produces 15,000 rads/150 mCi.[11] Pochin[11] has also estimated that three lung metastases, each 1 cm in diameter, with a total uptake of 0.5 percent of the dose would deliver 15,000 rads to tumor tissue. Scott et al.[12] quantitated uptake of ^{131}I in metastases in vivo and determined that one patient received 69,000 rads in one lobe of the thyroid gland and another patient received 26,000 rads to a metastasis in temporal bone/100 mCi.
7. About 85 percent of the nontarget background of ^{131}I is excreted, largely in the urine, within 2 to 3 days (7 mR/hour at 1 meter from body of patient when total body content has reached 30 mCi),[10] and the target concentration of ^{131}I is retained much longer (T½ b of 4 days).[11,13]

IS WELL-DIFFERENTIATED THYROID CANCER WORTH TREATING?

There is little point in discussing the treatment of well-differentiated thyroid cancer with radioactive iodine unless the reader is first convinced that well-differentiated thyroid cancer is worth treating.

Many physicians are not enthusiastic about treating well-differentiated thyroid cancer because they have read articles that state that this population of cancer patients, particularly young individuals, do very well without treatment.

One of the most commonly quoted articles is by Woolner et al.,[14] in *Thyroid Neoplasia,* published in 1968, on "1,181 cases followed for 40 years." These authors have presented survival tables showing that occult papillary carcinoma and intrathyroidal papillary carcinoma have a normal survival rate at 40 years. They also found a normal survival rate for noninvasive follicular carcinoma of the thyroid.

Careful review of their patients with intrathyroidal papillary carcinoma, however, reveals that eight died of their thyroid carcinoma. The average duration of life from surgery to death was 11 years. Obviously, these eight deaths from thyroid cancer should not endow a normal survival. It became evident that the authors had fitted their normal life table survival curve to three different populations. Our School of Public Health prepared a life table for normal survival of 300,000 females and 100,000 males starting at age 20 years and followed for 40 years. These were age- and sex-specific rates from the National Center for Health Statistics. Figure 7-1 shows that when this single normal survival curve for the population just described is fitted on to the two figures from the Mayo Clinic

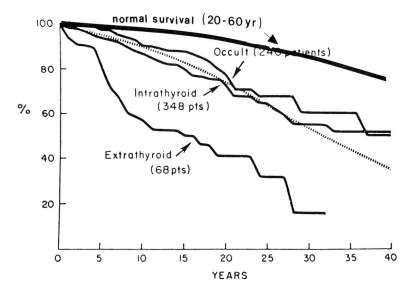

Fig. 7-1. Survival curves in patients with well-differentiated thyroid carcinoma. (Reproduced with permission from Woolner et al., *Thyroid Neoplasia,* 1968, with our Biostatics Department Life Table—normal survival curve—at top.)

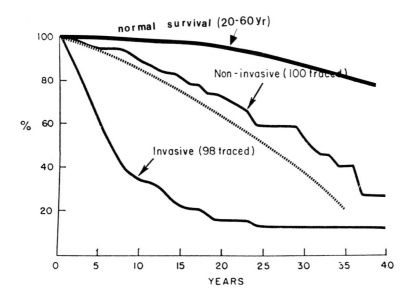

Fig. 7-2. Survival curves in patients with well-differentiated follicular carcinoma. (Reproduced with permission from Woolner et al., *Thyroid Neoplasia,* 1968, with our Biostatics Department Life Table—normal survival curve—at top.)

paper, that each of their cancer populations have subnormal survivals. The principal point to be made is that a normal survival curve must be exactly matched to the population with thyroid cancer being evaluated. It can not be matched to several different populations. Our sex and age populations of normals was chosen because in our paper on our first 8-year experience in the treatment of well-differentiated thyroid cancer in 57 patients,[2] the mean age of patients with colloid-producing well-differentiated thyroid carcinoma was 30 years (range of 3 to 63). Eighty-three percent of these patients were less than 50 years of age. The mean age of patients with no colloid production was 52 years (range of 14 to 86). Sixty-five percent of these patients were older than 50 years.

Using the normal survival curve of the Mayo Clinic, however, their articles stressed that the "extrathyroidal" well-differentiated papillary carcinoma of the thyroid did have a clearly subnormal survival rate. There was a 33 percent decrease in survival at 20 years. Of 38 cases having a biopsy only of the thyroid to lymph nodes, 16 patients died of thyroid cancer (42 percent). Of 68 patients traced who had adequate surgery, 10 died of thyroid cancer, a 16 percent death rate. In other words, this article clearly states that well-differentiated thyroid cancer does kill.

In the "noninvasive" follicular carcinoma group with a normal survival, there were 30 deaths from thyroid cancer. In other words, even the patients with slight to equivocal vascular invasion of well-differentiated follicular carcinoma did die of thyroid cancer.

Figure 7-2 from that article clearly indicates that well-differentiated follicular carcinoma that is "invasive" does kill. In this group, there were 51 deaths from thyroid cancer (52 percent) with a mean survival of 6 years.

Buckwalter and Thomas[15] have also presented normal survival curves simulating ours more than those from the Mayo Clinic, and they too have shown that well-differentiated thyroid cancer—both papillary and follicular—clearly kills.

Therefore, in answer to the first question, Is well-differentiated thyroid cancer worth treating?, there are adequate data demonstrating that because well-differentiated thyroid cancer clearly kills and decreases the survival rate, it is worth treating.

DOES SURGERY DECREASE THE DEATH RATE?

Data showing that adequate surgery does decrease the death rate have already been presented from the Mayo Clinic.[14] In "extrathyroidal" well-differentiated papillary carcinoma, of 38 cases having a biopsy only of the thyroid or nodes, 16 died of thyroid cancer (42 percent). Of 68 patients in the same pathological category traced, 10 died of thyroid cancer, a 16 percent death rate.

Thompson et al.,[16] from our institution have shown that between 1935 and 1955 with less aggressive surgery and less use of radioiodine postoperatively, in 255 patients there was a 12.5 percent mortality from papillary carcinoma and a 11.7 percent mortality from follicular carcinoma. From 1957 to 1972 with more adequate surgery, to be described, plus the routine use of ^{131}I postoperatively, the mortality from papillary cancer was 2.4 percent and the mortality from follicular cancer was 3.1 percent.

It should be stressed, however, that we do "adequate" surgery not only to decrease the death rate but to optimize the radioiodine uptake in metastases both for diagnosis and therapy. If adequate surgery is not done before doing the radioiodine uptake, metastases will be demonstrated in a smaller percentage of patients.

A lobectomy is done on the side of the clinical lesion and any visible lymph nodes are removed. These specimens are submitted for frozen section. If the frozen section shows thyroid cancer, an extracapsular lobectomy is done on the opposite side immediately. If one or more nodes are positive, a block dissection of nodes on that side is done without sacrifice of the sternocleidomastoid muscle, the jugular vein, or the spinal accessory nerve.

With our encouragement, many other large clinics are now doing a total extracapsular lobectomy on the side of the lesion but are leaving 1 or 2 grams of the opposite lobe. Figure 7-3 shows the before (a) and after (b) thyroid scans on a patient operated on by a visiting professor who demonstrated how he left "1 gram" of tissue in the opposite lobe. It is evident that there was radioactive iodine uptake in most of the left lobe area; the 24-hour radioiodine uptake was 9.6 percent. In our experience, this much remaining thyroid interferes with detecting metastases with radioactive iodine.

Another reason for removing the opposite lobe when cancer is found in one lobe has been described by Tollesfen et al.[17] In reviewing the literature he found a 5 to 7 percent occurrence rate of cancer in the opposite lobe with a minimum of cancer follow-up of 5 years. He found a 32 to 58 percent histopathologic demonstration of cancer in the opposite lobe.

Further evidence that adequate surgery is worthwhile was recently published

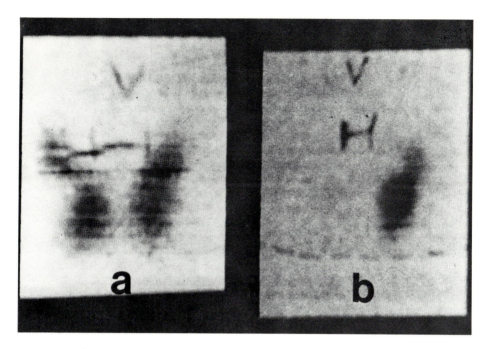

Fig. 7-3. Before (a) and after (b) scans of patient with a 1-gram thyroid tissue remnant in left lobe.

by Young et al.[18] They studied 576 patients in the Archives of Armed Forces Tumor Registry with well-differentiated thyroid carcinoma. Table 7-1 shows some of the important data.

It can be seen that there was a 15 percent recurrence rate of thyroid carcinoma after lobectomy and thyroid hormone administration, as compared to a 9 percent recurrence rate with "total thyroidectomy" and thyroid hormone. This difference was significant ($p < 0.5$).

Does surgery decrease the death rate? There are data to demonstrate that adequate surgery decreases not only the death rate but also the recurrence of well-differentiated thyroid carcinoma.

Table 7-1
Beneficial Effects of Surgery, ^{131}I Therapy, and
Thyroid Suppression after Surgery on
Well-Differentiated Thyroid Carcinoma

Recurrence Rate (%)	Treatment
32	Surgery only
11	Surgery + thyroid hormone
2.7	Surgery + ^{131}I ($p < 0.001$)
15	Lobectomy + thyroid hormone
9	"Total" thyroidectomy + thyroid hormone ($p < 0.05$)

(Reprinted with permission from J. Nucl. Med. 17:532, 1976.)

IS I-131 AFTER SURGERY EFFECTIVE?

The principal data on this problem are not only from Table 7-1, but are from our last follow-up article published in the *Journal of the American Medical Association*, 1970,[5] on 50 patients having surgery only as a control group, as compared to 263 patients with well-differentiated thyroid cancer having radioiodine after surgery. We also have recently presented[19,20] data on 36 patients treated with radioiodine for distant metastases. Leeper[9] has presented data from Memorial Hospital, New York City, on 46 patients with remote metastases.

In our article in the *Journal of the American Medical Association* in 1970,[5] we found that when we ablated uptake in the thyroid remnant, the death rate was decreased by a factor of 20 as compared to when we did not ablate uptake in the thyroid remnant.

For those who would rather not ablate uptake in the thyroid remnant, we observed that 15 out of 36 patients who had distant metastases from well-differentiated thyroid carcinoma did not have the metastases present at the time of the initial surgery. The mean duration of time between the original surgery and diagnosis in these 15 patients was 4.5 years (range of 1 to 9 years). Fortunately, in 14 out of 15 patients, the metastases were to lungs. But unfortunately in one patient the metastases were to bones. (We use a mean dose of about 150 mCi to ablate the uptake in the remnant.)

In the same article we showed that the death rate was four times lower when the uptake and lung metastases were treated with radioactive iodine until the metastases disappeared as compared to those patients not treated until metastases disappeared. We now routinely use 200 mCi for demonstrated uptake in lung and bone metastases.

In a recent article,[19] we confirmed our previous data that patients with metastases in bones generally have the worst prognosis. We were delighted to find, however, that there were no deaths in the first 5 years after treatment. There was also excellent palliation, often for years. In this same article we pointed out that most published series of patients with well-differentiated papillary and follicular carcinoma have a 90 percent survival of papillary carcinoma at 10 years and 80 percent survival of follicular carcinoma at 10 years, but these series included patients with distant metastases in only 4 to 20 percent of those with papillary carcinoma and only 10 to 50 percent of those with follicular carcinoma. In review of the literature, we found that when patients did develop distant metastases, their survival was only 25 percent at 5 years.

We reported in this article that our results in 36 patients with distant metastases are as good as the reported series where only about 10 to 20 percent of their patients had distant metastases. Our patients with lung metastases had a 92 percent survival at 5 years and a 87 percent survival at 10 years. Our patients with bone metastasis had a 100 percent survival at 5 years and 44 percent survival at 10 years.

Leeper[9] found that 100 percent of younger persons with papillary carcinoma were treatable. Only 47 percent of older persons with papillary carcinoma with distant metastases were treatable. He found 61 percent of young persons with follicular carcinoma and 47 percent of older persons with follicular carcinoma treatable. In the papillary carcinoma group with distant metastases, in 8 patients less than 40 years of age, all had metastases regress after radioiodine treatment. One later died of thyroid cancer. In the 17 patients older than 40 years with papillary thyroid carcinoma, 8 were treatable, only 1 responded. In the papillary carcinoma group of 6 young patients, 100 percent were alive at 5 years after ^{131}I treatment. In the older group of 7 with papillary carcinoma, only 14 percent survived 5 years, whereas 100 percent with follicular carcinoma survived 5 years.

WHEN RADIOACTIVE IODINE IN DISTANT METASTASES IS "ABLATED," ARE THESE PATIENTS PERMANENTLY CURED?

For years, we observed that if patients had negative scans at 1 year and 3 years after treatment, they "never" had a recurrence of uptake. We have now seen 6 patients with recurrent uptake out of 447 patients treated with radioiodine after surgery. The time period between the initial ablation of uptake and recurrence of uptake in metastases in these 6 patients was 6.2 years with a range of 3 to 15 years. The recurrence was always diagnosed by scan. In all 6 patients, a repeat treatment dose of ^{131}I caused a "repeat ablation."

Reference to Table 7-1 shows that although the use of thyroid hormone after surgery decreased the recurrence rate from 32 to 11 percent, the recurrence rate was decreased further when radioiodine was used after surgery, from 11 to 2.7 percent. This difference is significant ($p < 0.001$).

Therefore, data are accumulating to document that ^{131}I is effective after surgery.

SHOULD X-RAY TREATMENT BE USED?

In 1958 we published[21] that x-ray therapy should not be used until surgery and radioactive iodine have been used to treat as thoroughly as possible. We found that of 42 patients with well-differentiated thyroid cancer, 25 patients had had x-ray therapy before surgery plus [131]I. In 25 of these patients, we demonstrated good uptake in metastases, in 13 patients after a mean dose of 5050 rads ± 2630 rads of x-ray therapy.

When surgery and radioactive iodine were then used in these 13 patients, 11 experienced regression or disappearance of metastases. In the patients with pulmonary metastases, the metastases disappeared in 2 patients and decreased in size and number in 2. In patients with palpable metastases, the metastases disappeared in 4 and decreased in 3.

IS THE MORBIDITY OF TREATMENT REASONABLE?

Surgery

Thompson[22] published in 1970 on the complications of total thyroidectomy for thyroid cancer at our institution. During the 12-year period from 1957 to 1969 on

184 patients having a total thyroidectomy, he had accidental, temporary nerve paralysis in 4.8 percent of patients. There were no recurrent bilateral nerve paralyses. He had an incidence of temporary hypoparathyroidism of 22 percent. The permanent hypoparathyroidism rate was 1 percent. The accidental unilateral permanent nerve paralysis was 9.7 percent. The morbidity in this surgeon's hands since this study has markedly decreased, but it should be remembered that Dr. Thompson is not the "average" surgeon doing thyroid surgery.

131I

We have had no occurrence of leukemia or increased incidence of cancer in our 447 patients treated with radioactive iodine following surgery since 1947.

More recently, we have published information on 33 children that we have treated for thyroid cancer with radioactive iodine after surgery.[6] There has been no decrease in fertility and no increased incidence of birth history abnormality. The mean age of these children at treatment was 14.6 years with a range of 6 to 20 years. They were given a mean dose of 196 mCi of ^{131}I with a range of 80 to 691 mCi. They had a mean follow-up interval of 18.7 years with a range of 14 to 25 years. The cumulative absorbed radiation dose to the gonads in REMS was 8 to 69. Recently, Neel and coworkers[23] published their most recent follow-up of the Atom Bomb Casualty Commission in Japan. They calculated that the gametic doubling dose for chronic low-level radiation to the gonads is 150 to 200 REM for males and 125 REM for females.

Can treatment with radioactive iodine in a patient with widespread lung metastases cause deterioration of lung function from fibrosis? Rall et al.[24] answered "no" to this question. They showed that the treatment of lung metastases with radioactive iodine did not produce fibrosis with deterioration of lung functions, unless the patient had an uptake of 100 mCi or more of the radioactive iodine in his lungs. In our experience, with the present limitation by the Atomic Energy Commission of single treatment doses not larger than 200 mCi, it is impossible to achieve a dose of 100 mCi of radioactive iodine in the lungs of patients with lung metastases. The highest uptake we have found in the lungs was 15 to 20 percent of the therapeutic dose.

In answer to the question, "Is the morbidity of treatment reasonable?", the data indicate that the morbidity is reasonable, at the University of Michigan, in contrast to the death rate from untreated well-differentiated thyroid cancer.

WHAT ARE THE MOST COMMON CAUSES FOR FAILURE OF RESPONSE TO RADIOACTIVE IODINE?

I list the most common causes for failure of response to radioiodine as follows: (1) inadequate pretreatment surgery, (2) failure to take the patient off all thyroid hormone for a minimum period of 6 weeks, (3) lack of proof of adequate uptake of radioactive iodine (in the areas to be treated) immediately before the treatment is given, and (4) single treatment dose less than 150 mCi.

WHY STOP THYROID HORMONE BEFORE THE SCAN,
PERCENT UPTAKE, AND THERAPY?

It has now been demonstrated[25] that endogenous TSH developed by leaving the post-thyroidectomy patient off thyroid hormone for a minimum period of 6 weeks is better than the administration of endogenous TSH to a patient taking thyroid hormone. Off thyroid hormone, the serum TSH level rose without a plateau through 20 days of follow-up. The levels of endogenous TSH were as high as 200 μunits/ml at 20 days.

When the authors gave 10 units of bovine TSH daily, however, to patients on thyroid hormone, the serum level peaked at 2 to 6 hours and decreased by 50 percent by 8 to 10 hours. It should also be remembered that bovine TSH causes toxic reactions including death, antibodies that neutralize the effect of TSH, and considerable inconvenience and cost.

Recently Dr. James Sisson (*unpublished data* on 44 patients off thyroid hormone for 6 weeks) has shown that young people develop higher levels of TSH than older patients. He also showed that 7 out of 44 patients (15 percent) have surprising low levels of TSH. Perhaps some of these patients are continuing to take thyroid hormone without our knowledge. At any rate, we now routinely obtain serum TSH levels.

DOES STOPPING THYROID HORMONE ACCELERATE THE
GROWTH OF THYROID CANCER?

We have published[26] that thyroid cancer grew best in Fisher rats with well-differentiated thyroid cancer maintained on Na-1-thyroxine in very adequate doses throughout the entire 8-week period of tumor growth before sacrifice of the animals. The rats not maintained on adequate thyroid hormone showed the least tumor growth.

SHOULD THE PATIENT BE TREATED WITH A LOW-IODINE DIET
AND "IODIDE DIURESIS" BEFORE GIVING A THERAPY DOSE?

We have not carried out this procedure in the past, but now we believe it is indicated. If the extracellular iodide pool were significantly shrunken, the ^{131}I treatment dose would endow the smaller pool with a much higher specific activity for sampling by the thyroid carcinoma transport mechanism. After Pittman et al.[27] showed that radioiodine percent uptake normal values have fallen since 1947 with constantly rising dietary iodide intake, we found that the average daily iodide intake in the state of Michigan is 535 μg.[28]

Barakat and Ingbar[29] demonstrated an increased radioiodine percent dose uptake in the thyroid gland of a man acutely depleted of extracellular iodide with an iodide-deficient diet and diuretics. Hamburger[30] has simplified this procedure with less strenuous diuretics. Most recently, Goslings[31] demonstrated a mean doubling of the tumor dose from ^{131}I therapy as a result of a 5-day low-iodine diet.

The additional use of ethacrynic acid resulted in no enhancement of this dose. Powel[32] has presented evidence that the use of this low-iodine diet has resulted in ablation of the uptake in cervical lymph node metastases together with lung metastases in the majority of his patients with a single 100-mCi treatment dose of ^{131}I after use of the low-iodine diet.

ACKNOWLEDGMENT

We would like to thank the Biostatistics Department in the School of Public Health, University of Michigan, for their assistance with the Life Table.

REFERENCES

1. Beierwaltes, W. H.: Indications and contraindications for treatment of thyroid cancer with radioactive iodine. Ann. Intern. Med. 37:23–80, 1952.
2. Beierwaltes, W. H., Johnson, P. C.: Thyroid carcinoma treated with radioactive iodine: an eight year experience. J. Mich. Med. Soc. 55:410–419, 1956.
3. Haynie, T. P., Nofal, M. M., Beierwaltes, W. H.: Treatment of thyroid carcinoma with I-131: results at fourteen years. J.A.M.A. 183:303–306, 1963.
4. Haynie, T. P., Beierwaltes, W. H.: Hematologic changes observed following I-131 therapy for thyroid carcinoma. J. Nucl. Med. 4:85–91, 1963.
5. Varma, V. M., Beierwaltes, W. H., Nofal, M. M., et al.: Treatment of thyroid cancer: death rates after surgery, and after surgery followed by I-131. J.A.M.A. 214:1437–1442, 1970.
6. Sarkar, S. D., Beierwaltes, W. H., Gill, S. P., et al.: Subsequent fertility and birth histories of children and adolescents treated with 131-I for thyroid cancer. J. Nucl. Med. 17:460–464, 1976.
7. Harness, J. K., Thompson, N. W., Sisson, J. C., et al.: Differentiated thyroid carcinomas—treatment of distant metastases. Arch. Surg. 108:410–419, 1974.
8. Beierwaltes, W. H.: The treatment of thyroid carcinoma. In: Continuing Education Lectures of the Southeastern Chapter of the Society of Nuclear Medicine (From the proceedings of the annual meeting held at the Galt House, Louisville, Kentucky, October 13–16, 1976). Zippy Publishing Co., Atlanta, Georgia.
9. Leeper, J.: The effects of 131-I therapy on survival of patients with metastatic papillary or follicular thyroid carcinoma. J. Clin. Endocrinol. Metab. 36:1143–1152, 1973.
10. Rawson, R. W., Leeper, R. D.: Treatment of thyroid cancer with radioactive iodine. In: Nuclear Medicine, Ed. 2, W. H. Blahd (ed.). New York, McGraw-Hill Book Co., pp. 740–742, 1965.
11. Pochin, E. E.: Radioiodine therapy. In: The Thyroid, Ed. 3, S. C. Werner and S. H. Ingbar (eds.). New York, Harper & Row Publishers, pp. 467–475, 1971.
12. Scott, J. S., Halnan, K. E., Shimmins, J., et al.: Measurement of dose to thyroid carcinoma metastases from radio-iodine therapy. Br. J. Radiol. 43:256–262, 1970.
13. Thomas, S. R., Moran, H. R., Keriakes, J. G., et al.: Quantitative external counting techniques enabling improved diagnostic and therapeutic decision on patients with well-differentiated thyroid cancer. Radiology 122:731–737, 1977.
14. Woolner, L. B., Beahrs, O. H., Black, B. M., et al.: Thyroid carcinoma: general considerations and follow-up data on 1181 cases. In: Thyroid Neoplasia. New York, Academic Press, p. 51, 1968.

15. Buckwalter, J. B., Thomas, C. C., Jr.: Selection of surgical treatment for well-differentiated thyroid carcinoma. Ann. Surg. 176:565–578, 1972.

16. Thompson, M., Olsen, W. R., Hoffman, G. L.: The continuing development of the technique of thyroidectomy. Surgery 73:913–927, 1973.

17. Tollesfsen, H. R., Shah, J. P., Huvos, A. G.: Papillary carcinoma of the thyroid: recurrence in the gland after initial surgical treatment. Am. J. Surg. 124:468–472, 1972.

18. Young, E., Mazzaferri, E., Kemmerer, W., et al.: Effects of medical and surgical therapy on morbidity in papillary and/or mixed papillary-follicular thyroid carcinoma. J. Nucl. Med. 17:532, 1976 (Abst.).

19. Harness, J. K., Thompson, N. W., Sisson, J. C., et al.: Differentiated thyroid carcinomas—treatment of distant metastases. Arch. Surg. 108:410–419, 1974.

20. DeCosse, J. L., Beierwaltes, W. H., Brooks, J. R., et al.: Carcinoma of the thyroid. Arch. Surg. 110:783–789, 1975.

21. Carr, E. A., Jr., Dingledine, W. S., Beierwaltes, W. H.: Premature resort to x-ray therapy. A common error in treatment of carcinoma of the thyroid gland. Lancet 78:478–483, 1958.

22. Thompson, N. W., Harness, J. K.: Complications of total thyroidectomy for carcinoma. Surg. Gynecol. Obstet. 131:861–869, 1970.

23. Neel, J. V., Kato, H., Schull, W. J.: Mortality in the children of atomic bomb survivors and controls. Genetics 76:311–326, 1974.

24. Rall, J. E., Alpers, J. B., Lewallen, C. G., et al.: Radiation pneumonitis and fibrosis; a complication of radioiodine treatment of pulmonary metastases from cancer of the thyroid. J. Clin. Endocrinol. 17:1263–1276, 1957.

25. Hershman, J. M., Edwards, L.: Serum thyrotropin (TSH) levels after thyroid ablation compared with TSH levels after exogenous bovine TSH: implications for I-131 treatment of thyroid carcinoma. J. Clin. Endocrinol. Metab. 34:814–818, 1972.

26. Sisson, J. C., Beierwaltes, W. H.: The effect of thyroidectomy with and without thyroxine replacement on transplantable thyroid tumors in rats. Endocrinology 74:925–929, 1964.

27. Pittman, J. A., Dailey, G. F., Beschi, R. J.: Changing normal values for thyroidal radioiodine uptake. N. Engl. J. Med. 280:1431–1434, 1969.

28. Matovinovic, J., Child, M. A., Nichaman, M. Z., et al.: Iodine and endemic goiter. In: Endemic Goiter and Cretinism: Continuing Threats to World Health. WHO Scientific Publication #292: 67–94, 1974.

29. Barakat, R. M., Ingbar, S. H.: The effect of acute iodide depletion on thyroid function in man. J. Clin. Invest. 44:1117–1124, 1965.

30. Hamburger, J. I.: Diuretic augmentation of ^{131}I uptake in inoperable thyroid cancer. N. Engl. J. Med. 280:1091–1094, 1969.

31. Goslings, B. M.: Effect of a low iodine diet on ^{131}I therapy in follicular thyroid carcinomata. Proceedings of the Society of Endocrinology. J. Endocrinol. 30P: 40, 1975.

32. Powell, M.: Society of Nuclear Medicine (submitted for publication.)

Gerard N. Burrow and Stephen W. Spaulding

8
Role of Lithium in Radioiodide Therapy

An increased prevalence of goiter occurring in patients who were receiving lithium for affective disorders was the first indication that lithium had an antithyroid effect.[1] Investigation of the mechanism of goitrogenesis suggested lithium inhibited iodine release from the thyroid gland without significantly affecting other aspects of thyroid function.[2-4]

EFFECT OF LITHIUM ON THE THYROID

We studied the effect of lithium on thyroid hormone release from the gland using a method that obviates several of the technical difficulties in measuring hormone release[5] (Fig. 8-1). The thyroid gland was labeled with ^{125}I; ^{131}I-thyroxine was then injected intravenously and reuptake of iodide by the thyroid blocked. After equilibration, the ratio of protein-bound ^{125}I to protein-bound ^{131}I was calculated. This ratio compensated for the degradation and redistribution of ^{125}I-thyroxine release from the gland. With this method we were able to demonstrate that lithium inhibited thyroid hormone secretion in both hyperthyroid and euthyroid subjects.[6] Lithium also decreased the slope of the disappearance rate of exogenous ^{131}I-T_4, suggesting an additional peripheral inhibition of T_4 deiodination. These changes occurred with peak serum lithium concentrations that were within an acceptable therapeutic range (0.39 to 1.45 mEq/l). The biochemical mechanism whereby lithium inhibits the thyroid gland is not clear, but some evidence has suggested an inhibition of adenylate cyclase.[7]

The only therapeutic agent previously known to directly inhibit release of thyroid hormone was iodine. However, iodine interferes with subsequent radioiodine therapy and may also induce hyperthyroidism (Jod-Basedow).[8] Antithyroid agents which predominantly block organification of iodine produce clinical relief of thyrotoxicosis only after available stores of thyroid hormone are depleted. Although propylthiouracil also blocks the peripheral conversion of T_4 to T_3, a return to the completely euthyroid state takes weeks of therapy with this

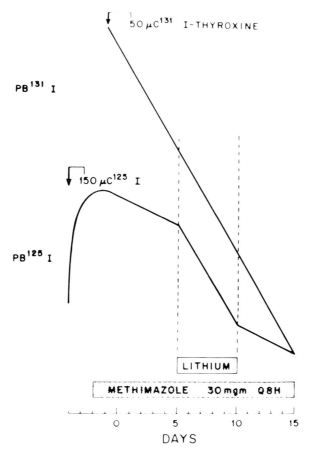

Fig. 8-1. Schematic representation of double-labeling to study effect of lithium on thyroid hormone secretion. (Reproduced with permission from Spaulding, S. W., Burrow, G. N., Bermudez, F. et al.: J. Clin. Endocrinol. 35:905, 1972.)

agent. Therefore, there was interest in lithium as a potential therapeutic agent in thyrotoxic individuals in whom a prompt decrease in thyroid hormone levels was desirable. However, since lithium did not block the absolute iodine uptake, the effectiveness of chronic lithium therapy might be diminished, due to continued accumulation of iodide by the thyroid. For prolonged therapy, one would infer that a thionamide would have to be used in conjunction with lithium.

LITHIUM THERAPY FOR THYROTOXICOSIS

To evaluate the role of lithium as an adjunct to thionamide treatment in hyperthyroidism, Turner and his colleagues[9] divided 63 thyrotoxic patients into three treatment groups. One group of 23 patients received lithium carbonate plus carbimazole while a comparable group of 20 patients were given carbimazole plus iodides. A third group of 20 patients received carbimazole alone. In patients

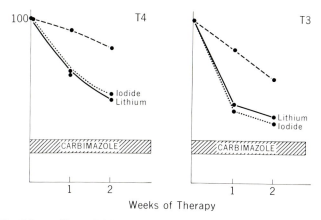

Fig. 8-2. Effect of lithium, iodides, and carbimazole on the serum T_4 and T_3 concentrations. (Modified from Turner, J. G., Brownlie, B. E. W., Sadler, W. A., et al.: Acta Endocrinol. (Kbh.) 83:86, 1976.)

treated with lithium, the mean serum T_4 fell 49 percent after 2 weeks of treatment, while the mean serum T_3 fell 57 percent. Similar results were obtained in patients who were given iodides in addition to carbimazole, while the results in 20 patients given carbimazole alone were less impressive (Fig. 8-2). A relatively low standard dose of lithium carbonate (750 mg daily) was used in an attempt to avoid lithium toxicity, and only 3 of 23 patients complained of symptoms such as polyuria and ataxia that could be attributed to the drug.

Lithium has been used as the sole agent in the initial treatment of hyperthyroidism. Twenty-four patients were randomly divided and received either lithium carbonate or 40 mg of methimazole daily.[10] The dose of lithium was adjusted to keep the concentration between 0.5 and 1.3 mEq/l. After 10 days of treatment, there was no difference in the mean decrease of serum thyroxine concentration between the two groups (38 percent). Of 11 patients treated with lithium, 8 complained of side effects such as tremor, nausea, and difficulty with accommodation.

Thyrotoxic patients have also been treated with lithium alone for prolonged periods of time with apparently good results.[11] Eleven thyrotoxic patients were treated with lithium alone for 6 months. They received 800 to 1200 mg of lithium daily in order to keep their serum lithium concentration between 0.5 and 1.5 mEq/l. On this regimen, 8 out of 11 patients became euthyroid 3 weeks after therapy, with a fall in the mean serum T_4 and T_3 by 35 percent of the original values. The lithium was discontinued after 6 months, and 7 patients relapsed 1 to 4 weeks after discontinuing the drug. Although based on previous data chronic lithium therapy alone would not have been expected to control thyrotoxicosis, it seems to have been effective in these patients.

LITHIUM VERSUS IODIDE

Both lithium and iodine inhibit thyroid hormone secretion with a consequent decrease in circulating levels of T_4 and T_3. Why a simple cation and a simple anion should have similar effects is not clear. It has been proposed that lithium may be acting through an increase on the intrathyroidal iodine content.[12] Although lithium decreases thyroid hormone secretion, it does not affect iodine uptake. Consequently, total intrathyroidal iodine content should increase during lithium therapy, and it is known that excessive quantities of iodine can inhibit both the synthesis and release of thyroid hormone. However, the acute administration per nanogram of iodine to patients on chronic lithium therapy enhanced their perchlorate discharge test, suggesting that at least the levels of iodide in the gland are probably not elevated.[13]

We examined the possible effects of increased iodide intake on the incidence of thyroid dysfunction in 10 patients who were receiving lithium.[14] Two of the patients became hypothyroid and a third had an increase in the serum TSH concentration without any change in serum T_3 or T_4. Interestingly, 1 patient developed hyperthyroidism while on lithium, probably secondary to the Iod-Basedow phenomenon. Although neither drug alone usually induces hypothyroidism in euthyroid patients, the two drugs appear to act synergistically perhaps by potentiating the disorder in intrathyroidal iodine metabolism.

LITHIUM TOXICITY

If lithium is to be used in the treatment of thyroid disease, it is important that the toxic effects do not outweigh the therapeutic benefits. The occurrence of toxicity is related to the plasma lithium concentration and rate of rise following administration. A therapeutic serum lithium concentration is usually between 0.6 and 1.3 mEq/l. Low-sodium diets potentiate the toxic effects of lithium. Acute toxicity is characterized by ataxia, vomiting, diarrhea, and eventually coma and convulsions. Symptoms of chronic toxicity that are likely to occur include nausea, vomiting, diarrhea, abdominal pain, and sedation. Problems in the nervous system include tremor, dysarthria, and mental confusion. The chronic use of lithium causes EKG changes and may cause cardiac arrhythmias and hypotension.

Lithium salts have a low therapeutic index, and any patient receiving lithium should have his serum lithium concentration monitored regularly. Whether the benefits outweigh the risks in treating thyroid disease depends on the specific case.

Polydipsia and polyuria may also occur in patients treated with lithium. The mechanism may involve inhibition of the action of antidiuretic hormone on renal adenylate cyclase. Radioactive iodide partitions itself between the thyroid and the urine. Thus, lithium-induced polyuria may lead to the increased urinary excretion of an administered dose of radioactive iodine with a corresponding decrease in the amount retained by the thyroid.

LITHIUM IN RADIOIODIDE THERAPY

Lithium therapy directly results in decreased thyroid hormone secretion without affecting the radioiodide uptake. Thus, a given dose of radioiodide administered to a patient on lithium should result in a larger dose of radiation deliv-

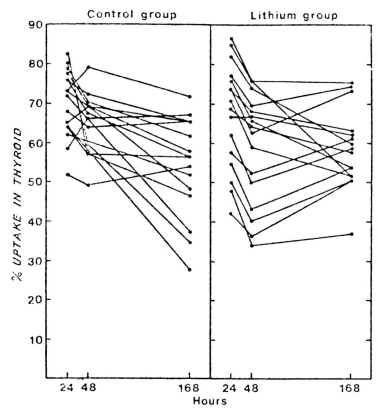

Fig. 8-3. Effect of lithium on the retention of ^{131}I within the thyroid gland. (Reproduced with permission from Turner, J. G., Brownlie, B. E. W., and Rogers, T. G. H. *Lancet* 1:614, 1976.)

ered than if the patient were not taking lithium. Sixteen thyrotoxic patients were treated with 400 mg of lithium daily for 1 week before and after the administration of 5 mCi ^{131}I.[15] The dose of ^{131}I retained by the gland was calculated and compared to that in 16 patients given ^{131}I without lithium. After the first 24 hours the mean dose retained was significantly greater in the lithium-treated group (Fig. 8-3).

The effectiveness of radioiodine treatment in functional thyroid carcinoma is compromised by limited uptake and rapid release. Lithium administration decreased the disappearance rate of ^{131}I from a metastasis of follicular thyroid carcinoma.[16] The increased ^{131}I retention would be expected to increase the therapeutic to toxic ratio of ^{131}I. However, a subsequent therapeutic dose of ^{131}I-iodine given with lithium was accompanied by an unexpected increase in blood ^{131}I and, therefore, in whole-body radiation, which resulted in significant bone marrow depression. It has been estimated that lithium therapy can increase the radiation dose of ^{131}I delivered to the thyroid tumor by several fold.[16]

Gershengorn and his colleagues[15] proposed the following regimen for the use of lithium as an adjunct to ^{131}I therapy for thyroid carcinoma:

1. Stimulate tumor uptake with endogenous or exogenously administered TSH.

2. Give sufficient lithium carbonate to maintain serum lithium levels between 0.6 and 1.3 mEq/l. Monitor!

3. Administer tracer dose of ^{131}I to perform dosimetry calculations followed by therapy dose.

4. Maintain lithium administration throughout the tracer and therapy periods.

SUMMARY

Lithium affects radioiodine therapy in several ways:

1. Lithium inhibits thyroid hormone release without affecting iodide transport.

2. This property can be used to increase the dose of radioactive iodine retained by the thyroid gland.

3. Lithium has a relatively low therapeutic to toxic effect ratio, so that serum lithium concentration must be carefully monitored.

4. Lithium therapy may occasionally be useful in the acute adjunctive management of hyperthyroidism.

5. Lithium may be particularly helpful as an adjunct to ^{131}I therapy in thyroid carcinoma where large amounts of radioactivity are administered.

REFERENCES

1. Schou, M., Amdisen, A., Eskjaer-Jensen, S., et al.: Occurrence of goitre during lithium therapy. Br. Med. J. 3:710–713, 1968.
2. Berens, S. C., Bernstein, R. S., Robbins, J., et al.: Antithyroid effects of lithium. J. Clin. Invest. 49:1357–1367, 1970.
3. Burrow, G. N., Burke, W. R., Himmelhoch, J. M., et al.: Effect of lithium on thyroid function. J. Clin. Endocrinol. 32:647–652, 1971.
4. Temple, R., Berman, M., Robbins, J., et al.: The use of lithium in the treatment of thyrotoxicosis. J. Clin. Invest. 51:2746–2756, 1972.
5. Wartofsky, L., Ransil, B. J., Ingbar, S. H.: Inhibition by iodine of the release of thyroxine from the thyroid glands of patients with thyrotoxicosis. J. Clin. Invest. 49:78–86, 1970.
6. Spaulding, S. W., Burrow, G. N., Bermudez, F., et al.: The inhibiting effect of lithium on thyroid hormone release in both euthyroid and thyrotoxic patients. J. Clin. Endocrinol. Metab. 35:905–911, 1972.
7. Wolff, J., Berens, S. C., Jones, A. B.: Inhibition of thyrotropin stimulated adenyl cyclase activity of beef thyroid membrane by low concentration lithium ion. Biochem. Biophys. Res. Commun. 39:77–82, 1970.
8. Vagenakis, A. G., Wong, C. A., Burger, A., et al.: Iodide-induced thyrotoxicosis in Boston. N. Engl. J. Med. 287:523–527, 1972.
9. Turner, J. G., Brownlie, B. E. W., Sadler, W. A., et al.: Successful treatment of thyrotoxicosis by lithium. Acta Endocrinol. (Kbh.) [Suppl.] 173:23, 1973.
10. Kristensen, O., Andersen, H. H., Pallisgaard, G.: Lithium carbonate in the treatment of thyrotoxicosis. Lancet 1:603–605, 1976.
11. Lazarus, J. H., Addison, G. M., Richards, A. R., et al.: Treatment of thyrotoxicosis with lithium carbonate. Lancet 2:1160–1162, 1974.

12. Burman, K. D., Dimond, R. C., Earll, J. M., et al.: Sensitivity to lithium in treated Graves' disease: effects on serum T_4, T_3 and reverse T_3. J. Clin. Endocrinol. Metab. 43:606–613, 1976.

13. Spaulding, S. W., Burrow, G. N., Ramey, J. N., et al.: Effect of increased iodide intake on thyroid function in subjects on chronic lithium therapy. Acta Endocrinol. (Kbh.) (in press).

14. Turner, J. G., Brownlie, B. E. W., Rogers, T. G. H.: Lithium as an adjunct to radioiodine therapy for thyrotoxicosis. Lancet 1:614–615, 1976.

15. Gershengorn, M. C., Izumi, M., Robbins, J.: Use of lithium as an adjunct to radioiodine therapy of thyroid carcinoma. J. Clin. Endocrinol. Metab. 42:105–111, 1976.

16. Briere, J., Pousset, G., Darsy, P., et al.: Interet de l'association lithium-iode [131] dans le traitement des metastases captantes du cancer thyroidien. Ann. Endocrinol. (Paris) 35:281–282, 1974.

Richard P. Spencer

9

Attempts to Reduce Whole-Body Radiation

In diagnostic nuclear medicine, we speak of the target to nontarget ratio (T/NT) of an administered radiopharmaceutical. The higher the activity in the target, and the lower that in the nontarget area, the better delineated is the image. However, the ratio becomes nondefined in the extreme. That is, when all activity is in the area of interest and none is in surrounding structures, the ratio then has zero in the denominator. Hence, we propose utilizing the inverse function, and calling it the "therapeutic whole-body radiation index."

$$TRI = \frac{\text{nontarget activity}}{\text{target activity}} \qquad (1)$$

This is a more realistic and usable expression, since it goes from a value of zero when all activity is in the target and none is outside (and the whole-body radiation is low), to a value of 1 when the material is equally distributed throughout the body. Only if the radioactive agent were specifically excluded from the target area would the ratio go above 1. The crucial question becomes: how do we obtain values of TRI as close to zero as possible? That is, how do we reduce radiation to the body while limiting it to the area of therapy? Several approaches will be discussed in turn.

Direct intralesional therapy. By this we mean the injection of a radioactive pharmaceutical directly into the lesion. This bypasses systemic pathways and, hence, limits the radioactive substance to the area of interest. Of course, after deposition occurs there may be loss from the region due to breakdown of the radiated tissue. Hence, the TRI, initially zero, may rise if there is escape of radiolabel from the region. An integrated TRI might, therefore, be an additional parameter worthy of investigation. In a later chapter in this volume, the topic of intralesional therapy is dealt with in greater detail.

Supported by U.S. Public Health Service Grant CA-17802 from the National Cancer Institute.

Indirect intralesional therapy. By this we mean introduction of the radioactive material into a lesion, but by other than direct injection. The most common method is by passing an arterial catheter and then injecting the therapeutic agent. For other than embolized or completely absorbed materials, there is escape from the region and a TRI higher than zero. The topic of catheter delivery of therapeutic agents is also dealt with later in the volume.

Isolated system. This is a variant of intralesional therapy, in which the lesion and surrounding segments are irradiated, but not the whole body. An example is limb perfusion, with collection of the effluent so that the radioactive material does not enter the general circulation. By specific pumping, it might be possible to extend this to individual organs.

Totally entrapped alpha or beta ray emitter. Even if direct or indirect intralesional therapy succeeded, some body radiation would occur if a gamma ray emitting radionuclide had been used. Hence, alpha ray and beta ray emitters are to be preferred with intralesional therapy. A small quantity of a gamma ray emitter could be administered in the therapeutic dose, in order to follow any escape of radiolabel from the lesion.

In other than intralesional therapy, the radioactive pharmaceutical passes through systemic pathways. Hence, there will be whole-body radiation exposure. How can this body radiation burden be minimized? As a specific example to illustrate the principles involved, we will use the thyroid gland.

Use of radioiodide in the therapy for hyperthyroidism, thyroid carcinoma, or euthyroid cardiac disease carried the undesirable effect of delivering radiation to other organs as well as the thyroid. Techniques for reducing the quantity of radioiodide needed for effective therapy would thus make a contribution to decreasing the body radiation burden. It is apparent that if all of a dose of radioiodide were taken up by the thyroid, and if none escaped, then the whole-body radiation dose would be minimized. Analysis of the factors involved in delivery of the radiation dose suggests ways in which this can be approached. The expression for the radiation delivered by an internally deposited emitter of weak beta rays is (using the classic notation):

$$D = K \cdot E_\beta \cdot C \cdot T\tfrac{1}{2} \tag{2}$$

where the radiation dose (D in rads) is given as a function of a constant (K), the average beta ray energy (E_β in mev), the concentration of radioiodide in the organ (C, in μCi/g), and the effective retention half-time (T½ in days) of radioiodide in the thyroid. Recall that the concentration of radioiodide in the thyroid can be expressed as:

$$C = Q \cdot U/W \tag{3}$$

where Q is the quantity of radioactive iodide given, U is the fractional uptake in the thyroid, and W is the thyroid weight. We now set a ratio between the radiation dose that would be delivered after (D_a) a radioactive medication was given for its effect on the thyroid, to that before (D_b) use of the radioactive medication.

$$\frac{D_a}{D_b} = \frac{Q_a \cdot U_a \cdot T\frac{1}{2}_a}{Q_b \cdot U_b \cdot T\frac{1}{2}_b} \cdot \frac{W_b}{W_a} \qquad (4)$$

Thus to keep a constant radiation dose to the thyroid ($D_a = D_b$) while reducing the quantity administered ($Q_a < Q_b$), we can manipulate only three factors (U, T, and W).

1. Uptake of radioiodide into the thyroid might be increased ($U_a > U_b$). This could possibly be accomplished by means of TSH administration, by iodide deprivation, or by having the patient on an antithyroid drug which is then discontinued, to utilize the "rebound phenomenon." Iodide deprivation has also been shown to be effective in increasing radioiodide uptake in follicular thyroid carcinoma.[1]
2. The thyroid retention half-time could be increased (that is, iodide might be kept in the thyroid for a longer period). This might be accomplished by use of the lithium ion, or by post-treatment administration of stable iodide to block egress. The lithium ion can also block egress of radioiodide from thyroid cancers.[2] This is further discussed in a later chapter. Vinblastine also inhibits thyroid secretion and is mentioned below.
3. The same dose of radioiodide is more effective as the size of the thyroid is reduced. Whether use of antimitotic agents or partial obstruction of the arterial inflow to the thyroid could accomplish such a reduction remains to be determined. The identical principle holds in tumor therapy. That is, systemic immunotherapy or chemotherapy is more effective when the tumor burden is small. Hence, reducing tumor size by vessel obstruction or intralesional therapy could precede other therapeutic modalities.
4. The radiation effect might be mimicked by chemical agents (that is, the amount of radioiodide might be reduced if a chemical agent were used). The synergistic effect of some antibiotics (such as adriamycin) and radiation is known[3] and a general discussion has appeared.[4] The use of "radiation sensitizers"[5] has to be worked on in order to find optimum combinations of chemotherapeutic agents and radiation so that the desired therapeutic goals are met while the radiation exposure is reduced. Vinblastine has been reported to inhibit thyroid secretion,[6] and hence it might have some effects similar to lithium (which blocks thyroid hormone egress).

The above discussion assumes a uniform biological response. There is insufficient evidence to allow us to draw firm conclusions as to the biological variability involved in the response to radioiodide. McCowen and associates[7] have suggested that lower doses of radioiodide (under 30 mCi) may be as effective as high doses (80 to 100 mCi) in thyroid ablation postsurgically in patients with thyroid cancer. Obviously, the lower the amount of radioiodide used, the lower the whole-body radiation dose.

When a medication which is to be used has two or more actions, each must be assayed in order to judge the net effect. For example, lithium is known to block iodide egress from the thyroid (desirable) but to sometimes decrease iodide uptake in the gland (undesirable), possibly by encouraging diuresis and iodide loss in the urine.[12] The equation for the radiation dose delivered can be recast into the form:

$$T\frac{1}{2} = \frac{D}{K \cdot E_\beta \cdot C} \qquad (5)$$

The reciprocal relationship between the effective retention T½ and the concentration of radioiodide in the gland (at a constant radiation dosage) can be appreciated. If the uptake is depressed by lithium to a value of $(1-p)$ then the $T^1/_2$ would have to be lengthened by more than $(1/1-p)$ to justify the use of the medication. For example, if the uptake value is depressed 20 percent by lithium, the value of $1 - p$ is $1 - 0.2$ or 0.8, and the $T^1/_2$ would have to be extended by at least $1/0.8$ or 1.25, in order to teach the "break even" point. There are thus possible techniques for reducing the quantity of radioiodide needed to irradiate the thyroid. Thus in turn would reduce the whole-body radiation exposure.

Radiation fractionation has been much discussed.[8] That is, the radiation can be delivered in multiple reduced doses rather than a single large dose. When this occurs, it is found that more total radiation has to be delivered, since some recovery or growth occurs during the individual radiation exposures. Does fractionation of the dose have a role to play in therapy with radioactive isotopes? This is difficult to document, since although external radiation can be turned on and off, there is less control over internally administered radionuclides. Perhaps the closest we can come to fractionated therapy with radionuclides, at the moment, are cases of individuals treated with reduced doses of radioiodide at intervals of 3 months or so for hyperthyroidism.

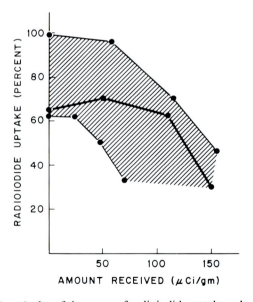

Fig. 9-1. A plot of the range of radioiodide uptake values, at 24 hours, in hyperthyroid patients. The values are given as a function of the total (sum of each therapy) radiation dose delivered to the thyroid, given in terms of ^{131}I μCi/g thyroid tissue. One typical case is shown; observe the fall in uptake values as higher radiation doses are given.

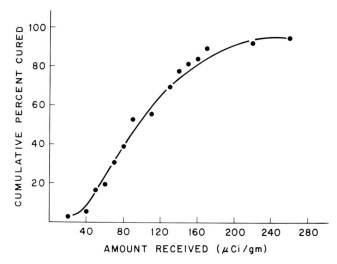

Fig. 9-2. A plot of the cumulative percent of patients cured of hyperthyroidism by "fractionated therapy" (that is, rendered euthyroid or hypothyroid), as a function of the total dose to the thyroid expressed in terms of μCi/g tissue.

We had the opportunity to examine a series of 39 patients treated with a "low-dosage" regimen at a community hospital.[9] A simple but illustrative way to present the data was to plot the value of the 24-hour radioiodide uptake as a function of the cumulative amount of radioiodide given (μCi/g). Figure 9-1 shows that, on the average, only when the cumulative dose was over 50 μCi/g did the uptake value fall. Such a plot could be made for other parameters such as the blood T_3 or T_4 values of the size of the thyroid gland. Such a compilation would be of use in determining the temporal relationship of the changes and how tightly coupled they are in these patients.

If we define "cured" of hyperthyroidism as being rendered euthyroid or hypothyroid, then a smooth progression can be seen, which increases with the dose of radioiodide given (Fig. 9-2). Such a curve, however, is difficult to handle. A simple transformation can be made, by casting the results in the form: percent cured/(100 percent cured). This is shown in Figure 9-3. Although many interpretations can be given to the data, it is clear that there is wide biological variability; "cures" occur, however, only at the higher doses (usually above 50 μCi/g thyroid). Are we justified in using this fractionated technique? Probably not. There are two reasons for saying this.

First, the "low-dosage" regime greatly prolongs the time needed to obtain relief of hyperthyroidism. Rapoport and coworkers[10] have commented on this point.

Second, there is no saving in radiation exposure. If we take the estimated radiation delivered to the thyroid glands by the "low-dosage" regimen, we end up with a plot that is shown on the left in Figure 9-4. However, if the results are corrected for the effects of fractionation, we end up with the plot on the right in Figure 9-4. It can be seen that we are down to the conventional doses of radioiodide. All we have done is to expend much time in curing the patient. The

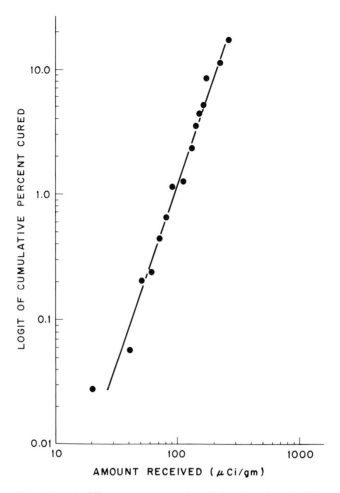

Fig. 9-3. A different representation of the data given in Fig. 9-2. The transformation: percent cured/(100-percent cured) is given on a logarithmic scale, as a function of the total dose to the thyroid (expressed in terms of μCi/g tissue), also on a logarithmic scale.

only argument we can see at the moment for a low-dosage regimen is the still inconclusive argument that late or delayed hypothyroidism might be reduced. The evidence thus far suggests that this is not the case.[11]

There is one other interesting approach to reducing the whole-body radiation dose. This is to rapidly remove the radionuclide when it has served its therapeutic purpose. In other words, the material is "flushed" or "displaced" from tissue when it has completed its role. This is but one example of a general phenomenon of "tissue displacement assay."[13] In effect, the displacement terminates the radiation exposure. As more specific compounds are devised, and their inhibitors developed, it may be possible to use tissue displacement of radiopharmaceuticals. We have discussed one case, the displacement of iodoaminopterin by more powerful (greater avidity) inhibitors of folate reductase.

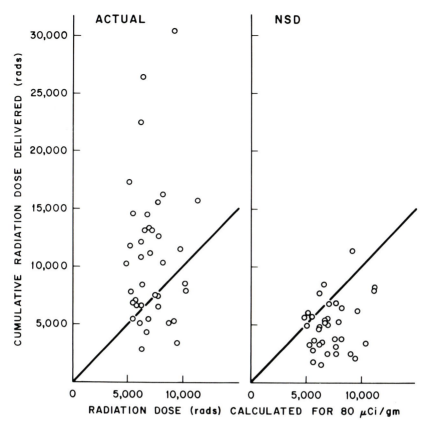

Fig. 9-4. A plot of the calculated radiation dose delivered to the thyroid by the individual doses summed (*left*), and after correction by the "nominal standard dose" formula (*right*).

REFERENCES

1. Goslings, B. M.: Effect of a low iodine diet on ^{131}I therapy in follicular thyroid carcinomata. J. Endocrinol. 64:30p, 1975.
2. Briere, J., Pousset, G., Darsy, P., et al.: Interet de l'association lithium-iode 131 dans le traitement des metastases captantes du cancer thyroidien. Ann. Endocrinol. (Paris) 35:281–282, 1974.
3. Greco, F. A., Brereton, H. D., Kent, H., et al.: Adriamycin and enhanced radiation reaction in normal esophagus and skin. Ann. Intern. Med. 85:294–298, 1976.
4. Nias, A. H. W.: Interactions of ionising radiation and cancer chemotherapy agents. Biochem. Pharmacol. 25:2117–2124, 1976.
5. Urtasun, R., Band, P., Chapman, J. D., et al.: Radiation and high-dose metronidazole in supratentorial glioblastomas. N. Engl. J. Med. 294:1364–1367, 1976.
6. Williams, J. A.: In vitro studies on the nature of vinblastine inhibition of thyroid secretion. Endocrinology 98:1351–1358, 1976.
7. McCowen, K. D., Adler, R. A., Ghaed, N., et al.: Low dose radioiodide thyroid ablation in postsurgical patients with thyroid cancer. Am. J. Med. 61:52–58, 1976.
8. Hethcote, H. W., McLarty, J. W., Thames, H. D., Jr.: Comparison of mathematical models for radiation fractionation. Radiat. Res. 67:387–407, 1976.

9. Spencer, R. P., Caride, V. J.: Analysis of sequential "low dosage" radioiodide therapy of hyperthyroidism. J. Nucl. Med. 16:572, 1975.

10. Rapoport, B., Caplan, R., DeGroot, L. J.: Low-dose sodium iodide I 131 therapy in Graves disease. J.A.M.A. 224:1610–1613, 1973.

11. Malone, J. F., Cullen, M. J.: Two mechanisms for hypothyroidism after ^{131}I therapy. Lancet 2:73–75, 1976.

12. Dousa, T. P., Barnes, L. D.: Lithium-induced diuretic effect of antidiuretic hormone in rats. Am. J. Physiol. 231:1754–1759, 1976.

13. Spencer, R. P.: Tissue displacement assay (TDA): a theoretical tool for following radiopharmaceuticals. Med. Hypoth. 1:150–151, 1975.

Sheldon S. Stoffer and Joel I. Hamburger

10

Avoiding Inadvertent Fetal Radiation Resulting from [131]I Therapy for Hyperthyroidism

Avoiding inadvertent fetal radiation from ^{131}I therapy for hyperthyroidism is really a two-part problem. The first essential is assuring that ^{131}I therapy is not administered to pregnant hyperthyroid patients. This is discussed in the first part of this chapter.

A second consideration is the definitive elimination of hyperthyroidism in women who plan childbearing. This will reduce the population at risk for inadvertent ^{131}I therapy during pregnancy. This is discussed in the second part of this chapter.

[131]I THERAPY IN PREGNANT HYPERTHYROID PATIENTS

Overview

Of 963 physicians surveyed to determine therapeutic attitudes and experience with inadvertent radioiodine therapy for hyperthyroidism during the first trimester of pregnancy, 116 physicians (of 517 responding) reported 237 patients. Therapeutic abortion was advised for 55 patients by 22 physicians. From the 182 remaining pregnancies there were two spontaneous abortions, two stillbirths, one neonate with biliary atresia, and one with respiratory distress. This complication rate was not greater than might be expected in a similar number of random pregnancies. Six infants had hypothyroidism (transient for one); four had mental deficiency. Three mothers had received radioiodine therapy in the second trimester. None of the six mothers had pregnancy tests prior to radioiodine therapy. Survey responses indicate that routine pregnancy testing prior to radioiodine therapy for patients in the childbearing age is not yet a standard procedure. It should be.

Survey of Physicians

Although it is well known that sodium iodide I-131 (^{131}I) therapy after the 12th week of pregnancy may result in a hypothyroid child,[1,2] clinical data regarding such administration in the first trimester are lacking. This information would be useful, since inadvertent ^{131}I administration is most likely to occur early in pregnancy. As thyroid consultants, about three or four times each year we are contacted by anxious physicians who have administered ^{131}I for hyperthyroidism only to discover subsequently that the patient had been a few weeks pregnant. The advisability of therapeutic abortion is the primary concern. The literature is remarkably silent on this point. Therefore, we have surveyed a large group of thyroidologists and endocrinologists in the United States to determine what they would recommend and what experience they have had with patients who inadvertently receive ^{131}I therapy for hyperthyroidism in the first trimester of pregnancy. We believe that the data from this survey permit certain limited conclusions which may be helpful to physicians faced with this dilemma.

We sent 963 letters of inquiry to members of the American Thyroid Association and the Endocrine Society, who were selected on the basis of our impression of the likelihood of their dealing with thyroid patients. The following questions were asked:

1. How many hyperthyroid patients have you seen who inadvertently received therapeutic doses of ^{131}I during the first trimester of pregnancy?
2. For these patients did you advise:
   a. therapeutic abortion, or
   b. observation, permitting the patient to carry to term?
3. If you permitted the patients to carry to term, what, if any, fetal or neonatal abnormalities were observed?

We deliberately did not request detailed information in our initial correspondence so as to encourage a maximum response.

Those physicians who reported fetal or neonatal abnormalities were asked these additional questions:

1. What was the estimated week of pregnancy at the time of ^{131}I therapy administration?
2. Was a urine pregnancy test done?
3. What was the date and dose of ^{131}I therapy?
4. If the infant was hypothyroid,
   a. Were thyroid function tests done on the newborn?
   b. At what age was the diagnosis of hypothyroidism made?
   c. Was there mental deficiency?
   d. What was the current age of the child?

The data obtained from these surveys constitute the basis for this report.

Results

THERAPEUTIC RECOMMENDATIONS OF THE SURVEYED PHYSICIANS

Of the 963 physicians surveyed, 517 (54 percent) responded. Of those responding, 116 had dealt with hyperthyroid patients who were inadvertently treated with ^{131}I while pregnant. The surprising total of 237 such patients was accumulated. For these patients 22 physicians (19 percent of those with experience) recommended therapeutic abortion for 55 (23 percent) of the pregnancies. The majority of physicians permitted the pregnant patients to carry to term.

MISCELLANEOUS FETAL AND NEONATAL COMPLICATIONS

There were two spontaneous abortions, two stillbirths, and 178 live births. One neonate had biliary atresia, and another had respiratory distress and possible neonatal hyperthyroidism. This small number of spontaneous abortions and fetal and neonatal abnormalities is no greater than might have been anticipated in a similar number of random pregnancies.[3]

HYPOTHYROIDISM AND MENTAL DEFICIENCY

Our initial survey revealed six hypothyroid infants, two of whom had been previously reported.[1,2] Five of these infants had permanent impairment of thyroid function, whereas for one the impairment was only transient. Two of the mothers received repeated doses of ^{131}I, beginning in the first trimester and extending into the second. A third mother was treated at 14 weeks. These three cases are included in this report primarily for comparative purposes.

Table 10-1 shows the relationship of the timing of ^{131}I therapy to subsequent hypothyroidism and mental deficiency. Three of the mothers whose infants had permanent hypothyroidism were clearly treated later than the first trimester, and for two of them (patients 1 and 2) multiple doses were given. A fourth infant was treated at about 12 weeks.

Table 10-1
Relationship of Timing of ^{131}I Therapy to Subsequent Hypothyroidism and Mental Deficiency

Time of Last Therapy Dose	Total ^{131}I Dose (mCi)	Est. Week of Preg.*	Urine Preg. Test Done	Age at Hypo. Diagnosis	Current Age	Mental Deficiency
Second trimester						
Patient 1†	150	26	No	1 year	11	Definite
Patient 2†	12.2	15	No	4 years	12	Definite
Patient 3	14.5	14	No	1.5 years	18	Definite
Late first trimester						
Patient 4	?	12	No	6 months	7	Definite
Patient 5‡	10	9	No	At birth transient	6	Possibly minimal
Mid first trimester						
Patient 6	?	6§	No	1 month	22	No

*If multiple doses, the time of the last dose is recorded.
†Patient received multiple doses of ^{131}I.
‡Infant was euthyroid by 1 year and remained so through age 6 years.
§This patient was treated over 22 years ago and precise timing of therapy and dose could not be obtained.

The mother of the infant with transient hypothyroidism received ^{131}I therapy early in the third month of pregnancy, and also was treated with propylthiouracil through the seventh month. At that time she was recognized as having rather severe hypothyroidism; the propylthiouracil was discontinued and supplemental triiodothyronine was given until term. The infant had transient hypothyroidism with recovery by 1 year of age; the euthyroid state had been maintained through the sixth year. It is impossible to assess the relative importance of the ^{131}I and the propylthiouracil in the etiology of the transient hypothyroidism experienced by this infant. Although the propylthiouracil was discontinued in the seventh month, the fetus may have had a more sustained suppression of thyroid function than the mother. Transient hypothyroidism following exposure to ^{131}I therapy is also a recognized event.[4]

The mother of the fifth infant with permanent hypothyroidism may have been treated no later than the sixth week of the pregnancy, although the timing is open to question since we could not obtain the exact date of the therapy, nor could we be certain that the infant was not premature. This mother was treated more than 22 years ago.

Four of the hypothyroid children also had definite mental deficiency. Three of the four mothers were treated in the second trimester of pregnancy, and the fourth was treated at 12 weeks. Furthermore, hypothyroidism was diagnosed at 6 months, 1 year, 18 months, and 4 years of age in these children. By contrast, for the two remaining infants the diagnosis was made at 1 month and at birth (the infant with transient hypothyroidism). Both the treatment of the mother late in pregnancy and the delay in diagnosis of hypothyroidism may have contributed in additive fashion to the development of mental deficiency in the former infants.

Three mothers of hypothyroid children clearly received ^{131}I therapy later than the first trimester, a fourth mother was treated late in the first trimester, and a fifth mother was treated at about 9 weeks. For these 5 cases, pregnancy would probably have been recognized had a urine pregnancy test been performed. The sixth and final mother was treated earlier in the first trimester. However, even for this mother a urine pregnancy test would probably have been positive.

USE OF PREGNANCY TEST

When this survey was planned we assumed that by this time everyone administering ^{131}I therapy would routinely perform a pregnancy test for patients in the childbearing years. Therefore, we did not request information on this point. Nevertheless, 22 physicians offered comments clearly indicating that our expectations were incorrect.

One physician (a radiotherapist) said that he administered ^{131}I therapy upon request of the attending physician and does not participate in the clinical evaluation. Another physician was not concerned because it was his understanding that the fetal thyroid does not concentrate ^{131}I in the first trimester, and later the diagnosis of pregnancy should be obvious. Three additional physicians considered themselves "lucky" that it had not happened to them. Five physicians felt secure since they do not treat patients less than 35 to 40 years of age. That this policy does not exclude pregnancy was brought home to us by a 42-year-old woman who was successful after attempting to become pregnant for the previous 15 years.

Eight physicians placed reliance on the menstrual or contraceptive history. One of our patients had been taking oral contraceptive medication, but in retrospect she had failed to take it regularly. Another had had regular menses, but the last one (2 weeks before the therapy) had been scanty. Only 4 of the 22 physicians indicated that they performed a pregnancy test routinely.

Discussion

The validity of data obtained by surveys of this type is always open to question. Obviously, many busy physicians will not take the time to respond. Others may respond from memory rather than review records in detail. Physicians who have had bad experiences may tend more to remember and report them, producing a possible bias in this direction. On the other hand, some physicians who have had unfavorable experiences may have preferred not to respond, out of concern for the current legal climate. Indeed, some of the respondents removed identifying data from their reply cards to preserve anonymity.

This overall problem is one which any given physician will not be likely to encounter more than a few times, even in a lifetime of practice. Therefore, a pooling of data seemed essential. The physicians to be surveyed were selected by one of us (J.I.H.) on the basis of personal knowledge of many of the physicians, derived from long-standing activity in the field of clinical thyroidology. The fact that 517 of the 963 physicians contacted actually responded is a reflection of both the appropriateness of the selection and the interest of the physicians in gaining further insight into this matter. Moreover, the large number of responses would seem likely to reduce one's concern for any particular bias. Accordingly, we believe that the data obtained are suitable for analysis both of the prevailing attitude toward therapeutic abortion in this predicament and of the results with those pregnant women who were advised to carry to term.

The data from this survey suggest that the majority of physicians do not recommend therapeutic abortion for pregnant patients who inadvertently received ^{131}I therapy in the first trimester of pregnancy. This conservative approach seems justified by the finding that the rate of fetal and neonatal abnormalities was no greater than that reported for uncomplicated pregnancies. It was disturbing to learn that 2 patients, both of whom had mentally defective hypothyroid infants, received repeated therapeutic doses of ^{131}I, in one instance as late as 26 weeks in the pregnancy (Table 10-1). Of perhaps greater concern was the discovery that urine pregnancy tests are still not performed routinely, even in major medical centers. When pregnancy testing is so simple, quick, and inexpensive, it is difficult to justify reliance on menstrual history or the reliability of the patient in employing contraceptive measures. To be sure, the test may be false-negative in the first few weeks of pregnancy, but the probability of fetal accumulation of ^{131}I is small during this period.[5] A false-negative test is much less likely between the eighth and tenth weeks of gestation, when the level of chorionic gonadotropin rises to its peak.[6] Thus, by a fortunate coincidence, just when the fetal thyroid begins to function in terms of ^{131}I concentration, the pregnancy test will be most strongly positive. The simple expedient of a routine urine pregnancy test for all women in the childbearing age group should virtually eliminate the danger of fetal hypothyroidism. As radioimmunoassay for serum chorionic gonadotropin, beta subunit,[7] becomes more generally available, it will be possible to detect even earlier stages of pregnancy.

For women who have had a false-negative urine pregnancy test with subsequent ^{131}I therapy, it seems reasonable to permit continuation of the pregnancy. Maternal serum levels of free thyroxine and thyroid-stimulating hormone should be carefully monitored to prevent hypothyroidism. Similar assays on the cord blood should be done, and the infant should probably be examined at 3-month intervals for the first 2 years and annually thereafter.

A final consideration still requires study. The radiation received by the fetus as a consequence of the post-therapy excretion of ^{131}I through the urine may possibly lead to the development of leukemia in the children years after birth. At least, this has been reported after other forms of radiation exposure to pregnant women.[8] It would seem proper to initiate a further study of as many of the "normal" infants as possible to settle this point.

Conclusions

1. Most authorities do not advise therapeutic abortion for women who have inadvertently received ^{131}I therapy early in the first trimester.

2. The data from the survey provide support for the safety of this position.

3. A urine pregnancy test should be performed routinely on all women in the childbearing age group prior to the administration of therapeutic doses of [131]I. A negative test, in conjunction with a normal menstrual history, provides reliable assurance that ^{131}I therapy will be safe.

ELIMINATING HYPERTHYROIDISM IN PROSPECTIVE MOTHERS

Overview

Of 32 pregnant hyperthyroid patients seen at the Northland Thyroid Laboratory, 20 patients had recognizable hyperthyroidism from 1 to 12 months ($\bar{x}$ = 4.6 months) prior to becoming pregnant. Successful definitive treatment with either ^{131}I or subtotal thyroidectomy could have eliminated the hyperthyroidism in these 20 patients, preventing this problem from complicating subsequent pregnancies. Other authors have reported that some women have been allowed two or even three pregnancies complicated by hyperthyroidism without employment of definitive treatment. Adequate forethought when treating hyperthyroidism in women likely to become pregnant in the near future may prevent a substantial portion of pregnancies complicated by hyperthyroidism.

Review of the Literature

Pregnancy complicated by hyperthyroidism is uncommon but continues to exact a fetal toll in terms of wastage and thyroid abnormalities.[9,10] The incidence of these complicated pregnancies could be reduced if definitive (^{131}I) rather than suppressive (antithyroid drugs) therapy were selected for hyperthyroid women who had plans for childbearing. For most hyperthyroid patients there is time for such a choice. For 20 of the 32 pregnant hyperthyroid women treated in our laboratory, the diagnosis of hyperthyroidism antedated the pregnancy. The same was true for 83 of 123 pregnancies culled from the recent literature.[9,11–14]

To assess the risks of this dual condition, and thus to determine how necessary it might be to prevent it, we reviewed 12 papers published since 1960 dealing with a total of 411 pregnancies in 364 women.[9–20]

In the first 20 weeks of pregnancy the fetal loss was 5 percent, not different from that expected in uncomplicated pregnancies. However, in the remaining 392 pregnancies from the 21st week of gestation there were 26 (6.6 percent) fetal and neonatal deaths, compared to an expected incidence of 1.6 percent.[15] By chi-square analysis, this is a significant increase ($p < 0.001$). The late gestational losses occurred in all reports with roughly equal frequency. By contrast, thyroid abnormalities which might be attributed to antithyroid drugs were discovered in 16 infants, six of whom were included in two papers by the same author.[10,18] Three reports including 96 pregnancies had no fetal thyroid abnormalities.[11,13,17]

Neither a 10.6 percent incidence of prematurity nor a 3.5 percent incidence of nonthyroidal congenital anomalies differed from that expected with uncomplicated pregnancies.

Maternal complications included two deaths, three episodes of thyroid crisis, six episodes of preeclampsia, and congestive heart failure in two patients.

In a recent seminar on this subject, concern was expressed for possible subclinical impairment of fetal intellect as a result of intrauterine exposure to antithyroid drugs.[19] There were no data on this point. However, it has been shown that the progeny of hypothyroxinemic mothers may have depressed intelligence quotients. Therefore, this is a potential risk of antithyroid drug overdosage in the mother.

It should be emphasized that the above results are from major medical centers where one would expect experienced physicians and the finest laboratory facilities. However, most patients with this problem may well be treated by physicians handicapped not only by less experience but also by more limited laboratory support. These physicians may do less well. One report compared the results for 20 women closely followed by the authors with 14 seen only in consultation, and followed through the majority of the pregnancy by the family physician.[20] In the latter group there were three infants with goiter and two stillbirths. Neither complication was seen in the pregnancies followed closely by the authors.

Even those with considerable success in the management of pregnant hyperthyroid patients should appreciate that antithyroid drugs present an added risk to the fetus which may be beyond the physician's control. Women do not always cooperate either in self-administration of medication or in returning for regular follow-up examinations. However, lack of concern or lack of foresight for this risk was demonstrated by the authors of 9 of the 12 papers reviewed, since they permitted women to have two and even three successive pregnancies while taking antithyroid drugs, rather than initiating definitive treatment after the first episode. All of our women who remained hyperthyroid after termination of pregnancy were treated with ^{131}I, and none has experienced a second episode of this dual condition.

[131]I treatment of hyperthyroid women who plan childbearing in the near future would seem likely to improve the fetal salvage rate, and eliminate antithyroid drug-induced goiter, without any appreciable increase in the risk of other fetal problems. Three recent reports deal with ^{131}I therapy for a total of 190 children with hyperthyroidism.[22-24] These patients subsequently had 193 pregnancies with no increase in fetal loss or anomalies. Indeed, two reports on the subsequent progeny of young patients treated with cancer doses of ^{131}I revealed no increase in these fetal complications.[25,26] These results are consistent with calculations indicating that ovarian radiation from ^{131}I therapy should not materially increase the risk of fetal anomalies.[27,28]

Some physicians still favor thyroidectomy for young hyperthyroid patients. Operative risks have been greatly reduced in recent years. However, there is no assurance that the enviable records achieved in the major medical centers can be duplicated in the average community hospital. Hypocalcemic crisis during delivery occurred in one woman who had been treated surgically earlier in the pregnancy.[17] Therefore, when definitive therapy is elected, the choice between ^{131}I and thyroidectomy must take into consideration the relative risks of the two treatments, and this may be influenced by the talent available in any given locale.

Neither method of definitive therapy is risk free. Hypothyroidism is a potential problem with serious reproductive implications. This may be avoided by the use of thyroid hormone, but again, patients may fail to cooperate. Still, the treatment of hypothyroidism is a far less formidable undertaking than the monitoring of antithyroid drugs during pregnancy.

In the final analysis, there is no risk-free method of dealing with the implications of hyperthyroidism for women in the childbearing years. Although use of antithyroid drugs may appeal to the conservative instincts of many physicians, our analysis suggests that definitive alternatives may be safer.

Conclusion

1. When pregnancy is complicated by hyperthyroidism there is an increased fetal loss after the 21st week of gestation.

2. The administration of antithyroid drugs during pregnancy may produce fetal goiter and hypothyroidism, even in the hands of experienced physicians.

3. The elimination of hyperthyroidism prior to pregnancy is a desirable goal, and one which may be advanced by the selection of definitive (our preference being for ^{131}I) rather than suppressive therapy for hyperthyroid women who contemplate childbearing.

ACKNOWLEDGMENT

We are deeply indebted to the hundreds of physicians who were kind enough to share their experience with us.

REFERENCES

1. Green, H. G., Gareis, F.J., Shepard, T. H., et al.: Cretinism associated with maternal sodium iodide ^{131}I therapy during pregnancy. Am. J. Dis. Child. 122:247–249, 1971.
2. Fisher, W. D., Voorhess, M. L., Gardner, L. I.: Congenital hypothyroidism in infant following maternal ^{131}I therapy. J. Pediatr. 62:132–146, 1963.
3. Means, J. H., DeGroot, L. J., Stanbury, J. B.: The Thyroid and Its Diseases, Ed. 3. New York, McGraw-Hill Book Co., p. 230, 1963.
4. Hamburger, J. I.: Hyperthyroidism—Concept and Controversy. Springfield, Ill., Charles C Thomas, p. 102, 1972.
5. Shepard, T. H.: Onset of function in the human fetal thyroid: bio-chemical and radioautographic studies from organ culture. J. Clin. Endocrinol. 27:945–958, 1967.
6. Catt, K. J.: An ABC of Endocrinology. Boston, Little, Brown & Co., p. 126, 1972.
7. Vaitukaitis, J. L., Braunstein, G. D., Ross, G. T.: A radioimmunoassay which specifically measures human chorionic gonadotropin in the presence of human luteinizing hormone. Am. J. Obstet. Gynecol. 113:751–758, 1972.
8. MacMahon, B.: Prenatal x-ray exposure and childhood cancer. J. Natl. Cancer Inst. 28:5, 1962.
9. Ayromlooi, J., Zervoudakis, I. A., Sadaghat, A.: Thyrotoxicosis in pregnancy. Am. J. Obstet. Gynecol. 117:818–823, 1973.
10. Mujtaba, Q., Burrow, G. N.: Treatment of hyperthyroidism in pregnancy with propylthiouracil and methimazole. Obstet. Gynecol. 46:282–286, 1975.
11. Herbst, A. L., Selenkow, H. A.: Hyperthyroidism during pregnancy. N. Engl. J. Med. 273:627–632, 1965.
12. Asper, S. P., London, F.: Thyrotoxicosis and pregnancy. Trans. Am. Clin. Climat. Assoc. 72:110, 1960.
13. Bokat, M. A.: Treatment of hyperthyroidism during pregnancy. Clin. Endocrinol. 2:236–243, 1968.
14. Talbert, L. M., Thomas, C. G., Holt, W. A., et al.: Hyperthyroidism during pregnancy. Obstet. Gynecol. 36:779–784, 1970.
15. Levy, R. P., Kopelson, M., Ryan, K. J.: Hyperthyroidism during pregnancy, editorial. N. Engl. J. Med. 274:165, 1966.
16. Howe, P.: Pregnancy and thyrotoxicosis. Br. Med. J. 2:817–822, 1962.
17. Worley, R. J., Crosby, W. M.: Hyperthyroidism during pregnancy. Am. J. Obstet. Gynecol. 119:150–155, 1974.
18. Burrow, G. N.: Neonatal goiter after maternal propylthiouracil therapy. J. Clin. Endocrinol. 25:403–408, 1965.
19. Werner, S. C.: Hyperthyroidism in the pregnant woman and the neonate. J. Clin. Endocrinol. 27:1637–1654, 1967.
20. Goluboff, L. G., Sisson, J. C., Hamburger, J. I.: Hyperthyroidism associated with pregnancy. Obstet. Gynecol. 44:107–116, 1974.
21. Man, E. B., Jones, W. S., Holden, R. H., et al.: Thyroid function in human pregnancy. Am. J. Obstet. Gynecol. 111:905–916, 1971.
22. Starr, P., Jaffe, H. L., Oettinger, L.: Later results of ^{131}I treatment of hyperthyroidism in 73 children and adolescents: 1967 followup. J. Nucl. Med. 10:586–590, 1969.
23. Hayek, A., Chapman, E. M., Crawford, J. D.: Long-term results of treatment of thyrotoxicosis in children and adolescents with radioactive iodine. N. Engl. J. Med. 283:949–953, 1970.
24. Safa, A. M., Schumacher, O. P., Rodriguez-Antunez, A.: Long-term followup results in children and adolescents treated with radioactive iodine (^{131}I) for hyperthyroidism. N. Engl. J.Med. 292:167–170, 1975.

25. Sarkar, S. D., Beierwaltes, W. H., Gill, S. P., et al.: Subsequent fertility and birth histories of children and adolescents treated with ^{131}I for thyroid cancer. J. Nucl. Med. 17:460–464, 1976.
26. Rosvoll, R. V., Winship, T.: Thyroid carcinoma and pregnancy. In: Thyroid Research, C. Cassano and M. Andreoli (eds.). New York, Academic Press, pp. 1042–1044, 1965.
27. Sobels, F. H.: Estimation of the genetic risk resulting from the treatment of women with [131]Iodine. Strahlentherapie 138:172–177, 1969.
28. Myant, N. B.: The radiation dose to the body during treatment of thyrotoxicosis by [131]I. Min. Nucl. 8:207–210, 1964.

Arnold M. Friedman

11
Radioastatine: Possible Uses
of a Heavy Halogen

INTRODUCTION

Several characteristics of short-lived alpha emitters make them attractive candidates for therapeutic use in nuclear medicine. Figure 11-1 is an illustration of a beta particle (0.6 mev) track (a) and an alpha particle (5.0 mev) track (b). As can easily be seen, the alpha particle track is much shorter and has a much greater ionization density. These considerations show that along their paths each 0.6-mev beta particle has a radiation density of 0.24 rads/g and each 5.0-mev alpha particle has a radiation density of 320 rads/g.

For many possible therapeutic uses, those radiation characteristics of alpha emitters (sharp localization of radiation, high radiation density, and high radiation level per particle) make these isotopes appear attractive.

Unfortunately, most of the alpha emitting isotopes which can be easily made are not very suitable. As is well known, the alpha emitters are clustered at the heavy end of the isotope chart. The only short-lived ones which can be made from common target materials are astatine (At) and polonium (Po) isotopes. Polonium is notorious for difficult chemical characteristics, whereas astatine is a halogen and has many chemical properties similar to those of iodine. In addition, one isotope of astatine, [211]At, has a convenient half-life, 7.2 hours, and no long-lived radioactive daughters.[1] One can produce [211]At by bombarding natural Bi with 20- to 28-mev alpha particles, a beam within the capability of many medical cyclotrons.

USES OF [211]AT

Most of the potential uses are based on the fact that organic compounds can be astatinated by the same techniques by which they can be iodinated. Thus one can bind astatine to proteins, enzymes, cells, and simple molecules. I will not go into the details of the reactions here but will note that the most common ones involved either the oxidation of At$^-$ to At$^+$, and subsequent substitution of the

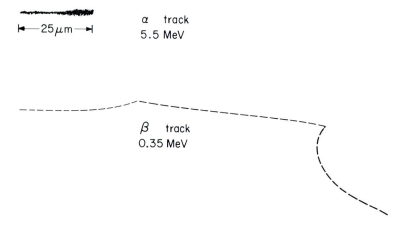

Fig. 11-1.   Alpha particle and beta particle tracks in emulsion.

latter species for a hydrogen atom, or the hydrolysis of a diazonium salt in the presence of At⁻. Table 11-1 illustrates these reactions and a convenient summary is given in ref. 2.

The most obvious uses for astatinated compounds would be in thyroid irradiation, tumor therapy, and antibody suppression. We will discuss each in turn.

THYROID IRRADIATION

Hamilton et al.[3] studied the thyroid uptake of ^{211}At in rats with results shown in Table 11-2. They also studied the effects of this uptake on the thyroid. In their experiments varying doses of astatine were injected as At⁻ ions, and the uptake of ^{131}I was measured in groups of animals at varying times subsequent to the At treatment. Some of their typical results are shown in Table 11-3.

As can be seen, there was a marked decrease in iodine uptake a year after the astatine treatment for all levels of astatine dosage. In addition, they also observed significant histological changes in thyroid tissue for all animals receiving at least 1.2 μCi/g of ^{211}At.

It is obvious that small dosages of ^{211}At can greatly modify thyroid functions.

Table 11-1
Typical Organoastatine Reactions

1. Oxidation reactions
   a. At⁻ + H_2O + lactoperoxidase + protein →
   b. At⁻ + chloramine −T + protein →
   c. At⁻ + H^+ + electrolysis
2. Substitution or addition reactions
   a. At⁻ + ClH—N≡N-protein + H^+ →
   b. At° + R—C≡C—R′ + H^+ →

Table 11-2

Uptake of $^{211}At^-$ and $^{131}I^-$ in Rat Thyroid

	$^{211}At^-$	$^{131}I^-$
% in thyroid	0.8	12.6
(%/g) in thyroid	50.6	811

However, before considering its potential use for thyroid therapy, one must evaluate the effects of ^{211}At on other organs since less than 1 percent goes into the thyroid itself.

TUMOR THERAPY

In his excellent review article[4] on the immunotherapy of cancer, Parker states that there may be several reasons for the failure of the immune system to destroy primary tumors. These include the difficulty for antibody to flow into the tumor; the saturation of sensitized lymphocytes by the large amounts of circulating antigen released by the tumor as soluble protein and fragmented and intact cells; possible release of blocking antibodies; and a low density of specific antigens on the surface of tumor cells.

In the case of this last effect, any increase in the cytotoxicity of the cancer antibodies would be of great help in destroying the cells. It has been postulated[4] that ^{211}At could be attached to the antitumor-specific antibody, and the alpha particles emitted after formation of the tumor-antibody complex could destroy the cell. Of course, the use of ^{211}At as a promoter of cytoxicity will be dependent on the ability to produce biologically stable, immunogenically competent antibody. As we will see, it has been shown that the complementary process of producing astatinated antigen has been accomplished. At present no astatinated antibodies have been produced; however, results obtained by Moolton et al.[5] show that target cells can be destroyed by diphtheria toxin conjugated to antibody directed to antigen on those cells.

Table 11-3

Postirradiation Thyroid Uptake of ^{11}I

$\mu Ci/g$ ^{211}At	% ^{131}I Uptake after 6 Days	% ^{131}I Uptake after 1 Year
0	9	7.4
0.4	—	2.6
0.6	—	3.0
0.8	4.1	1.6
1.2	1.3	0.2
1.5	0.3	—
1.8	1.3	—

ANTIBODY SUPPRESSION

Prolongation of allograft retention by reduction of the immune response causing graft rejection has long been a standard procedure. Unfortunately, the techniques used result in a general lowering of the immune defense mechanism and subsequent high risk of infection.

Many groups have attempted to specifically destroy those lymphocyte clones which will be responsible for the specific immune response to the donor cells. In principle, the donor antigens could be tagged with [211]At which would decay when

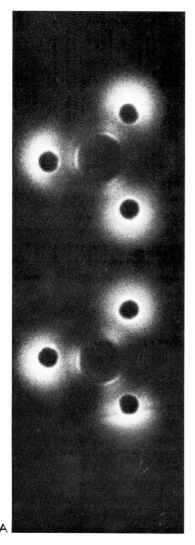 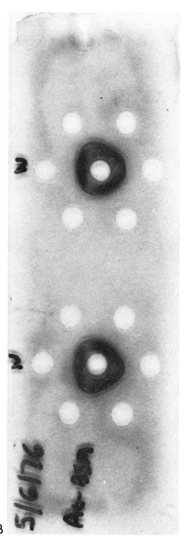

A   B

Fig. 11-2.   a. Autoradiograph of [211]At in immunodiffusion plate. **b.** Immunodiffusion plate with anti-BSA center, BSA in holes 1, 3, and 5, and BSA-para-iodo-benzoic-acid in holes 2, 4, and 6. (BSA, bovine serum albumin.) (Reprinted with permission of Internat. J. Nucl. Med. Biol.)

cloned by specific lymphocytes. The alpha particles emitted in the decay process would destroy the lymphocytes. Simple geometric considerations[6] show that if about 15 [211]At atoms are attached to the antigens bound to any lymphocyte, there will be greater than a 90 percent probability of cell destruction.

Attempts to label proteins with astatine using the standard protein iodination techniques have not produced an astatine-protein bond that is stable in vivo.[7,8] However, an in vitro immune "suicide" experiment by Neirinckx, Myburgh, and Smit[9] showed a high degree of selective suppression of the immune response. Myburgh and Smit[10] were able to extend the survival time of baboons with liver allografts from 12 days to 36 days using At-antigen complexes. However, they did not attempt to demonstrate a selective response.

The problem of biological stability was solved by Simonian et al.[11] These authors bound the astatine by diazonium hydrolysis into a charge-stabilized system and then conjugated the system as a heptene onto the protein. This procedure resulted in a chemically stable system as shown by the biological distributions. In addition, these At-heptene-protein compounds were found to be immunogenically competent.[12] Figure 11-2 illustrates the results of an immunodiffusion experiment obtained in ref. 12. Figure 11-2a is an autoradiograph of the immunodiffusion plate containing at At-heptene-protein compound; Figure 11-2b is a photograph of the same plate (stained to show the immunoprecipitation band of macroscopic heptene-protein and normal protein). As can be seen by comparing Figures 11-2a and 11-2b, there are no large immunogenic differences between the protein, heptene-protein, and At-heptene-protein compounds.

CONCLUSIONS

Alpha emitting isotopes such as [211]At have potential value in therapeutic nuclear medicine. However, there must be careful investigation of potential secondary damage to organs by nontargeted astatine. This is especially true since At-protein bonds seem to be more labile than I-protein bonds. New techniques[11] of binding astatine may ameliorate this problem.

REFERENCES

1. Lederer, M., Hollander, J., Perlman, I.: Table of Isotopes. New York, Wiley, 1967.
2. Meyer, G. J., Rosaler, K., Stocklin, G.: Preparation and high pressure chromatography of 5-astatouracil. Labeled Compounds and Radiopharmaceuticals 12:449–458, 1976.
3. Hamilton, J. G., Durbin, P. W., Asling, C. W., et al.: Metabolism of astatine. In: Peaceful Uses of Atomic Energy, Vol. 10. New York, United Nations, p. 173, 1956.
4. Parker, C. W.: The immunotherapy of cancer. Pharmcol. Rev. 25:325–342, 1973.
5. Moolton, F. L., Copperband, S. R.: Selective destruction of target cells with diphtheria toxin. Science 169:68–70, 1970.
6. Zalutsky, M. R., Friedman, A. M., Buckingham, F. C., et al.: Synthesis of a non-labile astatine-protein conjugate. Proceedings of the 1st International Symposium on Radiopharmaceutical Chemicals, Brookhaven, N.Y., 1976.
7. Borras, C.: Sc. thesis, University of Barcelona, Spain, 1974.

8. Aaij, C., Tchroots, W. R., Linden, L., et al.: Preparation of astatine labeled proteins. Int. J. Appl. Radiat. Isot. 26:25–30, 1975.

9. Neirinckx, R., Myburgh, R., Smit, J.: Labeling lymphocytes with [211]At and its applications. IAEA-SM 2:171–181, 1973.

10. Myburgh, J., Smit, J.: Enhancement and antigen suicide on the outbred primate. Transplant Proc. 5:597–600, 1973.

11. Simonian, S., Wainer, B., Friedman, A. M., et al.: Immunologically specific cell destruction. Fed. Proc. 35:334–335, 1976.

12. Friedman, A. M., Zalutsky, M., Wung, W., et al.: Preparation of a biologically stable, immunologically competent, astatinated protein. Int. J. Nucl. Med. Biol. 4:219–224, 1977.

SECTION III

Uses in Nonmalignant Diseases

Leonard Rosenthall

12

Use of Radiocolloids for Intra-Articular Therapy for Synovitis

Treatment of chronic synovitis by surgical synovectomy is not always successful as recurrences do occur with regeneration of the synovium; there is also a tendency to postoperative stiffness and limitation of motion.[1,2] Intraarticular injection of chemicals such as nitrogen mustard[3] and thiotepa,[4] although desirably less invasive, were not significantly successful.[5,6] The potential value of the intraarticular administration of colloidal radiogold ([198]Au) was discussed in 1958,[7] but the first published papers on its efficacy in the treatment of recurrent knee effusions did not appear until 1963.[8,9] Disadvantages of [198]Au are its gamma photon emissions, which do not contribute appreciably to local synovial irradiation but do augment total-body absorbed dose unnecessarily; and a rather substantial leak (in excess of 10 percent) from the joint cavity via the lymphatics to be deposited in the regional lymph nodes.[10,11] In the case of the knee joint, the most frequent site of application, deposition of [198]Au in the inguinal nodes leads to irradiation of the testis with a possible doubling of the natural risk of genetic damage.[10] Lymphocytes passing through the lymph nodes have been shown to develop chromosomal damage.[12–14] Circulation through the highly vascular inflamed synovium may also be a contributing factor to lymphocytic chromosomal damage.[12]

The small size of the [198]Au particle (Table 12-1) has been implicated as one of the factors responsible for the leak. To circumvent this, investigators have tried using colloid suspensions of other radionuclides. For the knee joint ^{90}Y and ^{32}P are presently in use in many centers as an alternative to [198]Au. They have the desirable physical characteristics of larger particle size, pure beta emission, and a greater tissue penetration of the beta particles than those of [198]Au (Table 12-1). Two other causes of colloidal particle leak from the synovial cavity have been suggested. These are synovial inflammation and joint movement. It has been shown that premedication with intraarticular hydrocortisone to reduce synovial hyperemia and bed rest decrease the frequency and amount of radiocolloid deposited in the regional nodes.[18,19]

Ideally, the penetration of the beta particles should be limited to the thickness of the synovium to avoid radionecrosis of cartilage and bone. Thus, in smaller

Table 12-1
Radiopharmaceuticals Used for Intra-Articular Therapy

Colloidal Radiopharmaceutical	Half-life (days)	Emission	Max. Energy of β (mev)	Range in Soft Tissue (mm)		Particle Size (mm)	Reference
				Max.	Mean		
(^{198}Au) Gold-198	2.7	β, γ	0.96	3.6	1.2	20–70	8, 9
(^{169}Er) Erbium-169 citrate	9.5	β	0.34	1.0	0.3	10–30	15
(^{32}P) ^{32}P-chromic phosphate	14	β	1.7	7.9	2.6	500–1000	16
(^{186}Re) Rhenium-186 sulfide	3.7	β, γ	0.98	3.6	1.2	5–10	15
(^{90}Y) Yttrium-90 silicate citrate resin	2.7	β	2.2	11.0	3.6	100	17

Table 12-2
Suggested Intra-Articular Radiocolloid Doses

Joint	Intraarticular Dose (mCi)				
	^{198}Au	^{32}P	^{90}Y	^{186}Re	^{169}Er
Knee	4–10	1–2	3–5	—	—
Hip	—	—	—	3	—
Shoulder	—	—	—	2	—
Elbow	—	—	—	2	—
Ankle	—	—	—	2	—
Wrist	—	—	—	1–2	—
Metacarpophalangeal	—	—	—	—	0.25–0.5
Proximal interphalangeal	—	—	—	—	0.25–0.5

joints such as the hips, shoulders, elbows, ankles, and wrists, rhenium-186 sulfide has been advocated and erbium-169 citrate recommended for metacarpophalangeal and proximal interphalangeal joints (Table 12-2).[15]

The energy absorbed in the synovium is difficult to calculate for the various treatment doses suggested (Table 12-2) because knowledge of the synovial surface area is imprecise. Inflamed synovium is hypertrophic and can be thrown into folds for a larger than normal surface area, but it can also hinder a uniform adsorption of the radiocolloid. Intraarticular fibrin also presents a surface for radiocolloid deposition which is not contributory to the radionuclide synoviolysis, and the degree of radiocolloid leak is variable. A very gross estimate is about 6000 to 8000 rads for the knee.[14] The treatment doses suggested are empirically derived and are designed to prevent cartilage necrosis and flexion deformities while attempting to minimize the failure rate of radiation synovectomy.

TREATMENT PROCEDURE OF KNEES

The patient is admitted to hospital at least 2 days prior to intraarticular radiocolloid treatment. Under local anesthesia in a sterile field, the knee is aspirated of fluid and then 50 to 100 mg of hydrocortisone is instilled into the cavity.

Two days later the radiocolloid in 5 to 10 ml saline is injected into the synovial cavity. If a pure emitter is used, such as ^{90}Y or ^{32}P, 1 or 2 mCi of ^{99m}Tc-sulfur colloid is added to the synovial cavity contents so that immediate and 24-hour post-treatment localization images can be obtained (Figs. 12-1 and 12-2). This is necessary to ensure that loculation in a blind pocket has not occurred as it could lead to soft tissue necrosis. It is perhaps more prudent to inject the ^{99m}Tc-sulfur colloid before the treatment dose to be sure loculation is not present. Before the needle is removed, a saline or air flush is made to preclude a deposit of radioactivity along the needle tract. Apply firm pressure to the knee after removing the needle to reduce local leakage.

The patient is then confined to bed rest for 48 hours.

The other joints, particularly the small articulations of the hands, may require

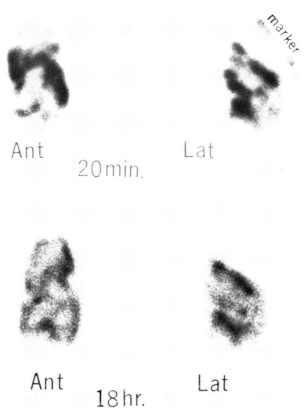

Fig. 12-1.   To visualize the distribution of radiocolloid in the
left knee, we added 2 mCi ^{99m}Tc-sulfur colloid to the 5 mCi
^{90}Y-silicate treatment dose. "Marker" indicates the sup-
rapatellar region. There is some redistribution of the
radiocolloid between 20 minutes and 18 hours post-dose.

fluoroscopic guidance and contrast injection to aid needle placement within the
synovial cavity. To simplify the procedure the steroid can be delivered with the
therapeutic dose of radiocolloid.

COMPLICATIONS

Transient fever and malaise may develop soon after intraarticular radiocolloid
treatment of the knees. A reactive synovitis has been reported to occur in about 30
percent of the patients[11] between a few hours and 2 weeks after treatment. This
reactive synovitis, which consists of increased pain and effusion, bears no relationship to the final outcome of treatment, and, in fact, these patients tend to have
a better end result than those who did not suffer this initial complication.[19] Other
sequelae of treatment may include radiation dermatitis of skin overlying the joint,
soft tissue reaction to radiocolloid deposited along the needle tract, and flexion

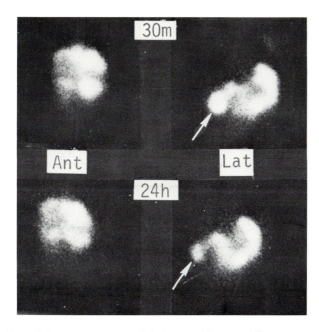

Fig. 12-2. Treatment of left knee with 1 mCi ^{32}P-chromic phosphate and 2 mCi ^{99m}Tc-sulfur colloid added for localization. Arrow points to a Baker's cyst. Only minor redistribution of radiocolloid is noted.

deformity and cartilage necrosis caused by too large a dose of radiocolloid. Two cases of knee joint rupture following radionuclide treatment have been reported.[21]

RESULTS

Symptomatic improvement following intraarticular delivery of radiocolloid usually occurs by 3 months and reaches a maximum at 6 months, but it is dependent in some measure on the stage of the disease and the thickness of the synovium. According to the anatomic staging of the American Rheumatism Association, stage I is no destructive changes by radiography; stage II is osteoporosis with or without slight bone destruction and minimal joint space narrowing; stage III is definite bone and cartilage destruction with joint space narrowing, joint deformity such as instability, and valgus deformity; stage IV is fibrous or bony ankylosis. Stage I patients benefited most in one series using ^{198}Au by 6 months showing a 54 percent excellent result; i.e., complete remission of effusion and pain, and a good result in 39 percent.[20] Stage II patients had a 42 percent frequency of an excellent result and 42 percent incidence of a good outcome. Stage III patients had an excellent and good outcome at 6 months of 40 percent and 14 percent, respectively.[20] At 1-year follow-up these values of improvement began to diminish. The benefit derived as a function of synovial thickness indicated an improvement in 90 percent of the patients with a thin synovium, of which 72 percent had an excellent result and 18 percent a good outcome. In contrast, 80 percent of the patients with a thick synovium had a favorable result, but only 16 percent could be classified as excellent.[20] A good to excellent result in the knees using the ^{90}Y colloids has been obtained in 66 percent of the patients unclassified with regard to anatomical staging or thickness of the synovium.[22,23]

Satisfactory results (good to excellent) were obtained in 33 percent of the shoulders, 53 percent of the elbows, 30 percent of the wrists and 43 percent of the hips 12 months after intraarticular [198]Au radiocolloid treatment.[22] The metacarpophalangeal joints treated with [169]Er-citrate yielded satisfactory results in 56 percent of the joints at 6 months and 36 percent at 12 months.[22] Proximal interphalangeal joints of the hand showed a satisfactory response to intraarticular [169]Er-citrate of 58 percent at 6 months and 68 percent at 12 months.[22]

In 29 patients with bilateral knee effusions and only one joint treated by radiation while the other joint served as control, at 6 months good to excellent results were achieved in 26 out of the 29 knees receiving intraarticular [198]Au, whereas a good response only was recorded in 5 of the 29 control knees.[20] A similar finding with ^{90}Y colloid has also been reported.[23]

A small series of cases were subjected randomly to either intraarticular radiocolloid treatment or surgical synovectomy. Relapse occurred in 3 out of the 10 irradiated knees and in 2 of the operated knees. Fewer of the irradiated knees were involved when generalized exacerbation of polyarthritis occurred.[24] The authors also conclude that both procedures are prone to failure in the presence of active generalized rheumatoid arthritis and extensive joint damage.

REFERENCES

1. Swett, P. P.: Synovectomy in chronic infectious arthritis. J. Bone Joint Surg. 5:110–121, 1923.
2. Goldie, I. F.: Synovectomy in rheumatoid arthritis: a general review and an eight year follow-up of synovectomy in 50 rheumatoid knee joints. Semin. Arthritis Rheum. 3:219, 1971.
3. Vaino, K., Julkunen, H.: Intraarticular nitrogen mustard treatment of rheumatoid arthritis. Acta Rheum. Scand. 6:25–30, 1960.
4. Flatt, A.E.: Intraarticular thiotepa in rheumatoid disease of the hands. Rheumatism 18:70–73, 1962.
5. Curry, H. L. F.: Intraarticular thiotepa in rheumatoid arthritis. Ann. Rheum. Dis. 24:382, 1965.
6. Ellison, M. R., Flatt, A.E.: Intraarticular thiotepa in rheumatoid disease: a clinical analysis of 123 injected MP and PiP joints. Arthritis Rheum. 14:212–222, 1971.
7. Ansell, B. M.: Early studies of [198]Au in the treatment of synovitis of the knee. Ann. Rheum. Dis. [Suppl.] 32:1–2, 1973.
8. Ansell, B.M., Cook, A., Mallard, J. R., et al.: Evaluation of intraarticular colloid gold, Au-198, in the treatment of persistent knee effusions. Ann. Rheum. Dis. 22:435–439, 1963.
9. Makin, M., Robin, R. C., Stein, J. A.: Radioactive gold in the treatment of persistent synovial effusion. Isr. Med. J. 22:107–111, 1963.
10. Topp, J. R., Cross, E. G.: The treatment of persistent knee effusions with intraarticular radioactive gold. Can. Med. Assoc. J. 102:709–714, 1970.

11. Virkkunen, M., Krusivs, F. E., Heiskanen, T.: Experiences of intraarticular adminis-
    tration of radioactive gold. Acta Rheum. Scand. 13:81–91, 1967.
12. de la Chapelle, A., Oka, M., Rekonnen, A., et al.: Chromosome damage after intraar-
    ticular injections of radioactive yttrium. Effect of immobilization on biological dose.
    Ann. Rheum. Dis. 31:508–512, 1972.
13. Stevenson, A. C.: Chromosomal damage in human lymphocytes from radioisotope
    therapy. Ann. Rheum. Dis. [Suppl.] 32:19–22, 1973.
14. Stevenson, A. C., Bedford, J., Dolphin, G. W., et al.: Cytogenetic and scanning study
    of patients receiving intraarticular injections of gold-198 and yttrium-90. Ann. Rheum.
    Dis. 32:112–123, 1973.
15. Ingrand, J.: Characteristics of radioisotopes for intraarticular therapy. Ann. Rheum.
    Dis. [Suppl.] 32:3–9, 1973.
16. Winston, M. A., Bluestone, R., Cracchiolo, A., et al.: Radioisotope synovectomy with
    ^{32}P-chromic phosphate—kinetic studies. J. Nucl. Med. 14:886–889, 1973.
17. Gumpel, J. M., Farran, H. E. A., Williams, E. D.: Use of yttrium-90 in persistent
    synovitis of the knee. Ann. Rheum. Dis. 33:126–128, 1974.
18. Gumpel, J. M., Williams, E. D., Glass, H. I.: Use of yttrium-90 in persistent synovitis
    of the knee. Ann. Rheum. Dis. 32:223–227, 1973.
19. Goode, J. D., Howey, S.: Effects of hydrocortisone on retention of ^{198}Au. Ann.
    Rheum. Dis. [Suppl.] 32:43–45, 1973.
20. Topp, J. R., Cross, E. G., Fam, A. G.: Treatment of persistent knee effusions with
    intraarticular radioactive gold. Can. Med. Assoc. J. 112:1085–1089, 1975.
21. Davis, P., Jayson, M. I. V.: Acute knee joint rupture after yttrium-90. Ann. Rheum.
    Dis. 34:62–63, 1975.
22. Menkes, C. J., Aignan, M., Galmiche, B., et al.: Le traitement des rhumatismes par les
    synovirothèse, choix des malades, choix des articulations, modalites practiques, re-
    sultats, indications, contre-indications. Rheumatologie [Suppl.] 2:61, 1972.
23. Bridgman, J. F., Bruckner, F., Eisen, V., et al.: Irradiation of the synovium in the
    treatment of rheumatoid arthritis. Q. J. Med. 42:357–367, 1973.
24. Gumpel, J. M., Roles, N. C.: A controlled trial of intraarticular radiocolloids versus
    surgical synovectomy in persistent synovitis. Lancet, 308:488–489, 1975.

William H. Beierwaltes

13
Therapeutic Implications of Adrenal Scanning Agents

ADRENAL IMAGING AGENTS

Figure 13-1 presents the chemical configuration of our imaging agents: Mark I, [131]I-19-iodocholesterol;[1-4] Mark II, 6-beta-19-norcholesterol;[5-11] and our current Mark III agent, ^{131}I-SKF 12,185[12-14] (in the figure labeled with ^{123}I), with which we have just imaged the dog adrenals.

RADIATION THERAPY WITH ADRENOCORTICAL IMAGING AGENTS: PAST, PRESENT, AND FUTURE

Radiation Responsiveness of Normal and Hyperplastic Endocrine Gland Tissue

It is well known that hyperplastic tissue is generally more susceptible than normal tissue to the necrotizing effect of ionizing radiation. Patients with polycythemia vera were not infrequently brought to low blood count values (red cells, white cells, and platelets) with as little as 3 mCi of ^{32}P, whereas Bertram Low Beer routinely gave 10 to 15 mCi of ^{32}P without serious effects on the bone marrow in women with carcinoma of the breast after mastectomy to irradiate any possible metastases that had implanted in the bone. Similarly, one may induce hypothyroidism in a patient with Graves' disease with as little as 3 mCi of ^{131}I, whereas occasionally one cannot ablate the uptake in a normal thyroid gland remnant in the treatment of well-differentiated thyroid carcinoma with 125 mCi.

ACTH EXCESS CUSHING'S DISEASE

For these reasons, we evaluated the effect of ^{131}I-19-iodocholesterol treatment of simulated ACTH excess Cushing's disease in dogs.[15] Three normal female

This research was supported in part by NIH Training Grant CA-09015-02, ERDA Contract No. EY-76-S-02-2031, and by the Nuclear Medicine Research Fund.

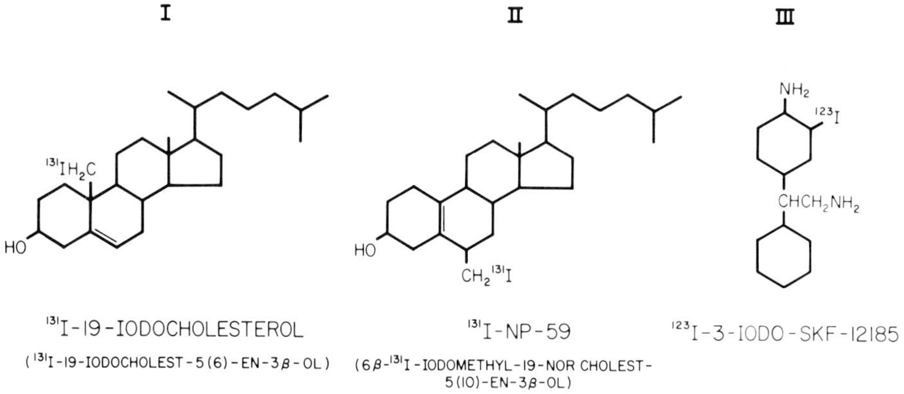

I   II   III

^{131}I-19-IODOCHOLESTEROL ^{131}I-NP-59 ^{123}I-3-IODO-SKF-12185

(^{131}I-19-IODOCHOLEST-5(6)-EN-3β-OL)   (6β-^{131}I-IODOMETHYL-19-NOR CHOLEST-
                                              5(10)-EN-3β-OL)

Fig. 13-1. Chemical structure of adrenal imaging agents: Mark I, ^{131}I-19-iodocholesterol; Mark II, 6 beta-19-norcholesterol; and Mark III, ^{131}I-SKF 12,185. (Reprinted with permission from Sem. Nucl. Med.)

dogs were given LD_{50} radiation doses of ^{131}I-19-iodocholesterol without producing gross or histopathologically demonstrable change of the adrenals at autopsy 3 months later. The adrenal cortices of three dogs were made hyperplastic (to simulate the adrenal cortex in Cushing's disease) with ACTH and three with metapyralone. In addition, these six dogs were given LD_{50} doses of ^{131}I-19-iodocholesterol. Three months after treatment the adrenal glands of the ACTH-treated dogs were not enlarged, the cortex was thicker than normal, and there were no changes attributable to irradiation. At 3 months, the metapyralone-treated dogs had enlarged adrenals, widening of the adrenal cortex, and no necrosis, or other changes attributable to irradiation. It was concluded that a therapeutic trial of ^{131}I-19-iodocholesterol in the treatment of Cushing's disease in humans was not indicated.

With the development of 6-beta-19-norcholesterol and the finding in dogs that there was a fivefold greater uptake in the adrenal cortices (without increased uptake in nontarget tissues),[5] we have calculated that the same 50 mCi dose to a dog will produce a radiation dose to the adrenal cortices of 7500 rads.

Well-differentiated thyroid cancer usually shows regression from ^{131}I treatment when the radiation dose reaches 5000 rads or greater.[16]

At present, therefore, we are inducing adrenocortical hyperplasia with metapyralone when simulating ACTH excess Cushing's disease. These dogs will each be treated with 50 mCi of ^{131}I-6-beta-19-norcholesterol.

ADRENOCORTICAL CARCINOMA

More recently, several authors[17-20] have demonstrated diagnostic localization of iodocholesterol in adrenocortical carcinoma metastatic to liver. Initially we demonstrated that whereas normal adrenal cortical tissue concentrated ^{131}I-19-iodocholesterol in a range of 0.1 to 0.2 percent dose/g,[21] adrenocortical carcinomas of two patients producing cortical excess concentrated only 0.0001–0.0004 and 0.001 percent dose/g, respectively. It is of interest in this regard that well-differentiated thyroid cancer, for all practical purposes, always concentrates ^{131}I less avidly than normal tissue.[22,23] The thyroid cancer with the highest functional activity reported[24] showed 40 percent of the concentrating ability shown by the normal thyroid gland (about 0.3 to 1.5 percent dose/g in normal thyroid gland). It seems reasonable, therefore, to search for adrenocortical carcinoma metastases in the human that concentrate 0.01 to 0.2 percent of the dose of ^{131}I-6 beta-19-norcholesterol per gram to evaluate the possible beneficial effects of therapy doses. Seabold et al.[19] have reported a patient with adrenocortical carcinoma percent dose per gram uptakes of 0.007 in metastases to liver and to vertebra as compared to 0.01 in the primary. The patient died from adrenocortical carcinoma and had been treated with OP-DDD.

ARE RADIOIODINATED CHOLESTEROLS IRREVERSIBLE ENZYME INHIBITIONS?

Our demonstrated ability to image the adrenal gland for as long as 23 days after a 2 mCi tracer dose of iodocholesterol suggests that the iodocholesterols have the same kinetics as irreversible enzyme inhibitors.[25-27] The advantage of a therapeutic dose of a beta radiation labeled irreversible enzyme inhibitor over pharmacologic doses of nonradiolabeled irreversible enzyme inhibitors in the treatment of carcinoma is that the radiation-induced necrosis will not allow the neoplasm time to develop alternate metabolic pathways to escape the unfavorable environment created by pharmacologic doses of a nonradiolabeled irreversible enzyme inhibitor.

BREAST AND PROSTATE CARCINOMA

We have called attention to the fact[26,27] that several enzymes that process steroids in the adrenal cortex also are found in carcinoma of the breast (and prostate). We have succeeded in synthesizing eight radiolabeled reversible enzyme inhibitors to several enzymes in the adrenal cortex of the rat, dog, and man.[12-14] Figure 13-2 presents our first successful radioiodine-labeled reversible enzyme inhibitor adrenal gland imaging in the dog.[14]

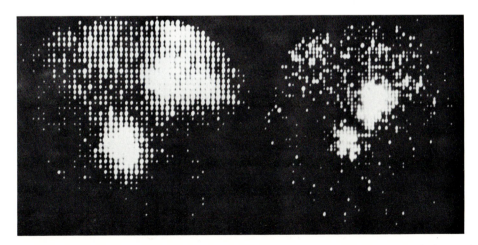

Fig. 13-2. Comparison of ^{131}I-SKF 12,185 (left) with ^{131}I-iodomethyl-6β-19-norcholesterol (right) in a dog's adrenal. (Reprinted with permission from J. Nucl. Med.)

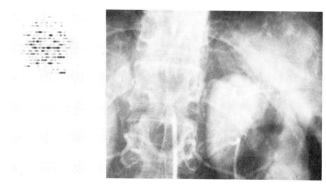

Fig. 13-3. Unilateral uptake of radiocholesterol in hyperfunctioning adrenocortical adenoma causing Cushing's syndrome. Treatment: surgical excision through right posterior approach. (Reprinted with permission from Lea & Febiger.)

DIAGNOSTIC AID OFFERED BY RADIONUCLIDE-LABELED ADRENAL IMAGING AGENTS IN TREATMENT OF ADRENAL GLAND DISEASES

Cushing's Syndrome

Differentiation of ACTH excess Cushing's disease from hyperfunctioning adrenocortical adenoma. If radionuclide adrenal imaging in a patient with Cushing's syndrome demonstrates uptake in one adrenal gland only (Fig. 13-3), surgical excision of an adenoma can be done without the use of the more traumatic and invasive venous catheterization studies.[28–31] If uptake is bilaterally equal (Fig. 13-4) and the percent uptake is greater than 0.28 percent of the administered dose in each adrenal gland,[28] the treatment is irradiation of the pituitary gland.

Detection and localization of adrenal remnant after "total" adrenalectomy[32,33] *adrenalectomy*[32,33] (Fig. 13-5). To date 9 of 11 patients (82 percent) had detectable

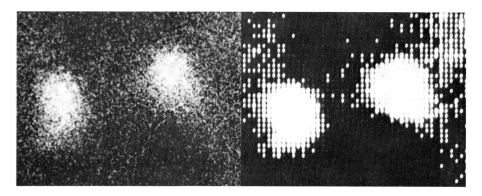

Fig. 13-4. Bilateral equal uptake of iodocholesterol in ACTH excess Cushing's disease. Treatment: pituitary irradiation. (Reprinted with permission from J. Clin. Endocrinol. & Metab.)

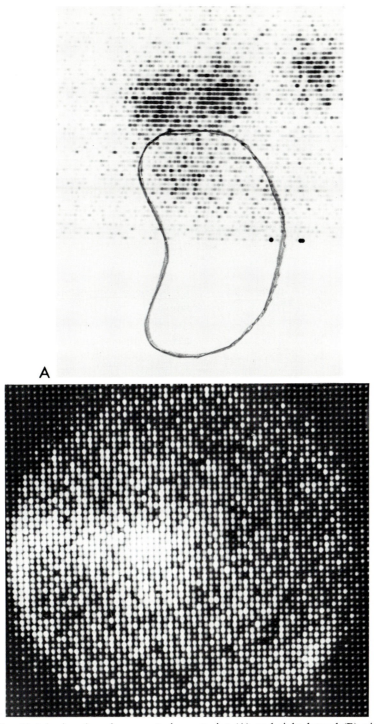

Fig. 13-5. Uptake in adrenal remnants in posterior (**A**) and right lateral (**B**) views, not detected by other techniques. Treatment: successful surgical removal through right posterior approach. (Reprinted with permission from Arch. Int. Med.)

adrenal remnants not detected by venography, arteriography, or venous sampling. Five of these patients had subsequent exploratory laparotomy, and in all five cases (100 percent) successful removal was accomplished with remission of Cushing's syndrome to date, with an average follow-up of 3.2 years.

Low-Renin Hypertension

Primary aldosteronism. If a patient with primary aldosteronism has an adenoma, the treatment is surgical, through a posterior approach. If the patient has micronodular or macronodular hyperplasia, the treatment is spironolactone. We have demonstrated[34-38] and others[39,40] have confirmed our findings that if dexamethasone suppression scanning demonstrates unilateral uptake of radiocholesterol, the adenoma can be removed surgically without resorting to an attempt at adrenal vein catheterization studies.

Figure 13-6 shows the three pathologic findings we have demonstrated with dexamethasone suppression radiocholesterol adrenal imaging in low-renin hypertension—both with and without primary aldosteronism[41] when we demonstrate adrenocortical abnormality with dexamethasone suppression scanning. When an adenoma (A) is found by unilateral uptake, the treatment is surgical removal through a unilateral posterior approach. When we find either macronodular hyperplasia (bilateral equal uptake early and late) or micronodular hyperplasia (suppressed uptake during first 3 days, then "breakthrough" equal imaging of both adrenals), the treatment is spironolactone.[38,41]

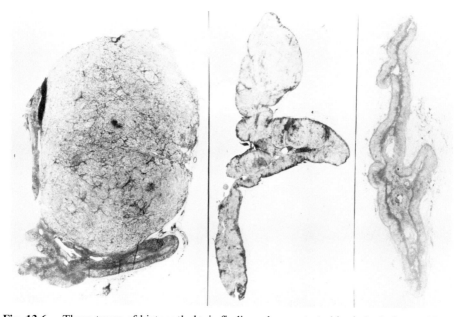

Fig. 13-6. Three types of histopathologic findings demonstrated by iodocholesterol imaging in low-renin hypertension, both with primary aldosteronism and in normal aldosterone low-renin hypertension when adrenocortical abnormality is demonstrated by dexamethasone suppression imaging. (See text for details.) (Reprinted with permission from J. Clin. Endocrinol. and Metab.)

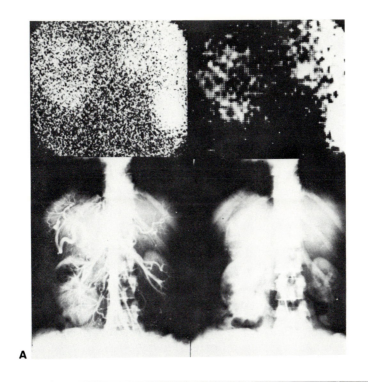

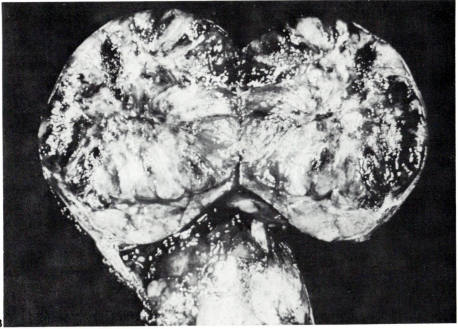

Fig. 13-7. *(Top and bottom.)* An adrenocortical carcinoma producing androgen. The left adrenal cortex is distributed over a much larger area due to the displacement of the normal adrenal cortex by the androgen secreting carcinoma in the left adrenal. There is no suppression of uptake in the right adrenal. (Reprinted with permission from Lea and Febiger.)

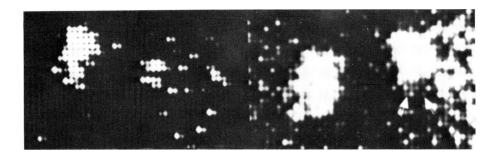

Fig. 13-8.   Two typical imaging patterns of pheochromocytoma for surgical resection. The pattern in patient #1 shows little uptake through any area of the right adrenal. The adrenal cortex has been stretched out by the pheochromocytoma so that the tumor is outlined by a bare trace of the adrenal cortex. The pattern in patient #2 (*right*) is more common; the lower one-half or two-thirds is truncated by the growth of the pheochromocytoma at the expense of the adrenal cortex. (Reprinted with permission from Elsevier/North Holland.)

Low-renin "essential" hypertension.   Our recent findings in low-renin "essential" hypertension cited above[41] are not unexpected since Gunnels et al.[42] found this same range of histopathology when they removed the adrenals in 32 patients with low-renin hypertension not due to aldosteronism. Although aldosteronism is the cause of hypertension in only 1 percent of patients with so-called essential hypertension, it is believed that up to one-third of all patients with "essential" hypertension have low-renin hypertension that is mineralocorticoid dependent.[42] It was of particular interest, therefore, when we found[41] a good blood pressure response to spironolactone in all patients with the macronodular pattern and in 3 of 5 with the micronodular pattern but a poor response in all 3 patients with normal suppression (no visible uptake in either adrenal through 10 days).

Adrenocortical Tumors with Androgen Excess

Androgen, like aldosterone (and unlike cortisol), does not shut off ACTH stimulation of the opposite adrenal or of the "normal" adrenal gland on the same side. An adenoma of the adrenal cortex secreting androgen as a cause of hirsutism and virilism would give the same unilateral uptake with dexamethasone suppression scanning as an aldosteronoma.

Figure 13-7 presents a radiocholesterol image of an adrenocortical carcinoma on the left secreting androgen with no suppression of uptake in the right adrenal gland. This type of metabolic determination of the type of neoplasm from the adrenal image cannot be discerned from ultrasound or CAT scanning.

Tumors of Adrenal Medulla

Radioactivity from radioiodinated cholesterol is found in the adrenal medulla in about one-half the concentration found in the adrenal cortex. As a result, pheochromocytoma detection is "cold spot" imaging.[43] Figure 13-8 shows two typical imaging patterns of pheochromocytomas and allows "lateralization" of the pheochromocytoma for surgical removal.

REFERENCES

1. Beierwaltes, W. H., Varma, V. M., Lieberman, L. M., et al.: Per cent uptake of radiolabeled cholesterol. J. Nucl. Med. 10:387, 1969.
2. Counsell, R. E, Renade, V. V., Blair, R. J., et al.: Tumor localizing agents. IX. Radioiodinated Cholesterol. Steroids 16:317–328, 1969.
3. Blair, R. J., Beierwaltes, W. H., Lieberman, L. M., et al.: Radiolabeled cholesterol as an adrenal scanning agent. J. Nucl. Med. 12:176–182, 1971.
4. Beierwaltes, W. H., Lieberman, L. M., Ansari, A. N., et al.: Visualization of human adrenal glands *in vivo* by scintillation scanning. J.A.M.A. 216:275–277, 1971.
5. Sarkar, S. D., Beierwaltes, W. H., Ice, R. D., et al.: A new and superior adrenal scanning agent: (NP-59). J. Nucl. Med. 16:1038–1042, 1975.
6. Basmadjian, G. P., Hetzel, K. R., Ice, R. D., et al.: Synthesis of a new adrenal cortex scanning agent, 6β-I-131-iodomethyl-19-norcholest-5(10)-en-3β-ol (NP-59). J. Labelled Compounds 11(3):427–434, 1975.
7. Kojima, M., Maeda, M., Ogawa, H., et al.: New adrenal scanning agent. J. Nucl. Med. 16:666–668, 1975.
8. Basmadjian, G. P., Hetzel, K. R., Ice, R. D., et al.: 6-I-131-iodomethyl-19-norcholest-5(10)-en-3-ol (NP-59). J. Nucl. Med. 16:514, 1975.
9. Sarkar, S. D., Ice, R. D., Beierwaltes, W. H., et al.: 6-I-131-iodomethyl-19-norcholest-5(10)-en-3-ol (NP-59) concentrates in the adrenal gland better than I-131-19-iodocholesterol. J. Nucl. Med. 16:565, 1975.
10. Kojima, M., Minoru, M.: Homoallylic rearrangement of 19-iodocholesterol. J.C.S. Chem. Comm. January 15, 1975.
11. Sarkar, S. D., Cohen, E. L., Beierwaltes, W. H., et al.: A new and superior adrenal imaging agent, NP-59: evaluation in humans. J. Clin. Endocrinol. Metab. 45:353–362, 1977.
12. Beierwaltes, W. H., Wieland, D. M., Ice, R. D., et al.: Localization of radiolabeled enzyme inhibitors in the adrenal glands. J. Nucl. Med. 17:998–1002, 1976.
13. Wieland, D. M., Kennedy, W. P., Ice, R. D., et al.: Radioiodinated pyridines— potential adrenocortical imaging agents. First International Meeting of Radiopharmaceutical Chemistry, Oak Ridge, Tenn., September, 1976.
14. Beierwaltes, W. H., Wieland, D. M., Mosley, S. T., et al.: Imaging the adrenal glands with radiolabeled inhibitors of enzymes. J. Nucl. Med. 14:200–203, 1978.
15. Anderson, B. G., Beierwaltes, W. H., Nishiyama, R. H. et al.: Effect of large doses of [131]I-19-iodocholesterol on metapyralone induced adrenal cortical hyperplasia in dogs. J. Nucl. Med. 16:928–932, 1975.
16. Scott, J. S., Halran, K. E., Shimmins, J., et al.: Measurement of dose to thyroid metastases from radioiodine therapy. Br. J. Radiol. 43:256–262, 1970.
17. Forman, B. H., Antar, M. A., Touloukian, J., et al.: Localization of a metastatic adrenal carcinoma using [131]I-19-iodocholesterol. J. Nucl. Med. 15:332–334, 1973.
18. Watanabe, M., Kamoi, I., Nakayama, C., et al.: Scintigraphic detection of hepatic metastases with ^{131}I labeled steroid in recurrent adrenal carcinoma. Case report. J. Nucl. Med. 17:904–906, 1976.
19. Seabold, J. E., Haynie, T. P., DeAsis, D. N., et al.: Detention of metastatic adrenal carcinoma using [131]-I-6-β-iodomethyl-19-norcholesterol total body scans. J. Clin. Endocrinol. Metab. 45:788–791, 1977.
20. Chatal, J. F., Carbonnel, B., Le Mevel, B. P., et al.: Uptake of [131]I-19-iodocholesterol by an adrenal cortical carcinoma and its metastases. J. Clin. Endocrinol. Metabol. 43:248–251, 1976.
21. Morita, R., Lieberman, L. M., Beierwaltes, W. H., et al.: Percent uptake of ^{131}I radioactivity in the adrenal from radioiodinated cholesterol. J. Clin. Endocrinol. Metabol. 34:36–43, 1972.

22. Fitzgerald, P. V., Foote, F. W.: The function of various types of thyroid carcinoma as revealed by the radioautographic demonstration of radioactive iodine (^{131}I). J. Clin. Endocrinol. 9:1153–1170, 1949.

23. Wollman, S. H.: Analysis of radioiodine therapy of metastatic tumors of the thyroid gland in man. J. Natl. Cancer Inst. 13:815, 1953.

24. Dobyns, B. M., Maloof, F.: The study and treatment of 119 cases of carcinoma of the thyroid with radioactive iodine. *J. Clin. Endocrinol.* 11:1323–1360, 1951.

25. Goldman, A. S.: Specific retention of an inhibitor of 3B-hydroxysteroid dehydrogenase in enzyme containing tissue of the rat. Endocrinology 86:678–686, 1970.

26. Ryo, U. Y., Beierwaltes, W. H.: Distribution of ^{14}C isoxazole in adrenals, ovaries, and breast carcinoma. J. Nucl. Med. 14:321–325, 1973.

27. Ryo, U. Y., Beierwaltes, W. H., Ice, R. D.: Enhancement of uptake with estradiol treatment of irreversible competitive enzyme inhibitor in the adrenal cortices and ovaries of rats with endocrine "autonomous" breast carcinomas. J. Nucl. Med. 15:187–189, 1974.

28. Thrall, J. H., Freitas, J. E., Beierwaltes, W. H.: Adrenal scintigraphy. Seminars in Nucl. Med. 8:23–42, 1978.

29. Moses, D. C., Schteingart, D. E., Sturman, M. F., et al.: Efficacy of radiocholesterol imaging of the adrenal glands in Cushing's syndrome. Surg. Gynecol. Obstet. 139:2–4, 1974.

30. Koral, K. F., Sarkar, S. D.: An operator-independent method for background subtraction in adrenal-uptake measurements. J. Nucl. Med. 18:925–928; 1977.

31. Lieberman, L. M., Beierwaltes, W. H., Ansari, A. N., et al.: Diagnosis of adrenal disease by visualization of human adrenal glands with [131]I-19-iodocholesterol. *N. Engl. J. Med.* 285:1387–1399, 1971.

33. Schteingart, D. E., Conn, J. W., Lieberman, L. M., et al.: Persistent or recurrent Cushing's syndrome after "total" adrenalectomy. Arch. Intern. Med. 130:384–387, 1972.

34. Freitas, J. F., Herwig, K. R., Cerney, J. C.: Preoperative localization of adrenal remnants: Efficacy of adrenal imaging. Surg. Gynecol. Obstet. 145:705–708, 1977.

34. Conn. J. W., Beierwaltes, W. H., Lieberman, L. M., et al.: Primary aldosteronism: preoperative tumor visualization by scintillation scanning. J. Clin. Endocrinol. Metabol. 83:713–716, 1971.

35. Conn, J. W., Morita, R., Cohen, E. L., et al.: Primary aldosteronism: photoscanning of tumors after [131]I-19-idocholesterol. Arch. Intern. Med. 129:417–425, 1971.

36. Conn, J. W., Morita, R., Cohen, E. L., et al.: Photoscanning of tumors in primary aldosteronism: Possible distinction from "idiopathic" aldosteronism. Presented at International Symposium on the Renin-Angiotensin-Aldosterone-Sodium System in Hypertension, September 30–October 4, 1971, Mount Gabriel Lodge, Quebec, Canada. In: Hypertension. Berlin, Springer-Verlag, pp. 299–312, 1972.

37. Conn, J. W., Beierwaltes, W. H., Cohen, E. L., et al.: Visualization of adrenal abnormalities by photoscanning after administration of radiocholesterol (Heath Memorial Lecture). In: Endocrine and Non-endocrine Hormone-Producing Tumors. Chicago, Year Book Medical Publishers, pp. 9–24, 1973.

38. Seabold, J. E., Cohen, E. L., Beierwaltes, W. H., et al.: Adrenal imaging with [131]-I-19-iodocholesterol in the diagnostic evaluation of patients with aldosteronism. J. Clin. Endocrinol. Metab. 42:41–51, 1976.

39. Hogan, M. J., McRae, J., Schambelan, M., et al.: Location of aldosterone-producing adenomas with [131]I-19-iodocholesterol. N. Engl. J. Med. 294:410–414, 1976.

40. Melby, J. C.: Solving the adrenal lesion(s) of primary aldosteronism. N. Engl. J. Med. 294:441–442, 1976.

41. Rifai, A., Beierwaltes, W. H., Freitas, J. E.: Adrenal scintigraphy in low renin "essential" hypertension. J. Clin. Nucl. Med. (in press).
42. Gunnels, J. C., McGuffin, W. L., Robinson, R. R., et al.: Hypertension, adrenal abnormalities and alterations in plasma renin activity. Ann Intern. Med. 73:901–911, 1970.
43. Sturman, M. F., Beierwaltes, W. H., Moses, D. C., et al.: Radiocholesterol adrenal images for the localization of pheochromocytoma. Surg. Gynecol. Obstet. 135:177–180, 1974.

Philip A. Bardfeld

14
Radionuclide Irradiation
of the Choroid Plexus
and Central Nervous System

In order for a radiopharmaceutical to be an effective radioablative agent in the CNS, it should fulfill the following requirements:

1. Relatively high uptake in target tissue
2. Minimal localization in nontarget tissue
3. An effective half-life in the target tissue that will permit adequate radioablation
4. Emission of particulate radiation with minimal gamma radiation in order to obtain maximal ablation of target tissue and avoid damage to contiguous normal structures
5. Mode of administration that will avoid or minimize systemic distribution

The radiopharmaceuticals included in the discussion of ablative agents are colloidal gold (^{198}Au), rhenium 188 (^{188}Re) as the perrhenate, and yttrium 90 (^{90}Y) as the chelate (^{90}Y-DTPA). The target tissues designated for ablation include the pituitary gland, the choroid plexus, sites of CNS leukemia, and metastatic neoplasms of the posterior fossa and spinal cord.

Destruction of the pituitary has been attempted using implants of radon, gold 198 seeds or pellets, and yttrium 90 rods or beads. The radioisotope was usually implanted through a transnasal approach. In general, the results of the neurosurgical techniques for pituitary ablation have been superior to the results obtained with radioisotopic transplants, and the latter have been abandoned.[1]

Initial attempts at radioablation of the choroid plexus began with the work of McClure and his group in 1955.[2] McClure instilled 4 to 8 mCi of colloidal gold 198 (^{198}Au) into the lateral ventricles of normal dogs and observed some concentration of ^{198}Au in the choroid plexus as determined by measurement of tissue activity. Interest had focused on the choroid plexus because of the major role played by this tissue in the formation of CSF and the hope that ablation of the choroid plexus would lead to amelioration of hydrocephalus.

With this goal in mind, Rish and Meacham[3] in 1967 studied the effects of intraventricular administration of 10 to 20 mCi of ^{198}Au into normal and hydrocephalic dogs. The dogs were made hydrocephalic by the injection of kaolin into the cisterna magna. A significant concentration of radioactivity was noted in the choroid plexus of each hydrocephalic dog within 3 to 10 days. The choroid plexus of the normal dog did not show any localization of [198]Au. Hemorrhagic necrosis and edema were also noted in the choroid plexus of the hydrocephalic dogs. The discrepancy between the uptake in normal and hydrocephalic dogs may have been due to a more prolonged contact time of the colloidal particles with the choroid plexus in the animals with hydrocephalus.

Weiss, Nulsen, and Kaufman[4] reported in 1972 on further studies of [198]Au in the kaolin model of hydrocephalus. A dose of 12 mCi of [198]Au was instilled into the lateral ventricles of each dog, and the animals were studied at serial intervals for periods up to 7 weeks. CSF flow was measured by a drip technique from a catheter inserted in a lateral ventricle.

A mean decrease in CSF flow of 32 percent was demonstrated after this treatment. A fall in intraventricular pressure was also noted. In four of the five animals which had air ventriculograms, a decrease in ventricular size and an increase in the thickness of the cortical mantle were observed. Histological studies showed a marked necrosis and vascular fibrosis in the choroid plexus, but serial scintiscans with a gamma camera revealed a diffuse distribution corresponding to the ventricles without any evident localization in the choroid plexus. The radioactivity per unit weight in the ependymal lining was almost one-half of that in the choroid plexus, and the activity in tissues 5 to 10 mm from the lining was 1 percent of the plexus activity.

The decay scheme of gold 198 is shown in Figure 14-1. Gold 198 has a physical half-life of 2.698 days and has both beta and gamma emissions. The most frequent beta energy is 0.962 mev and the most abundant gamma is 0.411 mev.

When judged by the criteria of an ideal ablative agent that were set forth at the

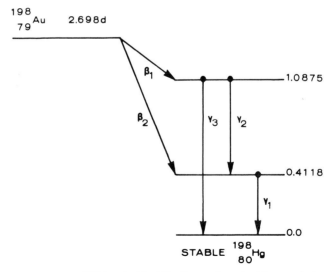

Fig. 14-1. Decay scheme of [198]Au (gold-198). (Reproduced with permission from J. Nucl. Med.)

beginning of this chapter, [198]Au has the advantage that it is a beta emitting radionuclide with a significant concentration in the choroid plexus. There are no published reports of the effective half-life of [198]Au in the choroid plexus. However, it is probably safe to assume that [198]Au will remain in the choroid plexus of the hydrocephalic animal for at least 2.7 days. Thus, the effective half-life of [198]Au in the choroid plexus would be satisfactory for ablation. The disadvantages of [198]Au are the presence of a moderately energetic gamma emission, which could damage contiguous normal brain tissue and constitute a health hazard to personnel in the immediate vicinity. Also, the concentration in the ependymal lining of hydrocephalic dogs would cause undesirable damage.

Another approach to the radioisotopic destruction of the choroid plexus was predicated on the ability of the choroid plexus to transport class VII anions out of the CNS. Initial attempts by Bernstein et al.[5] to ablate the choroid plexus of experimental animals with 100-mCi doses of ^{99m}Tc-pertechnetate suggested to us that it would be worthwhile to study the extraction of rhenium 188 by the choroid plexus. Rhenium 188 is produced from a tungsten 188 generator and decays with an energetic beta emission of 2.12 mev and a small percentage of gamma radiation (0.155 mev).[6] It has a physical half-life of 16.7 hours (Fig. 14-2).

We administered 200 μCi of rhenium 188 by ventriculocisternal perfusion to adult mongrel cats. We chose this mode of administration because it allowed the controlled delivery of a specific amount of radionuclide to the plexus by alteration of the perfusion time and it permitted us to determine the CSF formation rates (V_f), the CSF absorption rates (V_a), and the ventricular volumes (V_x) according to the method of Pappenheimer et al.[7] using blue dextran as an indicator of bulk flow. The choroid plexus of the lateral ventricle through which the perfusion was initiated concentrated rhenium 188 to a level 80 times that of the surrounding cortex and 26 times greater than the ingoing perfusion fluid[6] (Fig. 14-3). We demonstrated that the mechanism of rhenium 188 concentration in the choroid plexus involves active transport as well as simple diffusion of anion because pretreatment with perchlorate decreased the choroid plexus extraction and augmented the recovery of rhenium 188 in the cisternal outflow. The biological half-life of the radionuclide in the choroid plexus was 2 hours.[6]

Two weeks after the administration of 800-μCi doses of rhenium 188 to normal cats the CSF formation rate was 56 percent of the original, and at 4 months, it was 45 percent of the initial formation rate (Fig. 14-4).[6] Control cats perfused only

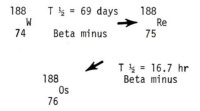

Fig. 14-2. Production and decay of [188]Re.

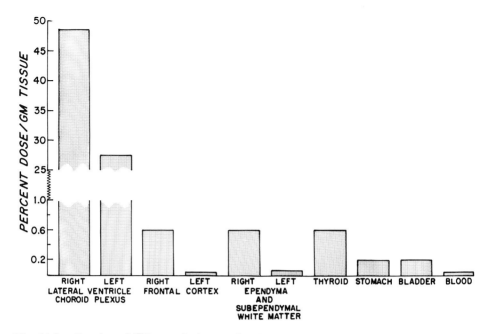

Fig. 14-3. Results of [188]Re perfusion study. (Reproduced with permission from Exptl. Neurol.)

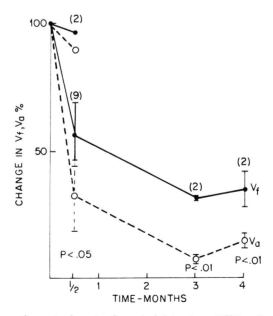

Fig. 14-4. CSF formation rates in cats after administration of [188]Re. (Reproduced with permission from Exptl. Neurol.)

with artificial CSF showed no change in formation rate after a 2-week interval. Histologic changes were also noted after [188]Re treatment. At 2 weeks the choroid plexus showed an increase in cellularity with round cells and polymorphonuclear leukocytes. At 3 and 4 months there was epithelial cell loss, cell vacuolization, and increased fibrosis.[6]

We were encouraged by these results to look at the effect of [188]Re in cats made hydrocephalic by the intracisternal injection of kaolin. At 10 days after kaolin injection, [188]Re was given to one group of cats in doses of 0.75 to 1.80 mCi by lateral ventricle to lateral ventricle perfusion.[8] Another group received doses of 4.6 to 5.1 mCi [188]Re by a single intraventricular injection.[7] Neither group showed diminution in the rates of formation or absorption of CSF or in the ventricular volumes, nor was there evidence of alteration in the thickness of the cortical mantle as shown by air ventriculograms (Tables 14-1 and 14-2). These observations were made at 2 to 4 weeks after treatment with [188]Re, and the animals were then sacrificed and the choroid plexuses were excised and studied. The gross pathologic and microscopic appearances of the choroid plexuses of the lateral, third, and fourth ventricles were similar in both the treated and untreated hydrocephalic animals. Tissue-to-medium ratios (T/M ratios) with $Na^{125}I$ were performed using choroid plexuses of normal, hydrocephalic, and [188]Re-treated cats. The T/M ratios were identical in both the normal and hydrocephalic group, but were significantly lower in the [188]Re-treated cats.[8]

Thus we have evidence that treatment did affect one parameter of choroid plexus function, i.e., the ability to selectively concentrate radioiodine from a medium. However, we do not know why the CSF formation rate, which is another measure of choroid plexus function, failed to show a reduction and why there was

Table 14-1

Effect of [188]Re Therapy Delivered by Ventricular Perfusion

Cat. No.	Dose and Duration	Pretreatment V_f ml/min	Pretreatment V_x ml	Post-treatment V_f ml/min	Post-treatment V_x ml	Weeks after Treatment
6601	1.54 mCi; > 5 hr	0.0120	17.3	0.0200	27.6	2
6595	2.00 mCi; > 8 hr	0.0042	11.8	0.0222	32.5	4
6602	1.75 mCi; > 8 hr	0.0201	13.4	0.0436	21.4	3
6605	0.75 mCi; > 8 hr	0.0173	21.3	0.0310	23.9	2
6630	1.80 mCi; > 8 hr	0.0146	9.7	No studies but autopsy showed no change in mantle		
Mean ± SEM		0.0134 ±0.0063	14.7 ±2.1	0.0292 ±0.0045	26.4 ±2.4	

(Reproduced with permission from Exptl. Neurol.)

Table 14-2
Effect of [188]Re Therapy Delivered by Single Intraventricular Injection

Cat. No.	Pretreatment			Post-treatment		
	Dose mCi	V_f ml/min	V_x ml	V_f ml/min	V_x ml	Days after Treatment
6713	5.1	0.0310	25.6	0.0428	33.3	24
17	4.6	0.0080	12.9	0.0313	33.0	23
6773	4.7	0.0050	8.4	0.03331	17.9	20
6774	4.6	0.0090	11.2	0.0163	29.8	18
Mean ± SEM		0.0132 ±0.0057	14.5 ±3.8	0.0309 ±0.0045	28.5 ±3.6	

(Reproduced with permission from Exptl. Neurol.)

no amelioration of hydrocephalus. These results can be explained by several factors:

1. The CSF formation rate in the kaolin-hydrocephalic cat may already be at a minimal level which is irreducible. There are many lines of evidence to support this explanation. For example, Hochwald et al.[9] have shown that the CSF formation rate is significantly lower than normal in kaolin hydrocephalic cats.
2. The choroid plexus might have been only partially ablated and the remnant might have been functioning at a normal or even supernormal level.
3. Extrachoroidal sites of CSF production might have assumed a more dominant role after radioablation of the choroid plexus, thus masking any initial reduction in the rate of formation that might have taken place.

As a radioablative agent, [188]Re does appear to have the advantages of high target-to-nontarget ratios and predominant beta emission. The effective half-life in the choroid plexus of about 2 hours may not be long enough for adequate ablation. However, it would be worthwhile to test the effect of [188]Re in an experimental model of hydrocephalus in which the morphology and function of the choroid plexus remain unaltered.

Beta emitting radionuclides have also been used to treat neoplastic lesions of the CNS. Yttrium 90 (^{90}Y) has a half-life of 64 hours and releases monoenergetic beta radiation at 0.93 mev (Fig. 14-5). No gamma rays are emitted by [90]Y. Smith and his coworkers[10] administered intrathecal doses of 1.0 to 8.7 mCi of ^{90}Y-DTPA to nine patients with CNS leukemia or CNS involvement in malignant lymphoma. Ytterbium 169 DTPA, which emits gamma rays of 177 and 198 kev, was administered simultaneously to permit external detection of the chelates. The clinical results were not successful. Three of the five cases that were available for follow-up had a relapse within 6 months. The absorbed doses to the brain and meningeal surfaces were adequate for therapy, but the faster clearance from the spinal subarachnoid space as compared to the intracranial CSF might have been responsible for the therapeutic failures.

D'Angio and his group[11] at the University of Minnesota and at Memorial Hospital developed a therapeutic method involving the intrathecal injection of

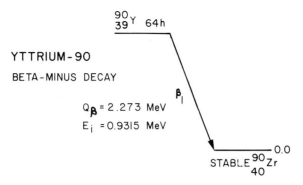

Fig. 14-5. Decay scheme of ^{90}Y. (Reproduced with permission from J. Nucl. Med.)

radiogold (^{198}Au) to treat metastatic seeding of the spinal leptomeninges from medulloblastoma and ependymoblastoma. After surgical excision of the tumor, the total neuraxis was subjected to 3000 to 4000 rads of external beam (^{60}Co) irradiation together with 1000 rads to the posterior fossa. Gold 198 was then given intrathecally at intervals of 6 weeks for an average of two treatments. The dose range was 10 to 15 mCi. Prior to the administration of ^{198}Au, myelography was performed with pantopaque to make sure that residual tumors at the spinal level had been eradicated, and, if not, additional radiotherapy was given. External monitoring was performed for several days after injection to ensure uniform distribution of the radionuclide. In addition, injection was done in a 15° head-down position, and a 90° position was maintained for 1 hour in order to avoid a sacral localization of the radiogold that would produce a "cauda equina" syndrome. The initial results with the use of ^{198}Au as a therapeutic adjunct were promising. Actuarial survival curves showed a 75 percent projected survival of 3 years or more. These data compared favorably with a 25 to 40 percent 5-year survival for patients with medulloblastoma who did not receive this form of treatment. However, intrathecal ^{198}Au has been abandoned by D'Angio's group because they ran into considerable transient morbidity and also encountered a cauda equina syndrome even when the head was tilted and two cases of cerebral ischemia due to fibrotic compression of the carotid arteries when the head-down position was used.

Gold 198 has also been used recently by Metz and his coworkers[12] to prevent spread of acute leukemia to the CNS.[11] Doses of 1 to 2 mCi of ^{198}Au were injected intrathecally, and it was reported that 23 of 26 children remained free of CNS metastases for a 3-month to 3-year period. No significant side effects were noted. However, there was no controlled study of other appropriate therapeutic modalities such as intrathecal methotrexate and/or external irradiation.

SUMMARY

1. Gold 198 (^{198}Au) has suitable beta emission, but its gamma radiation may lead to undesirable side effects.
2. The delivery of colloidal ^{198}Au into the ventricle of a hydrocephalic dog will

lead to improvement in the objective parameters of hydrocephalus, but the ependyma will receive too high a radiation dose.

3. The use of intrathecal colloidal ^{198}Au in medulloblastoma has been abandoned because of side effects, but its application in the prophylaxis of CNS leukemia requires a controlled study.

4. Rhenium 188 (^{188}Re) has a suitable beta and gamma emission.

5. A significant uptake of ^{188}Re occurs in the choroid plexus of the normal cat after ventriculocisternal perfusion, but the effective half-life in the choroid plexus is 2 hours.

6. Administration of ^{188}Re into the ventricle of a hydrocephalic cat (kaolin model) has no effect on ventricular size or CSF formation rate.

7. Further trials of ^{188}Re are warranted in an experimental model of hydro-cephalus which has a normal CSF formation rate.

8. Intrathecal ^{90}Y-DTPA has not been successful in the treatment of CNS leukemia.

REFERENCES

1. Escher, F., Ludi, R.: Hypophysektomie und radiogoldspeckung der hypophyse bei metastasierendem mammakarzinom. Schweiz. Med. Wochenschr. 91:709, 1961; as quoted in Silver, S.: Radioactive isotopes. In: Medicine and Biology Medicine, Ed. 2. Philadelphia, Lea & Febiger, p. 274, 1962.

2. McClure, C. C., Jr., Carothers, E. L., Hahn, P. F.: Distribution and pathology resulting from the intracerebral and intraventricular injection of radioactive gold and silver coated radiogold colloids. Am. J. Roentgenol. 73:81–87, 1955.

3. Rish, B. L., Meacham, W. F.: Experimental study of the intraventricular instillation of radioactive gold. J. Neurosurg. 27:15–20, 1967.

4. Weiss, M. H., Nulsen, F. E., Kaufman, B.: Selective radionecrosis of the choroid plexus for control of experimental hydrocephalus. J. Neurosurg. 36:270–275, 1972.

5. Bernstein, G. A., Fingerhut, A. G., Becker, D.: Pertechnetate in the treatment of hydrocephalus. J.Nucl. Med. 10:322, 1969 (Abst.).

6. Bardfeld, P. A., Shulman, K.: Transport and distribution of rhenium-188 in the central nervous system. Exp. Neurol. 50:1–13, 1976.

7. Pappenheimer, J. R., Heisey, S. R., Jordan, E. F., et al.: Perfusion of the cerebral ventricular system in unanesthetized goats. Am. J. Physiol. 203:763–774, 1962.

8. Bardfeld, P. A., Shulman, K.: Rhenium-188 therapy of experimental hydrocephalus. Exp. Neurol. 50:777–785, 1976.

9. Hochwald, G. M., Sahar, A., Sadik, A. R., et al.: Cerebrospinal fluid production and histological observation in animals with experimental obstructive hydrocephalus. Exp. Neurol. 25:190–199, 1969.

10. Smith, P. H. S., Thomas, P. R. M., Steere, H. A., et al.: Therapeutic irradiation of the central nervous system using intrathecal ^{90}Y-DTPA. Br. J. Radiol. 48:141–147, 1976.

11. Fuller, L. G. A., Rogoff, E., Deck, M., et al.: Recent experience with intrathecal radiogold for medulloblastoma and ependymoblastoma. A progress report. Am. J. Roentgenol. 122:75–79, 1974.

12. Metz, O., Stoll, W., Plevert, W.: Meningosis prophylaxe mit radiogold (^{198}Au) bei der leukamie im kindesalter. Dtsch. Med. Wochenschr. 102:43–46, 1977.

SECTION IV

Systemic Therapy

William D. Bloomer and S. James Adelstein

15

5-(^{125}I)-Iododeoxyuridine in Experimental Tumor Therapy

INTRODUCTION

Although the role of sealed radioactive sources in the treatment of cancer is well established, that of unsealed radionuclides has remained largely unrealized. Developing a strategy for treating cancer with unsealed radionuclide has many physical and biological constraints. In the first place, the radiopharmaceutical must be incorporated by tumor cells in high enough concentration to be toxic but without causing irreparable damage to normal tissues. Secondly, the radionuclide must deposit its energy within the tumor cell or preferably the sensitive targets of the tumor cell rather than the surrounding normal cells. In many ways, these requisites are met by the thymidine analogue 5-(^{125}I)-iododeoxyuridine (^{125}IUdR) in which the 5-methyl group of thymidine is replaced by ^{125}I. This substitution produces a compound which behaves remarkably like thymidine because both CH_3 and I have similar van der Waals' radii (Fig. 15-1).

A ^{125}I atom initiates its decay by capturing an inner shell electron resulting in a ^{125}Te nucleus with 35.5-kev excess energy. In 7 percent of disintegrations, a 35.5-kev photon is emitted; in the remaining 93 percent, an inner shell electron is ejected by internal conversion. These electron vacancies are filled by rearrangements of outer shell electrons, the resultant energy being released as characteristic radiation of ^{125}Te or as cascades of low-energy Auger electrons. Although the charge transfer associated with this electron release leaves ^{125}Te with a transient mean net charge of +9 in the gaseous state,[1] its importance in the condensed state is less clear.[2] Table 15-1 compares the yield of low-energy electrons from the decay of ^{125}I and ^{131}I. The decay of ^{131}I is by beta-minus emission and has a low yield of Auger and conversion electrons.

The local energy released from ^{125}I decay has a subcellular deposition and high specific ionization.[3] When ^{125}I is incorporated into DNA as ^{125}IUdR, marked

This work was supported by grants CA-12662 and CA-15523 from the National Cancer Institute and E(11/1)-4115 from the Department of Energy.

177

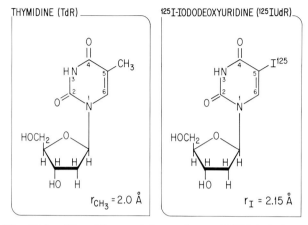

THYMIDINE (TdR) ^{125}I-IODODEOXYURIDINE (^{125}IUdR)

r_{CH_3} = 2.0 Å r_I = 2.15 Å

Fig. 15-1. Thymidine and its analogue 5-(^{125}I)-iododeoxy-uridine.

radiotoxicity has been observed in a number of systems using various endpoints: lethality, mutations, and DNA strand breaks in bacteria and phage,[4-6] diminished survival of prelabeled tumor cells assayed in vivo,[7] and lethality and chromosomal aberrations in cultured mammalian cells.[8-11] The intranuclear location of ^{125}I appears to be of paramount importance: ^{125}I is much less toxic if located extracellularly or bound to cell membranes as concanavalin-A.[12]

All these studies suggested that ^{125}IUdR might be efficacious in the treatment of certain tumors. The use of an ascites tumor model seemed promising because ^{125}IUdR could be incorporated directly from the peritoneal fluid before entering the general circulation where it is rapidly dehalogenated.[13] A pilot study using therapeutic doses of ^{125}IUdR in an experimental ascites tumor system indicated that the agent augmented median and absolute survival of treated animals.[14] Further studies in this same model identified the critical factors affecting treatment of 1-day ascites tumor cells.[15,16]

Table 15-1
Auger and Conversion Electrons for Iodine Isotopes

	Energy (kev)	No./Decay	Range (μm)
Iodine 125	30–35	0.2	18–20
	23–27	0.2	11–13
	2.9–3.7	2.2	0.3–0.4
	0.8	3.6	0.05
Iodine 131	46	0.03	28
	3.2	0.05	0.3
	0.9	0.12	0.06

TUMOR MODEL

A spontaneously arising ovarian carcinoma[17] has been maintained by serial intraperitoneal (ip) transplantation and used in its ascitic form in female C3HeB/FeJ mice (Jackson Laboratory). Median and absolute survival were determined after ip challenge of various tumor cell inocula (Fig. 15-2). Median survival was linearly related to the tumor cell inoculum between 10^3 and 10^7 cells. A sharp rise in median survival was observed with less than 10^3 cells and suggested that host defenses might be operating against these relatively small numbers of cells. Although tumor-associated antigens have been identified in this system,[18] rechallenge of tumor bearing mice successfully treated with ^{125}IUdR failed to show any modification of median survival. Even though it paralleled median survival, absolute survival was a less sensitive parameter because of the small number of long-term survivors.

The relatively long median survival of tumor bearing mice permits estimation of the degree of cell killing after treatment with ^{125}IUdR. If the median survival of animals given 10^7 tumor cells is 19 days but treatment prolongs it to 21 days, the animals died as though they had been injected with 10^6 cells, resulting in a one log killing of tumor cells (10^{-1} survival fraction). Similarly, if treatment prolongs median survival to 25 days, the animals died as though they had been injected with 10^4 cells, resulting in a three log killing of tumor cells (10^{-3} survival fraction).

Because ^{125}IUdR is a cycle active agent incorporated into DNA only during synthesis, it is important in planning treatment to know the parameters of the cell

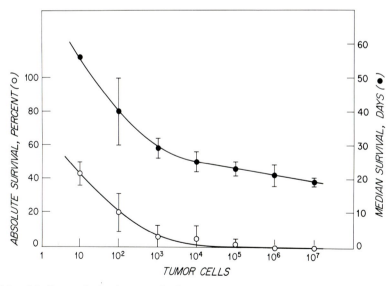

Fig. 15-2. Median and absolute survival ± standard deviation of untreated mice after ip injection of varying tumor cell inocula. The median survival after injection of 10 cells represents the pooling of data from 14 experiments in 6 of which fewer than half the animals died when followed for 150 days.

cycle. These were determined for 1-day ascites tumor cells by the percent labeled mitoses method. A single injection of ³H-thymidine was given 24 hours after tumor cell inoculation. Mice were then sacrificed at regular intervals and tumor cells prepared for autoradiography. Analysis of the percent labeled mitoses as a function of time after ³H-thymidine injection yielded a cell cycle time of 14.3 hours, DNA synthetic time of 5.8 hours, G_1 6.3 hours, G_2 1.7 hours, and mitosis 0.5 hours.[15] The growth fractiom can be estimated by analyzing the fraction of labeled cells after repeated injections of ³H-thymidine (labeling index.) For 1-day ascites cells, the growth fraction is > 0.95. In studies of other 1-day ascites tumors, the growth fraction also approaches unity, i.e., all cells are actively cycling and synthesizing DNA.[19–21]

¹²⁵IUdR and ¹³¹IUdR THERAPY

Carrier-free ¹²⁵IUdR or ¹³¹IUdR (New England Nuclear) was used. Doses of either agent were administered ip starting 24 hours after tumor cell inoculation. Because IUdR is rapidly dehalogenated in vivo, animal drinking water contained 0.1 percent potassium iodide to block thyroid uptake of released radionuclide. Although no gross acute or chronic toxicity was observed, studies were not undertaken to determine subtle toxicity to the bone marrow or gut. However, all animals that died had developed malignant ascites.

All 1-day ascites tumor cells can theoretically be labeled by choosing appropriate schema. One would expect to achieve optimal cell killing by lengthening the overall treatment to include several generation times, and in the absence of continuous infusion, by choosing an interval between treatments that is less than the DNA synthetic time. Fractionation schema whose interval between treatments exceeds the DNA synthetic time will not maximally label tumor cells. With a DNA

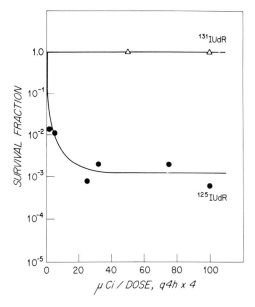

Fig. 15-3. Dose-response curve for ¹²⁵IUdR and ¹³¹IUdR therapy. Animals were treated every 4 hours for four doses starting 24 hours after the ip injection of 10⁵ tumor cells.

synthetic time of 6 hours, data from experiments using 4- and 12-hour intervals between dose fractions support this by showing no therapeutic efficacy for [125]IUdR administered at 12-hour intervals.[16]

In Figure 15-3, mice were treated with four doses of either [125]IUdR or [131]IUdR at 4-hour intervals and the survival fraction plotted as a function of the dose per treatment. [131]IUdR has no therapeutic efficacy in the range of doses examined. Treatment with [125]IUdR using the same regimen results in a rapid decrease in survival fraction to 10^{-3} at doses of 25 μCi per treatment with the curve being flat at higher doses.

Optimal conditions for [125]IUdR treatment were investigated by varying the number of treatments and the dose per treatment.[15] The use of four to seven sequential treatments at 4-hour intervals effectively lengthens the overall treatment time from one to two generation times. Although seven treatments are clearly more efficacious than four, the incremental reduction in survival fraction decreases with each additional treatment because fewer tumor cells remain viable to incorporate [125]IUdR. In Figure 15-4, mice were treated with seven doses of [125]IUdR at 4-hour intervals after the injection of 10^{6} tumor cells and the survival fraction plotted as a function of the dose per treatment. The survival fraction decreases rapidly to 10^{-5} at doses of 15 μCi per treatment and is flat at higher doses. Considering that the challenge was 10^{6} tumor cells, a survival fraction of 10^{-5} suggests that there exists a very small number of cells that are not cycling or have a very long generation time. Although one might have killed these few remaining tumor cells by increasing the number of treatments or by using continuous infusion, this might well have been done at the expense of causing serious bone marrow or gut toxicity.

Other studies showed that Na[125]I, Na[131]I, and nonradioactive IUdR had no antineoplastic activity when administered by similar treatment schema and in

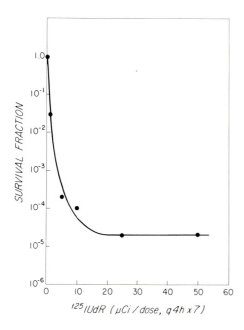

Fig. 15-4. Dose-response curve for [125]IUdR therapy of 1-day ascites tumor cells. Treatment was started 24 hours after the ip injection of 10^{6} tumor cells. Seven doses were given at 4-hour intervals. (Reproduced with permission from Nature 265:620–621, 1977.)

doses comparable to ^{125}IUdR.[14,16] Failure to observe x-ray sensitization in tissue culture at concentrations of IUdR that are toxic when applied as ^{125}IUdR supports the hypothesis that the antineoplastic activity of ^{125}IUdR is primarily due to the radiotoxicity of ^{125}I incorporated into DNA.[10] Nevertheless, in pharmacologic doses, nonradioactive IUdR is toxic in this experimental tumor model; however, the D_{37} values for IUdR and ^{125}IUdR differ by a factor of 10^5 when expressed on a weight basis.

CONCLUSION

^{125}IUdR has marked antineoplastic activity in this early ascites tumor model which is a propitious system in which to test the therapeutic efficacy of cell cycle active agents. In this model, a favorable therapeutic ratio is created by ip administration because the drug has direct access to tumor cells in the peritoneal cavity before entering the circulation. Rapid dehalogenation in the general circulation protects the normal cell renewal systems. The role for ^{125}IUdR in the treatment of solid tumors is problematic because drug access is less direct and the growth fraction less than unity. Nevertheless, the therapeutic potential of ^{125}I and other radionuclides whose decay results in a highly localized deposition of energy presents a challenge to design radiopharmaceuticals with high nuclear affinity.

REFERENCES

1. Carlson, T. A., White, R. M.: Formation of fragment ions from CH_3Te^{125} and $C_2H_5Te^{125}$ following the nuclear decays of CH_3I^{125} and $C_2H_5I^{125}$. J. Chem. Phys. 38:2930–2934, 1963.

2. Keough, G., Hofer, K. G.: Molecular consequences of the Auger effect: the fate of iododeoxyuridine following iodine-125 decay. Radiat. Res. 67:224–234, 1976.

3. Ertl, H. H., Feinendegen, L. E., Heiniger, H. J.: Iodine-125, a tracer in cell biology: physical properties and biological aspects. Phys. Med. Biol. 15:447–456, 1970.

4. Krisch, R. E.: Lethal effects of iodine-125 decay by electron capture in Escherichia coli and in bacteriophage T$_1$. Int. J. Radiat. Biol. 21:167–189, 1972.

5. Schmidt, A., Hotz, G.: The occurrence of double-strand breaks in coliphage T1-DNA by iodine-125 decay. Int. J. Radiat. Biol. 24:307–313, 1973.

6. Krisch, R. E., Ley, R. D.: Induction of lethality and DNA breakage by the decay of iodine-125 in bacteriophage T4. Int. J. Radiat. Biol. 25:21–30, 1974.

7. Hofer, K. G., Hughes, W. L.: Radiotoxicity of intranuclear tritium, ^{125}iodine and ^{131}iodine. Radiat. Res. 47:94–109, 1971.

8. Burki, H. J., Roots, R., Feinendegen, L. E., and Bond, V. P.: Inactivation of mammalian cells after disintegrations of ^{3}H or ^{125}I in cell DNA at −196°C. Int. J. Radiat. Biol. 24:363–375, 1973.

9. Burki, H. J.: Mammalian cells: damage in late replicating DNA as the most efficient cause of reproductive death. Exp. Cell Res. 87:277–280, 1974.

10. Bradley, E. W., Chan, P. C., and Adelstein, S. J.: The radiotoxicity of iodine-125 in mammalian cells. I. Effects on the survival curve of radioiodine incorporated into DNA. Radiat. Res. 64:555–563, 1975.

11. Chan, P. C., Lisco, E., Lisco, H., et al.: The radiotoxicity of iodine-125 in mammalian

cells. II. A comparative study on cell survival and cytogenetic responses to [125]IUdR, [131]IUdR, and [3]HTdR. Radiat. Res. 67:332–343, 1976.

12. Warters, R. L., Hofer, K. G.: Radionuclide toxicity in cultured mammalian cells. Elucidation of the primary site for radiation-induced division delay. Radiat. Res. 69:348–358, 1977.

13. Hughes, W. L., Commerford, S. L., Gitlin, D., et al.: Deoxyribonucleic acid metabolism in vivo: I. Cell proliferation and death as measured by incorporation and elimination of iododeoxyuridine. Fed. Proc. 23:640–648, 1964.

14. Bloomer, W. D., Adelstein, S. J.: Antineoplastic effect of iodine-125 labeled iododeoxyuridine. Int. J. Radiat. Biol. 27:509–511, 1975.

15. Bloomer, W. D., Adelstein, S. J.: 5-^{125}I-iododeoxyuridine as prototype for radionuclide therapy with Auger emitters. Nature 265:620–621, 1977.

16. Bloomer, W. D., Adelstein, S. J.: Therapeutic application of iodine-125 labeled iododeoxyuridine in an early ascites tumor model. Curr. Top. Radiat. Res. Q. 12:513–525, 1977.

17. Fekete, E., Ferringno, M. A.: Studies on a transplantable teratoma of the mouse. Cancer Res. 12:438–440, 1952.

18. Order, S. E., Donahue, V., Knapp, R.: Immunotherapy of ovarian cancer. An experimental model. Cancer 32:573–579, 1973.

19. Lala, P. K., Patt, H. M.: Cytokinetic analysis of tumor growth. Proc. Natl. Acad. Sci. U.S.A. 56:1735–1742, 1966.

20. Frindel, E., Valleron, A. J., Vassort, F., et al.: Proliferation kinetics of an experimental ascites tumour of the mouse. Cell Tissue Kinet. 2:51–65, 1969.

21. Tannock, I. F.: A comparison of cell proliferation parameters in solid and ascites Ehrlich tumors. Cancer Res. 29:1527–1534, 1969.

Klaus Mayer, K. S. Pentlow, R. C. Marcove, H. Q.
Woodard, A. G. Huvos, B. Chin, and J. S. Laughlin

16

Sulfur-35 Therapy for Chondrosarcoma and Chordoma

Gottschalk and Allen[1,2] demonstrated in 1952 that sulfur when injected intravenously as $Na_2{}^{35}SO_4$ is selectively taken up by chondrosarcoma. We confirmed the uptake in chondrosarcoma tissue and further demonstrated that there is also a preferential uptake of sulfur in chordoma, a polysaccharide-containing tumor.[3] Various attempts have been made to treat chondrosarcoma with this agent, but this approach was generally abandoned because the limited success was not justified by the severity of marrow toxicity.[4,5]

Bostrom[6], using as much as 1.735 Ci of ^{35}S-sulfate in seven doses over 7.5 months, reported control of pulmonary metastases and regression of osseous tumor tissue in one patient, without severe bone marrow depression. Follow-up was limited to 18 months[6].

In recent years, blood component preparation made platelet and granulocyte transfusion available, which permitted the administration of ever larger quantities of cytotoxic agents in other cancer and leukemia chemotherapy. Marrow suppression, even total bone marrow obliteration, with modern chemotherapy is transient, and patients are tided over with appropriate adjuvant transfusion therapy. Because it seemed possible to achieve tumor regression in chondrosarcoma with ^{35}S-sulfate, using larger doses than those employed by previous investigators, a further attempt was made to treat patients at Memorial-Sloan Kettering Cancer Center, where blood components for transfusion were readily available and there was abundant experience in management of the pancytopenic patient. The results are the subject of the present chapter.

MATERIALS AND METHODS

Patients were chosen who had histologically proved diagnoses of chondrosarcoma or chordoma in whom the tumors were actively growing and could not be completely removed surgically because of local extent or distant metastases. No cases were included who had recent treatment with cytotoxic agents or who had evidence of significant bone marrow depression from other causes. The majority of the patients had had previous unsuccessful attempts at control of their tumors by surgical resection, and some had had external irradiation. Written informed consent for the use of an experimental drug was obtained in all cases.

A test dose of about 0.2 mCi ^{35}S-sodium sulfate per kilogram of body weight was given intravenously and the concentration in blood and urine was followed for about a week. During this time an open biopsy of the tumor and one or more marrow aspirations were performed in order to obtain tissue samples for determination of ^{35}S uptake. Specimens of other tissues were also obtained for comparison with the tumor. If the selective uptake in terms of microcuries per gram of tumor tissue found per microcurie administered per gram of body weight (relative concentration, R.C.) was satisfactory, the patient was given a therapeutic dose of 5 mCi/kg. This was later increased to 6 mCi/kg. The treatment was repeated at intervals determined by the clinical and hematological response.

Laboratory

The ^{35}S was obtained from the Radiochemical Centre in Amersham, England. It was in the form of a sterile and pryogen-free solution of sodium sulfate in physiological saline, with a specific activity of at least 600 mCi/mg.

Two methods were used for the determination of radioactivity in biological material. When the activity was high, as in specimens of urine or tumor obtained shortly after therapeutic doses of ^{35}S, the specimens were placed in plastic vials and the Bremsstrahlen measured in a well-type scintillation counter. The counter was calibrated against a ^{35}S standard containing about 100 μCi. As the efficiency of this method is only about 10^{-4}, it could not be used when the activity was low, but was useful for preliminary screening. In the majority of cases, the tissue specimens were dissolved by incubation for 12 to 72 hours at 45°C in the solubilizer NCS (Amersham-Searle). When necessary, the solutions were decolorized with hydrogen peroxide followed by further incubation. Activity was then measured in a liquid scintillation counter. Quenching was determined by adding a known amount of standard ^{35}S solution to each sample and recounting it. The limit of detection by this method was about 10^{-4} μCi.

RESULTS

Biochemical Results

In harmony with previous investigators we found that from 70 to 90 percent of a dose of ^{35}S was excreted in the urine during the first 3 days after injection, that the initial uptakes in both tumor and bone marrow were high and approximately equal, and that the radionuclide was lost rapidly from marrow but was retained by tumor. At 1 day after injection the concentrations of ^{35}S in tumor and bone marrow were nearly equal and were about 5 times the concentrations in the body as a whole as indicated by excretion studies.

We obtained curves for the concentration of ^{35}S in whole blood for 1 to 2 weeks after most treatments. These were similar to those found by previous

Table 16-1

Sulfur 35 Activities in Specimens of Blood and Tissue

Tissue	No. Specimens	Time Summed (days)	Relative Concentration*		Cumulative Dose† (rads)
			Day 2	Final	
Whole blood	70	8	0.29	0.018	2.2
	97	16	0.29	0.011	2.4
Normal red marrow	6	70	1.4	0.018	33
Chondrosarcoma	18	70	1.2	0.33	129
	22	190	1.2	0.20	155
Chordoma	13	70	1.4	0.064	49
Normal cartilage		70	0.4	0.8	74
	8	190	0.4	0.4	135
Skin and subcutaneous tissue	14	70	0.20	0.021	10.5
Fibrous tissue	10	70	0.30	0.034	14.9
Muscle	12	70	0.10	0.027	6.8

(Reproduced with permission from J. Nucl. Med. 17(4):285, 1976.)

*Relative concentration = (μCi found/g tissue)/(μCi injected/g body weight). Corrected for physical decay.

†Normalized to an administered dose of 1 mCi/kg body weight.

investigators, especially Gottschalk et al.[7] In our series about 95 percent of the initial burden in blood was lost with a biological half-time (T_B) of 0.5 day, and most of the remainder with a T_B of about 6 days. The kinetics of material obtained by marrow aspiration did not differ greatly from those for blood during the first few days, but this appeared to be due to the large amounts of peripheral blood present in the specimens. In the small number of specimens of marrow obtained by biopsy in which there was little admixture of peripheral blood, it was evident that the retention in marrow was much greater than that in blood although considerably less than that in chondrosarcoma tissue.

Mean values for ^{35}S concentrations and integrated radiation doses are shown in Table 16-1. The radiation doses were computed by integration under the curves obtained by plotting against time the observed activities not corrected for physical decay, as described in ref. 3.

The initial uptake of ^{35}S in chordoma tissue was in the same range as that in chondrosarcoma. Long-term retention of ^{35}S in chordoma was considerably less than in chondrosarcoma.

In one case of chondrosarcoma in which the tumor was superficial, it was possible to localize it by external counting of Bremsstrahlen. Serial point counts showed that the ratio of activity over different parts of the tumor to that over symmetrical normal areas increased from 2.1 and 1.1 at 1 day post-injection to 3.0 and 2.3 at 32 days. This is additional evidence that ^{35}S is retained by tumor tissue for a substantial period of time.

Clinical Results

Table 16-2 depicts the six patients with chondrosarcoma who received therapeutic doses.

W. M. had shown progression of his disease. The course may have been slowed. Within 2 years he developed marrow hyperplasia which was terminally followed by a marrow resembling erythroleukemia. He had severe pancytopenia and major chromosome abnormalities consistent with radiation effect. At postmortem examination viable tumor was found.

C. K. had a striking regression of a fist-sized mass extending from the sacrum. The mass was biopsied and was found to consist of chondrosarcoma. Following ^{35}S therapy the mass disappeared entirely only to recur 4 months later. Subsequent therapy again caused regression of the tumor. At time of death the patient was pancytopenic, and postmortem examination revealed advanced chondrosarcoma, including pulmonary metastases.

R. T. is a young man with long-standing chondrosarcoma. He has had very slow progression of his disease and is the only one who is still alive at this time. He too has severe pancytopenia.

J. A. and D. O. were boys 12 and 13 whose tumors progressed unabated. In both, the tumors contained malignant osseous elements as well as malignant cartilage. They died within 6 and 3 months after treatment. Both were anemic. J. A. was leukopenic and D. O. was thrombocytopenic.

C. F. died within 4 months of treatment. When first seen she had advanced chondrosarcoma with pulmonary metastases and pleural effusions. No improvement can be claimed for this case. She too had anemia, but leukocytes and platelet counts were within normal limits.

The chordoma patients who received two or more therapeutic doses are tabulated in Table 16-3. Tumor regression could be ascertained objectively only in M. D. All except F. D. had hematologic abnormalities, and R. L. and M. D. had a terminal bone marrow consistent with acute myelocytic leukemia. M. D. also lost her red cell A and B antigens concurrent with the onset of the leukemic picture.

DISCUSSION

In chondrosarcoma, and to a lesser extent in chordoma, ^{35}S is initially concentrated in tumor tissue. In chondrosarcoma it is retained for a very long time. In one case of chondrosarcoma there was repeated clearly defined regression in tumor size with microscopic evidence of tumor necrosis. In the other chondrosarcoma patients there was also objective evidence of tumor regression or apparent decrease in progression of disease. In the chordoma patients the tumor retention of ^{35}S was less. In only one case was there objective regression of tumor mass.

The average tissue doses for an administered dose of 30 mCi/kg body weight are shown below. The method of calculation is given in ref. 3.

Chondrosarcoma	4650 rads
Chordoma	1470 rads
Normal cartilage	4050 rads
Bone marrow	990 rads

Table 16-2
Chondrosarcoma

| Patients | Sex/Age | Cumulative ^{35}S | | Number | | Clinical Time from: | | | | Hematology at Death/March 1977 | | | |
| | | mCi | mCi/kg | Dose | Wks.* | Death | | Alive | | | | | |
						Dx.	Rx.†	Dx.	Rx.	Bone Marrow	Hgb. g%	Wbc ×10³	Plt. ×10³
W.M.	M/51	4126	48.3	8	75	2 yrs.	2 yrs.	—	—	Hypercellular with many primitive cells. Slight differentiation, some clearly of erythroid series. Acute erythroid leukemia. Chromosomal abnormalities.	4.1	0.6	18.0
C.K.	F/56	2140	45.6	8	88	15 yrs.	3 yrs.	—	—	Markedly hypocellular section shows low-grade chondrosarcoma, abundant chondroid matrix.	10.1	1.7	33.0
R.T.	M/26	1550	28.3	5	66	—	—	10 yrs.	6 yrs.	Pancytopenia '75	11.6	2.0	47.0
J.A.	M/13	768	21.6	4	22	1 yr.	6 mo.	—	—	—	7.8	2.8	171
D.O.	M/12	388	10.7	2	5	4 mo.	3 mo.	—	—	—	7.2	18.5	35.0
C.F.	F/72	718	10.0	2	9	1 yr.	4 mo.	—	—	—	7.0	5.7	221

*Time from administration of first therapy dose to administration of last dose.
†Time from administration of first therapy dose.

Table 16-3
Chordoma

Patients	Sex/Age	Cumulative ³⁵S mCi	mCi/kg	Number Dose	Wks.*	Clinical Time from: Death Dx.	Rx.†	Alive Dx.	Rx.	Hematology at Death/March 1977 Bone Marrow	Hgb. g%	WBC × 10³	Plt. × 10³
H.S.	M/66	2823	37.6	7	64	8 yrs.	3 yrs.	—	—	Markedly hypocellular. Aplastic anemia	5.1	1.4	58.0
R.L.	M/63	1942	32.3	6	67	11 yrs.	5.3 yrs.	—	—	Hypocellular, ↓ myeloid series, ↑ in erythroid precursors. Terminal acute leukemia.	11.2	3.8	78.0
M.D.	F/75	1519	21.5	4	40	3.3 yrs.	3 yrs.	—	—	Myelomonocytic leukemia, ABO type change.	9.1	16.9	12.0
F. McE.	M/51	1106	13.2	3	44	6.5 yrs.	4.5 yrs.	—	—	Dysplastic erythroid hyperplasia.	8.0 10.0	4.0 2.2	6.0 22.0
P.P.	M/56	994	12.3	3	28	6.5 yrs.	1.3 yrs.	—	—	Sepsis, persistent thrombocytopenia; ↑ erythroid hyperplasia.	5.6	9.6	8.0
S.E.	M/71	824	12.4	2	15	3 yrs.	2.7 yrs.	—	—	—	10.6	5.0	13.4
F.D.	M/50	718	10.1	2	9	1 yr.	7 mo.	—	—	—	10.2	8.2	308

*Time from administration of first therapy dose to administration of last dose.
†Time from administration of first therapy dose.

From these calculations the effect on chondrosarcoma and lesser effect on chordoma are understandable. The radiation dose to hematopoietic marrow was also high. Bone marrow toxicity was found in all patients who received repeated therapy. The effect differed clinically from that due to cytotoxicity from chemotherapeutic agents. With the latter, the effect is more profound initially but also more transient and is usually accompanied by good marrow recovery within days or weeks. In most patients ^{35}S caused minimal effect with the first treatment but increased with each succeeding administration of the radionuclide, and there was further progression of thrombocytopenia, leukopenia, and lastly anemia. Not only was the prompt depression more profound after each dose, but subsequent recovery was less complete. In most cases the platelet counts remained above levels where bleeding is a major problem. The same is true for the leukopenia. With repeated treatments and dose accumulation, there was, however, no real recovery of the marrow. All patients developed a hypoplastic marrow, especially with respect to decrease in megakaryocytes or myelocytes. Three subjects, one with chondrosarcoma and two with chordoma, had increase in blasts in the marrow and terminally developed a picture consistent with leukemia. Two of these had several chromosome changes. Red cell morphology became abnormal in all. One of these patients concurrently lost A and B antigens on the red cells.

All chondrosarcoma patients are dead, except one. One showed unequivocal improvement. The others may have progressed more slowly, but the aplastic anemia was sufficiently devastating to limit further trials with this therapy only in the most advanced cases.

CONCLUSION

^{35}S-sulfate concentrates and is sufficiently retained in chondrosarcoma tissue to be an effective therapeutic agent. Long-range marrow toxicity is, however, of such severity to contraindicate its use. Unless a mechanism is found to protect the marrow during the first days after administration, this form of therapy must be used with great caution. The limited therapeutic results in chordoma are even more discouraging, and marrow toxicity does not justify its use except in the worst prognostic situation.

As a result of this therapy ^{35}S could be given in lower doses (Nilsonne), and as mentioned additional external radiation therapy can be added later if the patients' chondrosarcoma has progressed to the extremely advanced phase where one would accept the 25 percent leukemia complication.

REFERENCES

1. Gottschalk, R. G., Allen, C. H.: Uptake of radioactive sulfur by chondrosarcoma in man. Proc. Soc. Exp. Biol. Med. 80:334–339, 1952.
2. Gottschalk, R. G., Smith, R. T.: Chondrosarcoma of the hand. Report of a case with radioactive sulfur studies and review of literature. J. Bone Joint Surg. 45A:141–150, 1963.

3. Woodard, H. Q., Pentlow, K. S., Mayer, K., et al.: Distribution and retention of ^{35}S-sodium sulfate in man. J. Nucl. Med. 17:285–289, 1976.

4. Andrews, J. R., Swarm, R. L., Schlachter, L., et al.: The effects of one curie of sulfur 35 administered intravenously as sulfate to a man with advanced chondrosarcoma. Am. J. Roentgenol. Rad. Ther. Nucl. Med. 83:123–134, 1960.

5. Botstein, C., Marcus, N.: A case of recurrent chondrosarcoma of the maxilla treated unsuccessfully with sulfur 35. Am. J. Roentgenol. Rad. Ther. Nucl. Med. 94:798–806, 1965.

6. Bostrom, H., Edgren, B., Friberg, D., et al.: Case of chondrosarcoma with pulmonary and skeletal metastases after hemipelvectomy successfully treated with S-35 Sulfate. Acta Orthop. Scand. 39:549–564, 1968.

7. Gottschalk, R. G., Miller, P. O., Grantham, H. H., Jr.: Analysis of the disappearance of S^{35} from the blood of men, rats and mice. Radiat. Res. 25:295–308, 1965.

Rashid A. Fawwaz

17

Systematically Administered Compounds for Lymphatic Ablation

INTRODUCTION

Lymphatic tissue plays an important role in mediating the immune process responsible for homograft rejection.[1] Because of the marked vulnerability of the lymphocytes to irradiation,[2] internally administered radioisotopes have been used for the selective destruction of lymphoid tissue for control of homograft rejection.[3-7] Although this chapter is devoted primarily to a discussion of abrogation of homograft rejection utilizing internally administered radioporphyrins, other modalities for control of homograft rejection will be discussed briefly.

CURRENT RESEARCH ON HOMOGRAFT SURVIVAL IN OTHER INSTITUTIONS

Histocompatibility Typing

In recent years the prolongation of homograft survival has been due in large part to histocompatibility typing.[8] Improvements in tissue typing and computerized data centers will promote the future usefulness of this method. However, its widespread use is limited by the frequency of simultaneous donor/recipient compatibility. The problem of a recipient without a matched donor will remain.

Abolition or Modulation of Antigenic Expression in the Homograft Prior to Homotransplantation

Pretreatment of homografts with various agents such as tissue culture medium[9] or mucopolysaccharides[10] or concanavalin A[11] has been reported to result in loss

---

This work was supported in part under AEC Contract No. W-7405-ENG-48.

or modulation of antigenic expression. The clinical usefulness of these and similar methods for attenuation of cell surface antigenic determinants remains to be proven.

Induction of Immunologic Tolerance

In animals with a functioning mature lymphoid system, immunologic tolerance can be achieved in principle by either of two methods: First, immunologically competent lymphocytes capable of reacting to graft antigens may be destroyed while sparing immunologically immature and uncommitted lymphocytes. Upon maturation in the presence of the graft, the latter cells tolerate the graft in much the same manner of prenatally induced tolerance.[12] More recent evidence indicates that prenatal tolerance may be due to an immature reticuloendothelial cell system.[13] Antigens that are not processed by the reticuloendothelial cells are thought to act as tolerogens rather than immunogens. Thus according to this concept the induction of tolerance in the adult requires the destruction of mature competent lymphocytes and temporary inactivation of the reticuloendothelial cell system. Second, induction of specific immunologic tolerance in the adult experimental animal has followed administration of either repeated low doses or a single large dose of antigens.[14,15]

In the latter case, success has been limited predominantly to non-cell-mediated immunity even though the method should be applicable to cell-mediated immune reactions. In the former case, destruction of immunologically competent lymphocytes without concomitant destruction of immature uncommitted lymphocytes is not possible with presently available techniques. Methods for destruction of immunologically committed mature lymphocytes while simultaneously inactivating reticuloendothelial cell function have not been described.

Induction of Adaptation

Short-term disruption of immune reactivity using such immunosuppressive agents as azathioprine (Imuran®), antilymphocytic serum, extracorporeal blood or lymph irradiation may allow for the functional establishment of the homograft. By an as yet unknown adaptive process in the homograft, resistance to rejection may be observed despite the restoration of the body's immunologic reactivity. In experimental animals homograft adaptation has been documented in skin homografts[16] and after transplantation of tissues to privileged sites.[17] The degree of immunosuppression produced by presently available agents may not be sufficiently complete to allow for the establishment of an adaptive process in humans.

Total Destruction of Lymphoid and Hematopoietic Tissue Followed by Life-Saving Bone Marrow Transplants with Subsequent Organ Transplants from the Same Donor

Supralethal doses of x-irradiation administrated externally[18] or internally by the systemic injection of radioisotopes[6] can abrogate immunologic reactivity. Survival of irradiated animals depends on restoration of hematopoietic and immunologic function by bone marrow homografts. Since immunologic reconstitution is accomplished with donor lymphoid cells, other organ homografts from the bone marrow donor should be tolerated. Unfortunately, bone marrow homotransplants produce a "graft-versus-host" reaction which is often lethal to primates and man.[19] Improvements in elimination of competent lymphocytes from the bone marrow prior to homografting, and of therapeutic control of "graft-versus-host" reaction, may result in success of this method for homografting.[20,21] In man the radiation dose needed to abolish homograft rejection is relatively high and invariably causes irreversible damage to the gastrointestinal system.[22] This severely limits the clinical usefulness of the method.

THE USE OF SYSTEMATICALLY ADMINISTERED RADIONUCLIDES FOR CONTROL OF HOMOGRAFT REJECTION

Several methods for achieving long-term homograft survival utilizing systemically administered radionuclides have been advised. These are based on selective destruction of lymph nodes following administration of large doses of radioactive compounds which localize preferentially in reticuloendothelial cells. The intralymphatic route has been used for the administration of colloidal ^{32}P-chromic phosphate,[3] ^{198}Au-gold,[3] and aggregated protein particles labeled with ^{206}Bismuth or ^{111m}Ag-silver.[4] The intravenous route has been used for the administration of ^{131}I-iodo-labeled antigens.[5] Although these methods caused severe damage to lymphoid tissue with lymphopenia, homograft survival was not significantly prolonged.

Our interest in the use of radionuclides for control of homograft rejection stemmed from our investigation of radioactive metalloporphyrins as tumor scanning agents.[23] We noted in dogs and one human that the concentration of radioac-

Table 17-1

Fraction of Administered Radioactivity $\times$ 10^{-6} per Gram of Weight

Tissue	Average for 7 Dogs	Human
Muscle	9.2	1
Pancreas	21.4	—
Lung	54.7	—
Duodenal mucosa	73.5	—
Spleen	140	—
Kidney	987	—
Liver	908	—
Femoral marrow	163	11
Mesenteric lymph node	1230	62
Adrenal	290	—
Brain	4.5	—
Bone	6.5	—
Fat	16	2

(Reprinted with permission of J. Nucl. Med.)

Table 17-2

Fraction of Administered Radioactivity $\times$ 10^{-6} per Gram Weight

Tissue	5 mg ^{109}Pd-Protoporphyrin (Average of 3 Dogs)	120 mg ^{109}Pd-Protoporphyrin (Average of 3 Dogs)
Muscle	11	11
Liver	1900	1600
Kidney	514	600
Duodenal mucosa	75	100
Femoral marrow	420	380
Spleen	660	480
Popliteal lymph node	310	1300
Mesenteric lymph node	340	2340

(Reprinted with permission of J. Nucl. Med.)

tivity (from intravenously administered ^{58}Co-cobalt hematoporphyrin complexes) in lymph nodes was significantly higher than in bone marrow, intestinal mucosa, thymus, and other tissues (Table 17-1). Many of the cells contained in lymph nodes appear to be mature and committed in terms of their ability to react to foreign antigens.[24] Thus it was apparent that appropriately labeled radioactive metalloporphyrins might be used for selective lymphatic irradiation of immunologically committed peripheral lymphoid tissue. Subsequent regeneration of peripheral lymphoid tissue was expected to occur from lymphocytes present in the central lymphoid tissue (bone marrow and thymus),[25] which would be unaffected by the irradiation. We postulated that central lymphoid tissue would contain predominantly immature immunoincompetent lymphocytes able to tolerate homotransplants performed soon after irradiation.[26,27] We argued that subsequent maturation of lymphocytes in the presence of the homograft would result in im-

Table 17-3

Fraction of Administered ^{109}Pd-Hematoporphyrin $\times$ 10^{-6} per Gram Weight*

Tissue	Average of 3 Dogs	Ratio of Average Concentration in Tissue to Average Concentration in Muscle
Muscle	17.3	1
Liver	2300	135
Kidney	723	42.5
Duodenal mucosa	146	8.6
Femoral marrow	530	31.2
Spleen	593	35
Popliteal lymph node	1200	70.5
Mesenteric lymph node	2400	141

(Reprinted with permission of J. Nucl. Med.)
*5 mg of ^{109}Pd-hematoporphyrin mixed with 100 mg hematoporphyrin.

Table 17-4
Fraction of Administered Radioactivity $\times 10^{-6}$
per Gram Weight*

Tissue	Dog No. 1	Dog No. 2
Muscle	16	12
Liver	2100	2400
Right popliteal lymph node	1200	940
Left popliteal lymph node	1480	940
Mesenteric lymph node	550	3200

*Nine days after subcutaneous injection of homologous skin into
right lower hind leg.

munologic tolerance. We also argued that the high radiation dose delivered to the reticuloendothelial cells of the lymph node would interfere with their ability to process antigens normally. This would cause antigens to act as tolerogens.

A search for a suitable radioactive metal (short half-life, predominantly beta emitter, available in abundance, and strongly chelated by porphyrins) was initiated; [109]Pd-protoporphyrin complex was found to satisfy these requirements (Tables 17-2 and 17-3).[28]

It was of practical interest to determine whether an antigenically stimulated lymphocyte had a greater affinity for metalloporphyrin than a nonstimulated lymphocyte. Were this true, then best results might be obtained by administering the radioactive metalloporphyrin after sensitization with homograft. This would permit efficient elimination of lymphocytes specifically reactive to the antigens of the homograft. Our investigation showed that localization of radioactive metalloporphyrins in regional lymph nodes draining the site of antigen introduction was not dependent on the presence of antigenically stimulated lymphocytes (Table 17-4).

Because of the crucial role played by the paracortical area of the lymph node in mediating homograft rejection,[27] it was important to determine, within the lymph node, the exact anatomical site of localization of radioactive metalloporphyrin. It was felt that the radiation damage produced by the beta particle from [109]Pd (average tissue stopping power of 1 mm)[20] would be restricted to specific anatomical sites in the lymph nodes; i.e., those areas with the highest affinity for [109]Pd-protoporphyrin. Autoradiographic studies of the lymph nodes revealed that the radioactive metalloporphyrin concentrated in the reticuloendothelial cells of the sinusoids. The latter were most abundant in the medulla, less so in the paracortex, and least abundant in the cortex (Figure 17-1).

Thus it was apparent that lymphocytes present in the medulla and paracortex of the lymph node would be critically affected following the administration of large doses of radioactive metalloporphyrins. This was proven by the administration of 5 mCi/kg of [109]Pd-protoporphyrin to a dog; there was marked lymphocyte depletion in the medulla and paracortical area of the lymph node on histologic examination (Fig. 17-2). Except for the spleen, which showed lymphocyte depletion in the periarteriolar region, histologic examination showed that the other organs were not affected.

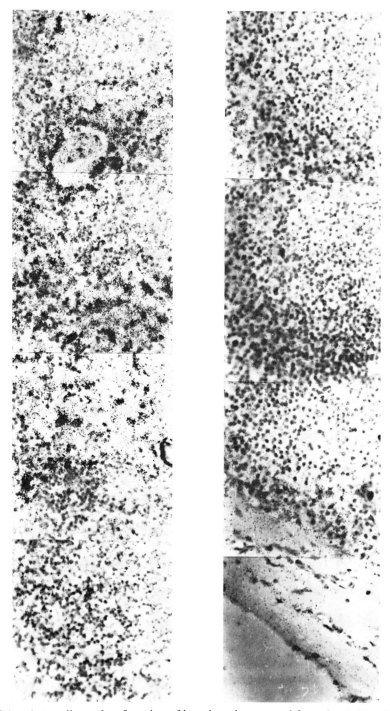

Fig. 17-1. Autoradiographs of section of lymph node removed from dog 1 day after intervenous administration of 500 μCi of ^{63}Ni-protoporphyrin. Figure sequentially shows regions of lymph node starting from capsule in the left uppermost panel to hilar medulla in the right lowermost panel. (Reproduced with permission from J. Nucl. Med.)

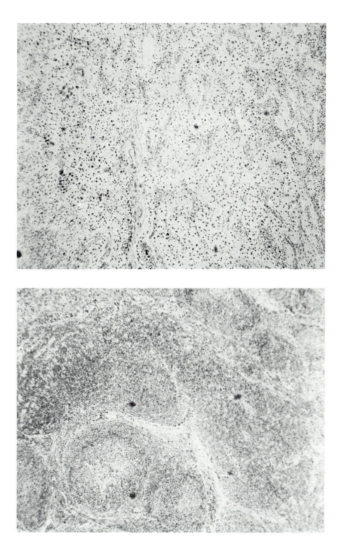

Fig. 17-2. Histologic section of mesenteric lymph node removed 1 day after administration of high-activity [109]Pd-protoporphyrin (*top*) and a similar section of mesenteric lymph node from normal control dog (*bottom*). (Reproduced with permission from J. Nucl. Med.)

In a preliminary test of the immunosuppressive efficacy of radioactive metalloporphyrins, skin homotransplants were performed on two dogs injected intravenously with 7.5 mCi/kg of [109]Pd-protoporphyrin. The skin homografts, whose donor origin in one case was verified by cytogenetic studies (Table 17-5), remain viable more than 13 months after homografting (Figs. 17-3, 17-4, and 17-5). The dogs remain in good health with no evidence of abnormalities in renal, hepatic, or hematopoietic functions.

To determine whether immunosuppression achieved with radioporphyrins is specific for a particular antigen and is not indiscriminate as might occur following

Table 17-5

Cytogenic Analysis*

Sex Chromosomes	Chromosomes per Cell			Cell Source
	< 78	78	> 78	
1 X	12	54	1	Homograft
2X	2	25	1	(100 cells)
?	2	3	—	
1 X	14	74	2	Male donor
2 X	—	—	—	(50 cells)
?	4	6	—	
1 X	4†	—	—	Female recipient
2 X	12	76	—	(50 cells)
?	4	2	2	

*Tabled entries are percentages of the total cells observed.
†Probably artifact due to random loss of chromosomes during slide preparation.

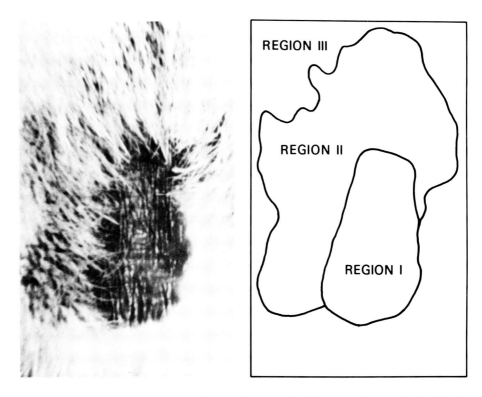

Fig. 17-3. Black pigmented donor skin (Region I) grafted into nonpigmented site of a dog injected with high-activity [109]Pd-protoporphyrin. In this dog pigment has spread (Region II) from homograft to surrounding originally nonpigmented skin of recipient dog. Region III is nonpigmented host skin.

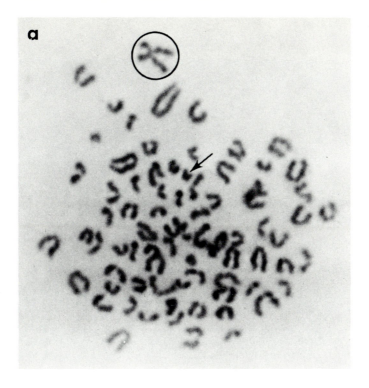

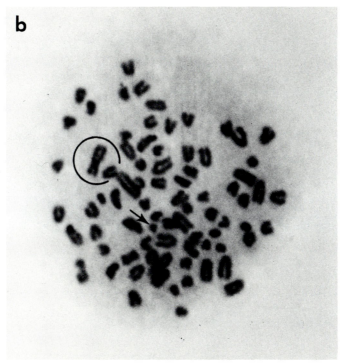

Fig. 17-4. Male chromosome pattern in two cells obtained from male donor skin homografted onto female recipient treated with [109]Pd-protoporphyrin. Circled chromosome is X chromosome and arrow indicates Y chromosome.

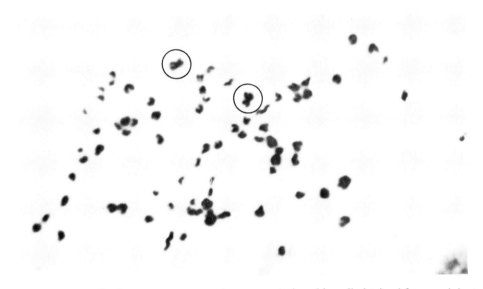

Fig. 17-5. Female chromosome pattern in representative skin cell obtained from recipient female dog at site near male homograft. Two X chromosomes are circled. (Reproduced with permission from J. Nucl. Med.)

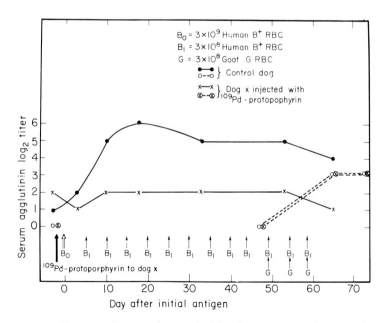

Fig. 17-6. Pattern of serum hemagglutinin titer response in control and [109]Pd-protoporphyrin-treated dogs, injected initially with human red cells and subsequently with goat red cells.

a generalized immune weakness, the following study was conducted. A dog was injected with human red cells beginning 3 days after the administration of 7.5 mCi/kg of [109]Pd-protoporphyrin. Subsequently, human red cell injections were repeated twice a week for 10 weeks. In the same dog goat red cells were injected beginning 7 weeks post-porphyrin administration and repeated twice a week for 2 weeks. At 10 weeks after initiation of the experiment, there was no elevation in human red cell hemagglutination titers. However, goat red cell hemagglutination titers were substantially elevated (Fig. 17-6).

These preliminary results obtained with [109]Pd-protoporphyrin as immunosuppressive agents are encouraging and warrant further investigation. Clearly there is need for significant refinement of the method such that damage to tissues not directly involved in mediation of homograft rejection is minimized. Artificial lipid vesicles carrying suitable radionuclides[30] and synthetically tailored radioporphyrins[31] are two potentially promising approaches to this problem.

SUMMARY

Preliminary studies in dogs indicate that the intravenous administration of radioporphyrins causes selective destruction of peripheral lymphoid tissue and allows for survival of skin homografts. These results suggest that further investigation with radioporphyrins for control of homograft rejection is warranted.

REFERENCES

1. Gowans, J. L.: The role of lymphocytes in the destruction of homografts. Br. Med. Bull. 21:106–110, 1965.
2. Casarett, A. P.: Radiation Biology. Englewood Cliffs, N.J., Prentice-Hall, p. 179, 1968.
3. Chiba, C., Kondo, M., Rosenblatt, M., et al.: The selective irradiation of canine lymph nodes by means of intralymphatic injection of [32]P. Transplantation 5:232–240, 1967.
4. Wheeler, J. R., White, W. F., Calne, R. Y.: Selective lymphopenia by use of intralymphatic [198]Au and splenectomy. Br. Med. J. 2:339–342, 1965.
5. Matthews, C. M. E., Dempster, W. J., Copros, C., et al.: The effect of bismuth 206 irradiation in survival of skin homografts. Br. J. Radiol. 37:306–310, 1964.
6. Winchell, H. S., Pollycove, M., Loughman, W. D., et al.: Homotransplantation studies in dogs following selective radioisotopic lymphatic ablation. J. Nucl. Med. 7:416–423, 1966.
7. Weber, M. M.: Allograft survival following antibody suppression with radio iodine labeled antigen. Transplantation 5:1198–1203, 1975.
8. Patel, R., Michkey, M. R., Terasaki, P. I.,: Serotyping for homotransplantation. XVI. Analysis of kidney transplants from unrelated donors. N. Engl. J. Med. 279:501–506, 1968.
9. Maugh, T. H.: Tissue cultures: Transplantation without immune suppression. Science 181:929–931, 1973.
10. Toledo-Pereyra, L. H., Simmons, R. Najarian, J.: Modification of immunogenicity on kidney allografts treated with acid mucopolysaccharides. Surg. Forum 26:331–332, 1975.

11. Simmons, R. L., Rios, A., Toledo-Pereyra, L. H., et al.: Modifying the immunogenicity of cell membrane antigens. Am. J. Clin. Pathol. 63:714–734, 1975.
12. Billingham, R. E., Brent, L., Medawar, P. D.: Actively acquired tolerance of foreign cells. Nature 172:603–606, 1953.
13. Weigle, W. O.: Immunologic unpresponsiveness. Adv. Immunol. 16:61–114, 1973.
14. Dresser, D. W.: Specific inhibition of antibody production II. Immunology 5:378–388, 1962.
15. Dresser, D. W.: Specific inhibition of antibody production I. Immunology 5:161–168, 1962.
16. McKenzie, I. F. C., Koene, R. A. P., Winn, H. J.: Evidence for adaptation of skin grafts in enhanced irradiated mice. Transplantation 13:661–663, 1972.
17. Woodruff, M. F., Woodruff, H. G.: The transplantation of normal tissue with special reference to auto- and homografts of thyroid and spleen in the anterior chamber of the eye and subcutaneously, in guinea pigs. Phil. Tans. 234:559–582, 1950.
18. Micklem, H. S., Loutit, J. F.: Tissue Grafting and Radiation. New York, Academic Press, 1966.
19. Simonsen, M.: Graft-versus-host-reactions. Their natural history and applicability as tools of research. Prog. Allergy 6:349–467, 1962.
20. Dickie, K. A., J. L. M., Van Hooft, Van Bekkum, D. W.: The selective elimination of immunologically competent cells from bone marrow and lymphatic cell mixtures. Transplantation 6:562–570, 1968.
21. Ledney, G. D.: Antilymphocytic serum in the therapy and prevention of acute secondary disease in mice. Transplantation 8:127–132, 1969.
22. Casarett, A. P.: Radiation Biology. Englewood Cliffs, N.J., Prentice-Hall, p. 189, 1968.
23. Fawwaz, R. A., Winchell, H. S., Frye, F., et al.: Localization of ^{58}Co and ^{65}Zn-hematoporphyrin in canine lymph nodes. J. Nucl. Med. 10:581–585, 1969.
24. Croos, A. M., Leuchars, E., Miller, J. F. A. P.: Studies on the recovery of the immune response in irradiated mice thymectomized in adult life. J. Exp. Med. 119:837–850, 1964.
25. Metcalf, D.: The Thymus. New York, Springer-Verlag, p. 27, 1966.
26. Park, B. H., Biggar, W. D., Good, R. A.: Paucity of thymus-dependent cells in human marrow. Transplantation 14:284–286, 1972.
27. Miller, J. F. A. P.: The thymus and transplantation immunity. Br. Med. Bull. 21:111–117, 1965.
28. Fawwaz, R. A., Hemphill, W., Winchell, H. S.: Potential use of ^{109}Pd-protoporphyrin complexes for selective lymphatic ablation. J. Nucl. Med. 12:231–236, 1971.
29. Oort, J., Turk, J. L.: A histologic and autoradiographic study of lymph nodes during the development of contact sensitivity in the guinea pig. Br. J. Exp. Pathol. 46:147–154, 1965.
30. National Academy of Sciences. National Research Council Publication 1133. Nuclear Science Series Report No. 39, p. 249, 1964.
31. McDougal, I. R., Dunick, J. K., McNamee, M. G., et al.: Distribution of fate of synthetic lipid vesicles in the mouse. A combined radionuclide and spin label study. Proc. Natl. Acad. Sci. U.S.A. 71:3487–3491, 1974.
32. Fawwaz, R. A., Hambright, P., Valk, P., et al.: The distribution of various water soluble radioactive metallo-porphyrins in tumor bearing mice. Bioinorg. Chem. 5:87–92, 1975.

Gordon L. Brownell, Robert G. Zamenhof,
Brian W. Murray, and Glyn R. Wellum

18
Boron Neutron Capture Therapy

INTRODUCTION

Boron Neutron Capture Therapy

There are two important focal points in the advance of cancer therapy. The first is the continued improvement in methods for preventing or controlling metastatic spread. The second is the control of the group of locally recurrent tumors that do not have distant metastases. This latter group comprises about one-sixth of all cancers[1] and is an area in the treatment of neoplastic disease where a technique such as boron neutron capture therapy (BNCT) might make a significant impact.

The technique of BNCT for the treatment of brain tumors depends on the selective loading of a tumor with a ^{10}B-enriched boron compound and subsequent irradiation of the brain with thermal or epithermal neutrons. The neutron capture reaction, ^{10}B(n,α)^{7}Li, releases an alpha particle and a recoiling ^{7}Li ion with an average total kinetic energy of 2.33 mev. These charged particles have a range in tissue of less than 10μm, which is comparable to or less than a cell diameter. Consequently, the radiation dose distribution due to these particles follows the boron distribution in the irradiated tissue even to the cellular level. BNCT, therefore, combines the attractive features of both external beam and internal radioisotope therapy to deliver a large differential dose to boron-loaded tumor cells interspersed within healthy tissue. Although our efforts at the Massachusetts Institute of Technology (MIT) and the Massachusetts General Hospital (MGH) have been directed toward the treatment of brain tumors, tumors in other parts of the body could in principle be treated by neutron capture therapy.

This work has been supported in part by NIH Grants CA 07368 and CA 19665; U.S. Energy Research and Development Administration Grant E(11-1)-3334; and National Institute of Health postdoctoral training grant CA 09076 (to R.G.Z.).

Clinical Aspects of BNCT of Brain Tumors

The annual incidence of deaths in the United States due to cancers of all types was estimated in 1972 at 345,000.[2] Of these cancers, approximately 3 percent constitute tumors of the central nervous system.[3] Since the vast majority of central nervous system tumors originate in the brain, the annual death rate due to primary brain tumors may be estimated at 10,000. In a review of over 15,000 intracranial tumors culled from several reports, the incidence of gliomas ranged from 31 to 49 percent of all brain tumors.[3] Since astrocytomas grades I to IV represent from 72 to 89 percent of all gliomas, the annual deaths in the United States due to astrocytomas may be estimated at 3000.

High-grade astrocytomas, often referred to as glioblastoma multiforme, are characterized by rapid growth and poor prognosis. These tumors consist of a main tumor with "fingerlets" of neoplastic cells infiltrating the surrounding healthy brain tissue. The cells of the tumor fingerlets are usually well vascularized while the cells of the main tumor mass may be anoxic or even necrotic.[4] Even with surgical removal of the main tumor mass, the neoplastic cells comprising the fingerlets often constitute foci of tumor regrowth (W. H. Sweet, *personal communication*).

These characteristics of glioblastoma multiforme have frustrated attempts at their treatment using currently available therapeutic modalities. The most effective therapy procedure for glioblastoma multiforme reported to date involves a combination of surgery and photon irradiation for which a 13 percent 3-year survival rate has been reported.[5]

History of BNCT

Neutron capture therapy for the treatment of cancer was first suggested by Locher in 1936.[6] During the early 1940s, several workers investigated this technique in animals using various boron and lithium compounds.[7-9] Sweet and Javid[10] first demonstrated that certain boron compounds would concentrate in human brain tumor relative to normal brain tissue, and subsequent studies led to clinicals trials of BNCT at Brookhaven during 1951 and 1952,[1,2] and at the MIT research reactor during 1961 and 1962.[13]

To alleviate the consequences of the rapid attenuation of thermal neutrons in scalp, skull, and brain tissue, investigators carried out the second therapy trial in the following way. A craniotomy was first performed on each patient to remove the main tumor mass. Two to three weeks following this first procedure, a second craniotomy was performed to reflect the scalp, skull, and dura in order to expose the tumor bed directly to the incident neutrons. The thermal neutrons were collimated into the region of the tumor bed using a ^{6}Li-loaded collimator. In spite of these procedures to improve the neutron flux-depth distribution, the results of this clinical trial were uniformly discouraging. Subsequent histologic studies indicated that radiation necrosis in normal brain had occurred primarily as the result of radiation damage to the walls of capillaries and small arterioles within the irradiated cerebral tissue.[13,14] The principal reason for the failure of these early trials was the lack of a boron compound which would give rise to a high sustained concentration within the tumor while its concentration in the blood dropped to a low level.[14] Over the past several years, a concerted effort at the MGH has been made to develop a boron compound with such pharmacokinetic characteristics[15–18,41]

Clinical Trials in Japan

In 1968 Hatanaka and coworkers[19–21] initiated a clinical trial of BNCT in Japan. The boron compound used by Hatanaka, $Na_2B_{12}H_{11}SH$, which had been originally developed at the MGH,[15] was synthesized in a purified ^{10}B-enriched form for clinical use by Shionogi and Co., Osaka, Japan. To date Hatanaka has reported the treatment of 12 brain tumor patients, including 8 cases of glioblastoma multiforme. The patients were divided into three categories: those having previously received surgery and photon irradiation, those having previously received surgery alone, and two glioblastoma multiforme patients with no prior treatment. Of these 12 patients, only the 2 patients in the last category are alive and well, some 70 months after a single treatment by BNCT (H. Hatanaka, *personal communication*).* The apparent success of the treatment of these 2 patients with verified glioblastoma multiforme has increased the enthusiasm for a renewed trial of BNCT at the MIT reactor therapy facility.

DEVELOPMENT AND ASSESSMENT OF BORON COMPOUNDS

Initial attempts to produce high tumor-to-normal brain boron concentration ratios were predicated on the reduction of the blood-brain barrier at the site of a glioma. Encouraging results were obtained using water-soluble compounds such as borax, sodium pentaborate, *p*-carboxyphenylboronic acid, and sodium decahydrodecaborate.[17,22–24] Following the 1961 to 1962 clinical trial of BNCT, it was realized that in order to minimize radiation damage to the endothelial cells comprising the blood vessel walls, high tumor-to-blood boron concentration ratios were desirable. Two materials which showed considerable promise in this respect when tested in tumor-bearing mice were reported to be $B_{12}H_{11}SH^{2-}$ and $B_{10}Cl_8(SH)_2^{2-}$,[15] the former of these being to date the most extensively studied compound for BNCT for gliomas. Much of the continuing interest in $Na_2B_{12}H_{11}SH^{2-}$ stems from the encouraging results of Hatanaka's work, described above. In an attempt to discover boron compounds with superior pharmacological properties, investigators at the MGH have studied the tissue distributions of a number of derivatives of the thiol $B_{12}H_{11}SH$ using rats bearing a subcutaneous tumor of glial origin.[18] Of particular interest are compounds possessing a linked borane cage structure such as $B_{12}H_{11}SSB_{12}H_{11}^{4-}$ and $B_{12}H_{11}SOSB_{12}H_{11}^{4-}$.[18,25]

Boron compounds to be evaluated for their applicability in BNCT are screened using the rat tumor model described above. Up to 50 mg of B per

---

*Note: The survival of Hatanaka's two gliolastoma multiforme cases treated by BNCT is currently 80 months. In addition, Hatanaka has treated eight additional patients in the past year by BNCT, with encouraging results.

kilogram of body weight is administered intravenously in a single dose. The animals are then sacrificed at different time intervals (up to about 1 week after boron administration) and their tissues analyzed for boron content.[26] The boron-containing tissues of primary importance are tumor and blood, the boron concentration in normal brain usually being negligibly low. The potential therapeutic efficacy of a boron compound is strongly dependent on the tumor-to-blood boron concentration ratio. The higher this ratio, the more favorable will be the subsequent dose distribution between the tumor cells and the microvascular endothelium.[27]

Although the macroscopic boron distribution within tumor tissue has received more attention in evaluating a particular boron compound's potential for use in BNCT, the microscopic boron distribution also plays a crucial role in such an evaluation. This is due to the short (5 to 10μm) path lengths of the $^{10}B(n,\alpha)^7Li$ reaction products in tissue. For example, a boron compound which is not taken up within tumor cells probably will not be as effective in destroying such cells as one which is. It is clear, therefore, that in the assessment of the expected efficacy of any boron compound for the treatment of tumors by BNCT, knowledge of the distribution of boron at the cellular level is critically important. Such information may be obtained using autoradiographic techniques, and in particular, neutron-induced alpha autoradiography. This technique is currently being perfected in our laboratory in order to determine the microscopic distribution of ^{10}B in tumor samples obtained from patients administered $Na_2B_{12}H_{11}SH$.

Much of the effort to produce boron compounds with improved tissue distribution properties has relied on the blood-brain barrier phenomenon in normal brain to achieve high tumor-to-brain boron concentration ratios. An alternative approach involves the use of tumor-specific antibodies.[17,28-33] In its simplest form this would require a number of boron-containing molecules to be coupled to a tumor antibody preparation in a manner which would not inhibit the tumor-binding properties of the antibodies. The superficial simplicity of this approach has led to several reports of boron compounds being linked to proteins, particularly immunoglobulins. However, an analysis of such an approach has indicated that unless tumor antibodies having a relatively high antibody-antigen association constant are used, and unless the antigen site density on the tumor cells is high, tumor-to-blood boron concentration ratios significantly better than for the best existing blood-brain barrier compounds will not be achieved.[8,42]

At the present time it appears that the compound $Na_2B_{12}H_{11}SH$ remains the first choice for clinical use in view of its availability, ^{10}B enrichment, and pharmacological properties.

DOSIMETRY

BNCT presents many challenging problems in the area of radiation dosimetry; the reasons for this are as follows. First, the radiation components include thermal, epithermal, and fast neutrons, externally incident and neutron-induced gamma rays, and heavy charged particles from the $^{10}B(n,\alpha)^7Li$ reaction. The spatial distribution of these different radiation components depends on a variety of different transport mechanisms. Second, since the irradiated target dimensions are small with respect to characteristic relaxation lengths, the radiation fields are substantially affected by the proximity of boundary surfaces and incident sources. The accurate description and measurement of the radiation fields near boundaries and sources requires transport theory based calculational methods and precise experimental modeling. Third, since the different radiation components exhibit different RBEs, the distributions for each dose component must be determined separately in order to estimate total RBE dose distributions. Fourth, the microdosimetry of the ^{10}B(n,α)^{7}Li reaction at the cellular level and the uncertainty in the maximum tolerable dose to healthy tissues at risk complicate the estimation of the tissue-sparing effectiveness of BNCT. Over the past 3 years at MIT, a number of calculational and experimental dosimetry studies of BNCT have been performed. Some of the conclusions from these studies are briefly summarized.

Transport Calculations

Neutron energy optimization for BNCT has been investigated since an epithermal rather than a thermal neutron beam may be required to obtain a deeper penetration of boron capture dose in tissue.[34] Using a one-dimensional transport code called ANISN, investigators have shown a monoenergetic 37-ev epithermal neutron beam to be close to optimal for this type of therapy[27,35] since the neutron KERMA in tissue is minimum at this energy.[36] Figure 18-1a shows dose-depth curves computed for such an epithermal neutron beam incident upon a tissue equivalent head phantom. The ''nitrogen'' component of the dose results from thermal neutron capture by nitrogen (^{14}N(n,p)^{14}C*), whereas the induced gamma dose results principally from neutron capture by hydrogen (^{1}H^{1}n,γ)^{2}H). The sum of these two components constitutes the boron-free tissue dose distribution labeled ''O.'' Dose distributions are also shown for tissue loaded with ^{10}B in concentrations of 10 to 160μg ^{10}B g^{-1}. Figure 18-1b shows a similar set of curves for a pure thermal neutron beam. Although it possesses a less favorable dose distribution, this type of beam is a more realistic choice for BNCT. Figure 18-1c shows the dose-depth curves computed for the original MIT Reactor (MITR-I) therapy beam. Note the large incident gamma dose component and the substantial fast neutron dose component (shown by the difference between the ''nitrogen'' and the ''particulate'' dose). The incident gamma and fast neutron contamination has been greatly reduced in the new MIT Reactor (MITR-II) therapy beam which is discussed below.

An advanced multidimensional Monte Carlo radiation transport code has also been used to investigate the radiation fields within a more realistic model of the human head.[37] These calculational studies have underlined the importance of reducing the incident gamma dose component and have indicated the sensitivity of the radiation fields to boundary effects and neutron beam diameter.

Neutron Flux Distributions

The thermal neutron flux distribution has been measured within a tissue-equivalent head phantom irradiated in the MITR-I medical therapy beam. Figure 18-2 shows the experimentally derived thermal neutron isoflux curves obtained using dilute gold activation foils. These data show excellent agreement with the

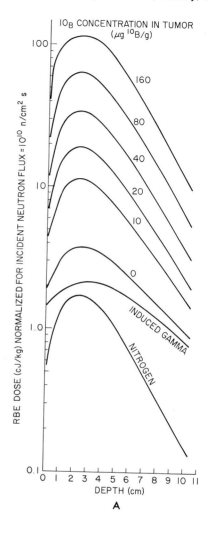

Fig. 18-1. (*Right, and facing page.*) Computed RBE dose-depth curves in a rectangular head phantom irradiated with parallel beams of incident neutrons and gamma rays. For these curves, RBE dose = (1.0)X (gamma ray dose in rads) + (2.0)X (nitrogen dose and fast neutron dose in rads) + (3.7)X (^{10}B(n,α) ^{7}Li dose in rads). (**a.**) 37ev neutron beam; (**b.**) thermal neutron beam; (**c.**) MITR-I therapy beam. (Reprinted with permission from Zamenhof R. G., Murray B. W., Brownell G. L., et al., Med. Phys. 2:47, 1975.)

Monte Carlo calculations described above.[37] The target boundaries and the beam diameter have a considerable effect on the thermal neutron relaxation length. Although the relaxation length in a semi-infite slab is about 2.7 cm,[38] this is reduced to about 1.7 cm for the head phantom shown in Figure 18.2.

As part of our radiation biology studies, a number of young adult beagles were recently irradiated using the MITR-II therapy beam. A phantom head modelled in paraffin wax was used to calibrate the incident neutron flux, while the flux-depth distribution was measured with dilute gold foils. The results are shown in Figure 18-3, from which it can be seen that the measured thermal neutron relaxation length has been reduced to 1.2 cm.

Microdosimetry

BNCT is dependent on the microscopic ^{10}B distribution and concentration in tumor, blood, and normal tissue. Therefore, the calculation of the ^{10}B radiation

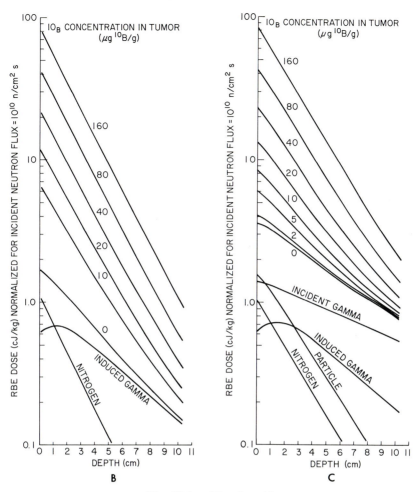

Fig. 18-1. (Continued.)

dose to tumor cells and vasculature requires a microdosimetric approach.

Figure 18-4 shows a cross section of a capillary of the human brain. Assuming the ^{10}B to be distributed uniformly throughout the lumen, it is clear that a significant fraction of the ^{10}B(n,α)^{7}Li energy released within the lumen will not be absorbed by the capillary wall. A Monte Carlo calculation has been performed to assess the magnitude of this effect.[39] The results of this study, summarized in Figure 18-5, show that for an 8-μm lumen diameter and a 0.25-μm capillary wall thickness, only about 32 percent of the total ^{10}B dose is delivered to the capillary wall. Figure 18-6 shows the results of a similar Monte Carlo calculation which indicates that for ^{10}B uniformly distributed within a spherical 10μm diameter isolated tumor cell, about 80 percent of the energy released is absorbed by the cell. One may conclude, therefore, that even if the ^{10}B concentrations in blood and tumor cells are equal, the ratio of tumor cells-to-endothelial cell ^{10}B dose will be significantly greater than unity.

A second approach to the microdosimetry of BNCT is the "point hit" con-

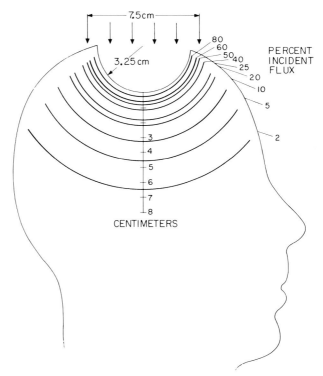

Fig. 18-2. Measured thermal neutron isoflux curves in a gelatin-based tissue equivalent head phantom. Dilute Au (3%) in Al foils were enplaced and the phantom was irradiated with the MITR-I therapy beam.

cept. Monte Carlo calculations have been carried out to investigate the probabilities for inactivation of endothelial cell nuclei resulting from direct hits by alpha and ^{7}Li particles produced by ^{10}B(n,α)^{7}Li reactions in the blood.[37] Figure 18-7 shows the results of these calculations, plotted as the probability of survival (zero hits) versus macroscopic ^{10}B RBE dose level. Contrary to earlier assumptions, it can be seen that larger blood vessels such as arterioles are not less vulnerable to ^{10}B radiation damage than are small capillaries. The histopathologic findings in the brain tissue of patients treated in the second BNCT clinical trial seem to support this conclusion.[13] At the present time, not enough is known about the damage mechanisms involved in boron neutron capture therapy to determine if either of the above models reasonably represents the true radiobiologic damage process.

MITR-II NEUTRON THERAPY FACILITY

Figure 18-8 shows a diagram of the recently redesigned MITR-II research reactor. The Medical Therapy Facility, located immediately below the reactor core, has been designed specifically for BNCT. The features of this facility include

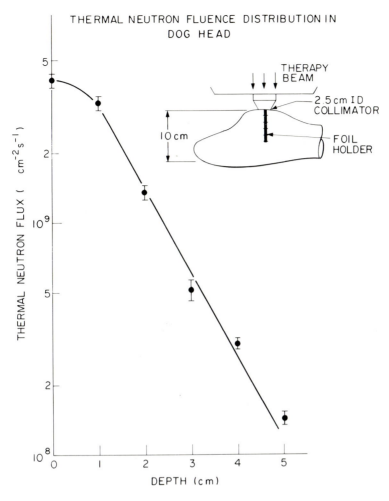

THERMAL NEUTRON FLUENCE DISTRIBUTION IN
DOG HEAD

Fig. 18-3. Measured thermal neutron flux-depth curve in a paraffin wax dog head phantom exposed to the MITR-II therapy beam.

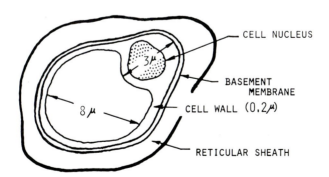

Fig. 18-4. Cross section of a typical brain capillary showing a single endothelial cell and surrounding structures. (Reprinted with permission from Deutsch O. L. and Murray B. W., Nucl. Technol. 26:320, 1975.)

213

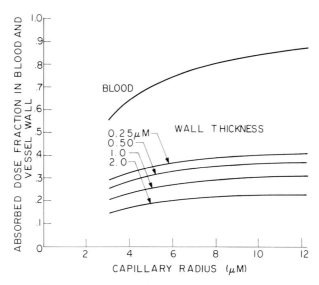

Fig. 18-5. Monte Carlo calculated alpha particle and ^{7}Li ion absorbed dose fractions to capillary wall and blood pool. All ^{10}B (n, α) ^{7}Li reactions occur within capillary lumen. (Reprinted with permission from Rydin R. A., Deutsch O. L., and Murray B. W., Phys. Med. Biol. 21:134, 1976.)

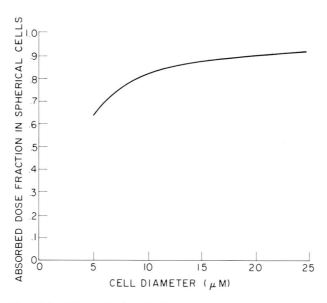

Fig. 18-6. Monte Carlo calculated alpha particle and ^{7}Li ion absorbed dose fraction to a spherical cell uniformly loaded with ^{10}B. (Reprinted with permission from Rydin R. A., Deutsch O. L., and Murray B. W., Phys. Med. Biol. 21:134, 1976.)

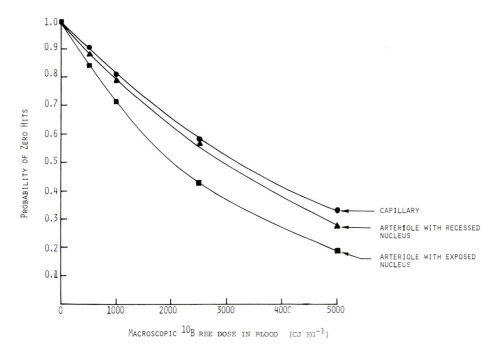

Fig. 18-7. Monte Carlo computed probabilities for survival of endothelial cell nuclei in the wall of a 8-μm diameter capillary, recessed in the wall of a 60-μm diameter arteriole, and partially exposed in the lumen of a 60-μm arteriole. RBE = 3.7. (Reprinted with permission from Deutsch O. I. and Murray B. W., Nucl. Technol. 26:320, 1975.)

(1) an aseptic environment for surgical procedures, (2) operation independent of other reactor functions, and (3) several fail-safe controls to ensure the safety of the patient. The redesigned reactor core and beam portal contain (1) a larger volume of heavy water moderator to reduce the fast neutron component, (2) a raised light water shutter tank to reduce the incident gamma ray component, (3) a boral-shrouded graphite reflector beneath the light water shutter to increase the thermal neutron flux in the beam, and (4) increased neutron and gamma ray shielding around the portal to reduce background radiation. All of these features combine to produce a superior beam for BNCT. In addition to the redesign of the portal, current studies are being conducted to determine the optimum thickness of a bismuth plug to be placed in the beam aperature in order to maximize the thermal neutron flux-to-incident gamma ray dose ratio. Beneath the patient portal, a lithium-loaded patient collimator (not shown in Fig. 18-8) confines the thermal neutrons to the exposed tumor bed. Preliminary measurements of the new beam immediately beneath the patient collimator have yielded the following parameters: (1) a gold-cadmium ratio of 250, (2) a thermal neutron flux of about 4×10^9 cm^{-2} s^{-1}, and (3) an incident gamma ray exposure rate of about 0.085 R s^{-1}. The previous MITR-I therapy beam had a gold-cadmium ratio of 22, and an incident gamma ray dose rate about nine times the present dose rate for the same incident thermal neutron flux.[43]

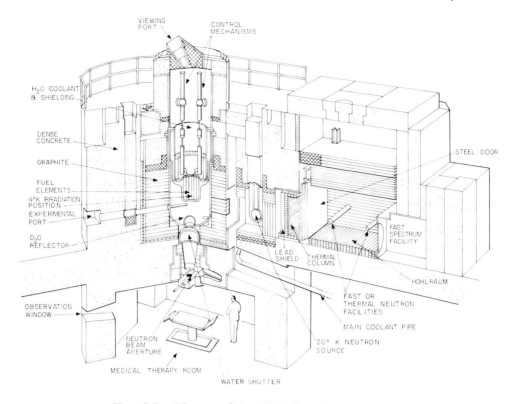

Fig. 18-8. Diagram of the MITR-II nuclear reactor.

PRECLINICAL ANIMAL IRRADIATIONS

In an attempt to estimate the maximum dose that may be safely administered to a patient undergoing BNCT, investigators have carried out two series of dog irradiations at the MIT reactor Therapy Facility. The first series was carried out in 1972 and 1973 using the MITR-I therapy beam, whereas the second series was conducted during January of 1977 using the improved MITR-II therapy beam. Six young adult mongrel dogs (first series) and six colony-bred beagles (second series) were infused with varying amounts of $Na_2B_{12}H_{11}SH$ prior to neutron irradiation of their intact brains. The boron compound was supplied in [10]B-enriched form by Shionogi and Co. A scalp reflection and a small trephine hole through the skull were made for each dog in the first series, whereas only a scalp reflection was made for the dogs in the second series.

In the first series, only one dog (R-6) developed any substantial cerebral ischemia following these procedures. The pertinent information for the irradiation of the two dogs receiving the highest doses in the first series is shown in Table 18-1. It would appear that for a thermal neutron fluence of $1.25 \times 10^{13} cm^{-2}$ and a blood [10]B concentration of $23.6\ \mu g\ {}^{10}B\ g^{-1}$, some ischemia can be induced in normal healthy brain tissue. Nevertheless, it is difficult to arrive at firm conclusions regarding the results of the first series since the incident gamma and fast neutron dose components constituted a substantial portion of the total dose.

Table 18-1
Pertinent Dose Information on Dog Irradiation
Studies Using the MITR-I Neutron Therapy Beam

Dog No.	R-6	R-7
^{10}B concentration in blood (μg/g)	23.6	10.5
Incident thermal neutron fluence (cm^{-2})*	1.25×10^{13}	1.34×10^{13}
Incident γ-dose (rads)*	1020	1020
Nitrogen and induced γ-dose (rads)*	680	730
Nonthermal neutron dose (rads)	340	340
^{10}B dose (rads)*	2210	1030
Total dose to blood (rads)*	4250	3120
Postirradiation life prior to sacrifice (months)	16.5	25.0
Neuropathologic observations	Some cerebral ischemia	No cerebral ischemia

*Tissue surface.

The dogs irradiated in the second series have not yet been sacrificed. Figure 18-9 indicates the various background dose components and the ^{10}B $(n,\alpha)^7$Li dose as a function of ^{10}B concentration in the blood for an incident thermal neutron fluence of 1×10^{13} cm^{-2}. Since the brain size in these animals is rather small, the incident and induced gamma doses are nearly uniform throughout the brain whereas the nitrogen and ^{10}B doses are strongly dependent on depth. In Figure 18-9 the thermal neutron and ^{10}B doses are calculated for the incident tissue surface, and the incident gamma exposure rate of 0.13 Rs^{-1} was before beam optimization.

PRETHERAPY PATIENT STUDIES

A study is currently being conducted at MIT-MGH to determine the boron concentrations in tumor and blood of glioma patients who have been administered the compound Na$_2$B$_{12}$H$_{11}$SH. Between 10 and 24 hours prior to their scheduled tumor resection, the compound is administered by intracarotid infusion at a dose level of about 30 mg of boron per kilogram of body weight. Blood samples are taken at subsequent intervals and several samples of the excised tumor are analyzed for boron content and examined histologically. In the patients studied the measured tumor boron concentration has varied considerably from sample to

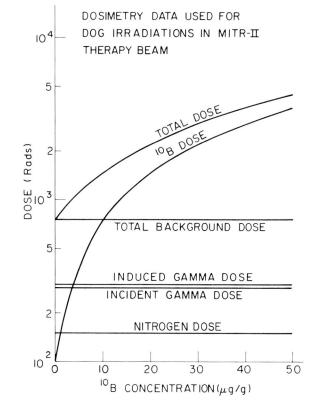

Fig. 18-9. Tissue surface dose components to boron-free and boron-loaded tissue exposed to the MITR-II therapy beam to a neutron fluence of 1×10^{13} cm^{-2}.

sample, and regional tumor-to-blood boron concentration ratios from 0.6 to 3.0 have been observed. Hatanaka has reported a tumor-to-blood boron concentration ratio averaged over several patients of somewhat above 3.0.[20] These tumor and blood samples were obtained immediately prior to the BNCT irradiation which was performed several days after the initial craniotomy. The tumor samples obtained in this manner may have been better perfused and consequently may have attained higher boron concentrations than in the case of the MGH studies.

PROPOSED CLINICAL TRIAL AT MIT-MGH

Preclinical studies currently in progress at MIT-MGH are aimed at answering two important questions. The first concerns the neutron fluence that can be delivered to boron-loaded brain tissue and blood before unacceptable radiation effects occur in normal brain. The second is the question of adequate tumor-to-blood ^{10}B concentration ratios. Data obtained from the recent dog irradiations together with the experience of Hatanaka in Japan will help to resolve the first problem, whereas the pretherapy patient studies currently being conducted at MIT-MGH will indicate what tumor-to-blood ^{10}B concentration ratios can be expected. From the results of the microdosimetry studies discussed earlier, a ^{10}B tumor-to-blood ratio of unity may be adequate for therapeutic effect. Moreover, ^{10}B tumor-to-blood ratios measured on gross tumor specimens may correspond to higher ^{10}B tumor-to-blood ratios on a cellular level; it is hoped that the neutron-induced alpha autoradiography studies will elucidate this aspect.

Following the completion of these investigations and authorization from the appropriate committees and agencies, a series of patients with high-grade astrocytomas and with no prior therapy will be selected for BNCT. These patients will first undergo a resection of the main tumor mass. After approximately 2 weeks are allowed to permit the blood-brain barrier to be reconstituted, each patient will be administered ^{10}B-enriched $Na_2B_{12}H_{11}SH$ at a dose level of about 30 mg of ^{10}B per kilogram of body weight several hours before the scheduled irradiation. Blood samples will be obtained during the period between the boron infusion and the irradiation and will be rapidly analyzed for ^{10}B content at the MIT reactor using a recently developed neutron activation technique.[40] From these data a blood boron clearance curve will be constructed which will allow the determination of the appropriate incident neutron fluence to be delivered.

SUMMARY

Recent developments in the areas of radiation dosimetry, boron chemistry, and nuclear ^{10}B assay methods, together with the encouraging reports of the clinical application of BNCT in Japan, have heightened the enthusiasm at MIT-MGH for a renewed clinical trial of BNCT to treat glioblastoma multiforme patients. A boron compound has been developed which provides not only high tumor-to-normal brain but also acceptable tumor-to-blood boron concentration ratios. In this respect this compound ($Na_2{}^{10}B_{12}H_{11}SH$) differs markedly from previously used boron compounds. Dosimetry studies show that with this compound adequate dose distributions may be obtained on a macroscopic level, while even more favorable dose distributions are expected at the cellular level. A recent redesign of the MIT reactor Medical Therapy Facility has resulted in a therapy beam having markedly improved physical characteristics. Preclinical dog studies and pretherapy patient studies are currently under way to provide data on the tolerance of normal brain to boron neutron capture radiation, and on the ^{10}B tumor-to-blood concentration ratios which might be expected in glioblastoma multiforme patients.

Success in the treatment of glioblastoma multiforme may lead to the application of neutron capture therapy to other tumors.

ACKNOWLEDGMENTS

We gratefully acknowledge the enthusiastic support of Dr. W. H. Sweet and Dr. H. Hatanaka. Much of the progress in our physical studies would not be possible without the guidance and collaboration of Professors R. A. Rydin and O.

L. Deutsch. We also gratefully acknowledge the assistance of Dr. A. Takeuchi, Dr. J. G. Fox, Dr. M. Shalev, and J. R. Messer in our animal irradiation studies. We would like to thank Dr. H. Otsuka (Shionogi Research Laboratory) for supplying the boron compound.

REFERENCES

1. Cohen, L., Awschalom, M.: The cancer therapy facility at the Fermi National Accelerator Laboratory, Batavia, Illinois: a preliminary report. Appl. Radiol. 5:51, 1976.
2. Powers W. E.: Introduction. In: Conference Proceedings on Particle Accelerators in Radiation Therapy. Los Alemos Scientific Laboratory, LA-5180, p. 4., 1972.
3. Kennedy, B. J.: Chemotherapy of brain tumors. In: Cancer Chemotherapy II, I. Broadsky, S. B. Kahn, and J. H. Moyer, (eds.). New York, Grune & Stratton, p. 227, 1972.
4. Maker, H. S., Lehrer, G. M.: Experimental factors in the structure, metabolism, and growth of glial tumors. In: *Experimental Biology of Brain Tumors,* M. K. Wolff, E. G. Paoletti, and D. Paoletti, (Eds.). Springfield, Ill., Charles C. Thomas, p. 521. 1972.
5. Bouchard, J.: Radiation therapy in the management of primary brain tumors. Ann. N.Y. Acad. Sci. 159:563, 1969.
6. Locher, G. L.: Biological effects of therapeutic possibilities of neutrons. Am. J. Roentgenol. 36:1, 1936.
7. Kruger, P. G.: Some biological effects of nuclear disintegration products on neoplastic tissue. Proc. Natl. Acad. Sci. U.S.A. 26:181, 1940.
8. Zahl, P. A., Cooper, F. S., Dunning, J. R.: Some *in vivo* effects of localized nuclear disintegration products on a transplatable mouse sarcoma. Proc. Natl. Acad. Sci. U.S.A. 26, 589, 1940.
9. Zahl, P. A., Cooper, F. S.; Localization of lithium in tumor tissue as a basis for slow neutron therapy. Science 93:64, 1941.
10. Sweet, W. H., Javid, J. J.: The possible use of neutron capturing isotopes such as boron-10 in the treatment of neoplasms. I. Intracranial Tumor. Neurosurgery 9:200, 1952.
11. Farr, L. E., Sweet, W. H., Robertson, J. S., et al.: Neutron capture therapy with boron in the treatment of glioblastoma multiforme. Am. J. Roentgenol. 71:279, 1954.
12. Farr, L. E., Haymaker, W., Konikowski, T., et al.: Effects of alpha particles randomly induced in the brain in the neutron capture treatment of intracranial neoplasms.
13. Asbury, A. K., Ojemann, R., Nielsen, S. L., et al.: Neuropathologic study of fourteen cases of malignant brain tumors treated by boron-10 slow neutron capture therapy. J. Neuropathol. Exp. Neurol. 31:278, 1972.
14. Brownell, G. L., Murray, B. W., Sweet, W. H., et al.: A Reassessment of Neutron Capture Therapy in the Treatment of Cerebral Gliomas. Proceedings of the Seventh National Cancer Conference, p. 827, 1973.
15. Soloway, A. H., Hatanaka, H., Davis, M. A.: Penetration of brain and brain tumor. VII. Tumor-binding sulfhydryl boron compounds. J. Med. Chem. 10:714, 1967.
16. John, K. C., Kaczmarczyk, A., Soloway, A. H.: The alkylation and acylation of $B_{10}H_9NH_3^-$. J. Med. Chem. 12:54, 1969.
17. Soloway, A. H.: Chemical aspects of neutron capture therapy. In: Radionuclide Applications in Neurology and Neurosurgery, Y. Wang and P. Paoletti (Eds.). Springfield, Ill., Charles C Thomas, 1970.
18. Tolpin, E. I., Wellum, G. R., Dohan, F. C., Jr., et al.: Boron neutron capture therapy of cerebral gliomas II. Oncology 32:223, 1975.

19. Hatanaka, H., Sano, K.: A revised boron neutron capture therapy for malignant brain tumors. I. J. Neurol. 204:309, 1973.

20. Hatanaka, H.: A revised boron neutron capture therapy for malignant brain tumors. II. J. Neurol. 209:81, 1975.

21. Hatanaka, H., Sweet, W. H.: Slow neutron capture therapy for malignant tumors—its history and recent development. In: Proceedings of the IAEA International Symposium on Advances in Biomedical Dosimetry. Vienna, IAEA, p. 147, 1975.

22. Brownell, G. L., Soloway, A. H., Sweet, W. H.: Boron capture therapy. In: Modern Trends in Radiotherapy I, T. J. Deeley and C. A. P. Wood (Eds.). London, Butterworths, 1967.

23. Easterday, O. D.: Second Boron *ad hoc* Meeting on Neutron Capture Therapy, New York City, September, 1959.

24. Soloway, A. H.: Boron compounds in cancer therapy. In: Progress in Boron Chemistry I, H. Steinberg and M. C. McCloskey (Eds.). New York, Pergamon Press, 1964.

25. Wellum, G. R., Tolpin, E. I., Soloway, A. H.: et al.: Synthesis of μ-(disulfido)bis(undecahydro-closo-dodecaborate)(4−) and of a derived free radical. Inorg. Chem. (in press).

26. Soloway, A. H., Messer, J. R.: Determination of hydrolytically stable boron hydrides in biological materials. Analt. Chem. 36:433, 1964.

27. Zamenhof, R. G., Murray, B. W., Brownell, G. L., et al.: Boron neutron capture therapy for the treatment of cerebral gliomas I. Med. Phys. 2:47, 1975.

28. Bale, W. F., Spar, I. L.: Studies directed toward the use of antibodies as carriers of radioactivity for therapy. In: Advances in Biological and medical Physics, Vol. 5, Lawrence; J. H. and Tobias, C. A. Eds., Academic Press, New York, 1957.

29. Hawthorne, M. F., Wiersema, R. J., Takasugi, M.: Preparation of tumor-specific boron compounds. 1. *In vitro* studies using boron-labelled antibodies and elemental boron as neutron targets. J. Med. Chem. 15:449, 1972.

30. Tolpin, E. I., Wong, H. W., Lipscomb, W. N.: Binding studies of boron hydride derivatives to proteins for neutron capture therapy. J. Med. Chem. 17:792, 1974.

31. Wong, H. S., Tolpin, E. I., Lipscomb, W. N.: Boron hydride derivatives for neutron capture, antibody approach. J. Med. Chem. 17:785, 1974.

32. Mallinger, A. G., Jozwiak, E. L., Jr., Carter, J. C.: Preparation of boron-containing bovine γ-globulin as a model compound for a new approach to slow neutron therapy of tumors. Cancer Res. 32:1947, 1972.

33. Sneath, R. L., Jr., Soloway, A. H., Dey, A. S.: Protein-binding polyhedral boranes. J. Med. Chem. 17:796, 1974.

34. Fairchild, R.: Development and dosimetry of an epithermal neutron beam for possible use in neutron capture therapy. Phys. Med. Biol. 10:491, 1964.

35. Engle, W. W.: A User's Manual for ANISN, a One-Dimensional Discrete Ordinates Transport Code with Anisotropic Scattering. New York, Report K-1693, Union Carbide Corporation, 1967.

36. Ritts, J. J., Solomito, M., Stevens, P. N.: Calculation of neutron fluence-to-KERMA factors for the human body. Nucl. Appl. Technol. 7:89, 1969.

37. Deutsch, O. L., Murray, B. W.: Monte Carlo dosimetry calculation for boron neutron capture therapy in the treatment of brain tumors. Nucl. Technol. 26:320, 1975.

38. Reactor Physics Constants, 2nd Ed., Report ANL-5800, Argonne National Laboratory, p. 30, 1963.

39. Rydin, R. A., Deutsch, O. L., Murray, B. W.: The effect of geometry on capillary wall dose for boron neutron capture therapy. Phys. Med. Biol. 21:134, 1976.

40. Murray, B. W., Deutsch, O. L., Zamenhof, R. G., et al.: New approaches to the dosimetry of boron neutron capture therapy at MIT-MGH. In: Biomedical Dosimetry. Vienna, IAEA, p. 179, 1975.

41. Tolpin, E. I., Wellum, G. R., Berley, S. A. The synthesis and chemistry of mercaptoundecahydro-closo-dodecaborate (2−). Inorg. Chem. Submitted.
42. Wellum, G. R., Zamenhof, R. G., Tolpin, E. I. Boron neutron capture therapy of cerebral gliomas III. Oncology. In press.
43. Murray, B. W., Deutsch, O. L., Brownell, G. L. The MITR-II medical therapy facility. In: Proceedings of the Third Symposium on Neutron Dose Symmetry in Biology and Medicine. Munich, IAEA, in press.

Tuhin K. Chaudhuri

19
Role of ^{32}P in Polycythemia Vera and Leukemia

INTRODUCTION

Lawrence started ^{32}P therapy in leukemia in 1936. Three years later he and his colleagues extended the same therapeutic modality to polycythemia vera. Since then, ^{32}P therapy in polycythemia vera has become increasingly popular and, to many physicians, ^{32}P remains the best therapy for polycythemia vera. With the discovery of various chemotherapeutic agents for treating leukemia, the role of ^{32}P in the therapy of this disease has become less common. The prognosis in acute leukemia tends to remain poor irrespective of therapeutic regimen. ^{32}P has not offered any advantage over chemotherapy in the treatment of chronic leukemia. In leukemia, trials with new and ever-changing antitumor drugs continue with the understandable hope for a better drug.

The role of ^{32}P, on the other hand, in treating the polycythemia vera patient remains increasingly important. Accumulating evidence leaves little doubt that ^{32}P therapy prolongs the life of polycythemia vera patients to a great extent. The major concern during the past years has been the leukemogenic effect of radiation therapy in patients with polycythemia vera. With the advent of various chemotherapeutic agents in the treatment of leukemia, trial has continued to also evaluate their effectiveness in the treatment of polycythemia vera. As a result, during the past two decades the use of ^{32}P in polycythemia vera has been relatively reduced with the hope of finding a better agent in the therapy for this disease. However, the attempt so far has been disappointing.

Major problems of comparing data in the literature arise from the fact that many cases initially described as polycythemia vera were not really polycythemia vera; some of these were secondary polycythemia and some were other forms of myeloproliferative disease. The incidence of polycythemia vera is relatively low, about 5 new cases per million per year,[20] or 1000 new cases per year in the United States, or less than 1 case per specialist physician per year. This precludes a meaningful study by a single group within a short period of time. Many of the accurately diagnosed polycythemia vera cases did not receive a controlled therapeutic regimen. To overcome this, several specialized polycythemia clinics were established. Involvement with one such clinic in Donner Laboratory, with the leadership of Dr. John Lawrence, created an opportunity for me to see a few cases every week and study them closely with other interested physicians such as Drs. Les Hollander, Steve Landaw, Myron Pollycove, Donald Van Dyke, Saul Winchell, and others. Since then, I have treated a few more cases with ^{32}P, with the help of my colleagues in the Nuclear Medicine and Hematology Departments in Iowa. Experience to date has been rewarding.

Under the leadership of Dr. Louis Wasserman, a Polycythemia Vera Study Group (PVSG) was formed in 1967. The role of the PVSG in unfolding many unknown areas related to polycythemia vera has been and will continue to be of tremendous importance to the medical community. To date, this group has registered more than 420 cases of genuinely diagnosed polycythemia vera and randomized them equally in three therapeutic groups: phlebotomy, ^{32}P therapy, and chemotherapy. Many of the ^{32}P and chemotherapy group patients are supplemented by phlebotomy. Available data from the study group are mentioned or referred to in appropriate places throughout the chapter.

The major questions discussed in this chapter are listed below:

1. What criteria should we follow to correctly diagnose polycythemia vera?
2. Is simple venesection enough for all polycythemia vera cases?
3. How does ^{32}P therapy compare with chemotherapy in terms of longevity and quality of life?
4. What is the leukemogenic role of ^{32}P in polycythemia vera, and how does this compare with the chemotherapeutic agents?
5. What is the role of ^{32}P as a therapeutic agent in chronic leukemia?

CORRECT DIAGNOSIS OF POLYCYTHEMIA VERA

It has been recognized that individuals with increased red blood cells, hemoglobin, or hemotocrit can be classified mainly into three groups: (1) polycythemia vera, (2) secondary polycythemia, and (3) relative polycythemia. We are concerned with the first group, polycythemia vera, sometimes referred to as primary polycythemia or polycythemia rubra vera. This entity is now regarded as a chronic neoplastic disease of the bone marrow characterized by varying degrees of proliferative activity of the erythroleukothrombopoietic cell lines derived from the primitive cells. The disease progresses from a benign orderly proliferation of marrow cells with an initial erythrocytosis, through a "spent phase" associated with myelofibrosis and myeloid metaplasia, frequently associated with a blood picture resembling that of chronic myelocytic leukemia. Various stages of the erythropoietic marrow distribution pattern in polycythemia vera can be shown by ferrokinetic studies and total-body scanning[1-3] with radioactive iron (Fig. 19-1). An accelerated malignant phase may eventually supervene, with an increasing leukocytosis consisting of primitive white cells, a progressive anemia, severe thrombopenia, and enlarging painful spleen and liver. This terminal picture of acute leukemia is seen with increasing frequency as the polycythemia vera patients are now reaching a normal or near normal survival. During the early stages,

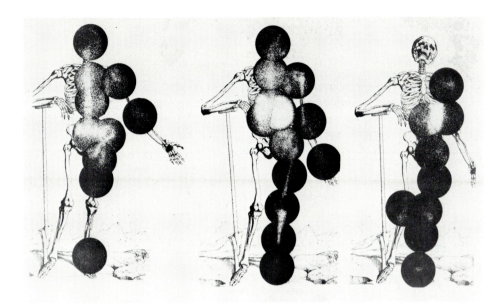

Fig. 19-1. ^{52}Fe-Whole-body scans showing erythropoietic marrow distribution in: (**a**) a hemopoietically normal adult (*left*); (**b**) a patient with myeloid metaplasia with extramedullary hemopoiesis (*middle*); and (**c**) a patient with "burnt out" stage of polycythemia vera (*right*). (Reprinted with permission from Prog. Atomic Med. 2:65, 1968.)

in addition to erythrocytosis, leukocytosis, and thrombocytosis, the laboratory findings include increased leukocyte alkaline phosphatase, blood urate, and serum B_{12}. Normal arterial saturation is one of the key factors in differentiating polycythemia vera from secondary polycythemia. Criteria established by the Study Group[4] in uniformly diagnosing polycythemia vera are shown in Table 19-1.

Table 19-1
Criteria Established by the Polycythemia Vera Study Group
for the Diagnosis of Polycythemia Vera

Category A	Category B
1. Total red cell mass	1. Platelet > 400,000/mm³
Male ≥ 36 ml/kg	2. WBC > 12,000/mm³
Female ≥ 32 ml/kg	(no fever or infection)
2. Arterial O_2 saturation ≥ 92%	3. ↑ Leukocyte alkaline phosphatase
3. Splenomegaly	(no fever or infection)
	4. ↑ Serum B_{12} (> 900 pg/ml)
	on unbound B_{12} binding capacity

Criteria for polycythemia vera   → $A_1 + A_2 + A_3$
                                              or
                         $A_1 + A_2 +$ any 2 of Category B

IS PHLEBOTOMY ENOUGH?

Phlebotomy

Phlebotomy is useful in those indolent cases in which occasional procedures (500 ml every few months) can control the erythrocytosis. Initially, repeated phlebotomies every other day may be necessary. Rapid reduction in the blood volume may prevent serious hemorrhagic or thromboembolic episodes temporarily in those patients susceptible to such complications. Phlebotomy is also useful in those occasional patients in whom the platelet or white cell counts are normal or below normal and myelosuppressive drugs (chemotherapy or ^{32}P) are contraindicated.

Although phlebotomy alone is a simple method of treatment in polycythemia vera, there are certain disadvantages to consider. Phlebotomy does not have an

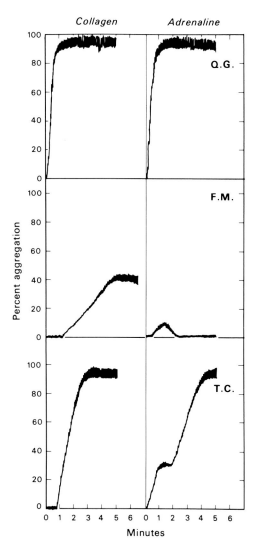

Fig. 19-2. Platelet aggregation with collagen and adrenaline in: (**a**) a normal individual (T. C.); (**b**) a polycythemia vera patient with a history of recent hemorrhage into her right eye (F. M.); and (**c**) a polycythemia vera patient with past history of thrombosis (Q. G.).

effect in managing patients with thrombocytosis (over one million platelets) or painful splenomegaly.

The principal causes of morbidity and mortality in untreated polycythemia vera are related to hemorrhage and thrombosis.[5] Increased blood viscosity, related to elevated hematocrit, and thrombocythemia are felt to contribute to these hemorrhagic and thrombotic states. In a limited series, we have shown that thrombotic or hemorrhagic episodes in polycythemia vera are associated with the nature of platelet aggregation defect.[6]

This series consisted of 17 cases. All patients studied fulfilled the diagnostic criteria for polycythemia vera. Two of these patients showed delayed and diminished aggregation in response to epinephrine and collagen (Fig. 19-2). One of these patients had a recent severe hemorrhage into her right eye. Three additional patients had accelerated platelet aggregated on exposure to collagen or epinphrine (Fig. 19-2). One of these patients had a past history of thrombosis and one had symptoms of impending basilar artery occlusion. The remaining patients had normal platelet aggregation studies. There was no apparent correlation between platelet aggregation defects and peripheral blood cell values or treatment regimen.

The few patients studied suggest a possibility that patients having an increased thrombotic tendency may have an increased platelet aggregation on exposure to collagen and epinephrine or those who have a tendency to hemorrhage may have diminished platelet aggregation on such exposure. If such is the case, platelet aggregation studies may be useful in determining the form of therapy in patients with polycythemia vera. Thus, the patients with defective platelet aggregation should be considered for an early myelosuppressive therapy rather than the phlebotomy alone.

In some cases progressive erythremia may be difficult to control with venesection alone. Repeated phlebotomies usually result in depletion of iron stores, with symptoms of iron deficiency such as anorexia, lassitude, dysphagia, and glossitis. In some cases, pruritus and hyperuricemia are not alleviated by phlebotomy.

Myelosuppressive Therapy

Most patients require myelosuppressive drug therapy (either chemical or radiation) when the disease process is complicated by one or more of the following:[7]

1. Erythrocytosis uncontrollable by phlebotomy alone.
2. Excessive thrombocytosis with platelet counts approaching one million.
3. Extramedullary hematopoiesis with painful spleen, hypersplenism, abdominal pain, or splenic infarct.
4. Persistent symptoms such as pruritus or hyperuricemia not controlled by phlebotomies, allopurinol, or antihistamine.
5. Cardiovascular problems contraindicating frequent phlebotomies.

Two kinds of myelosuppressive therapy may be considered: drugs and radiation. Although, among the drugs, hydroxyurea, procarbazine, pipobroman, dibromomannitol (DBM), and pyrimethamine (Daraprim®) have been tried with various frequency, time has shown that the alkylating group is more useful. Of the

Table 19-2
Physical Properties of ^{32}P

Half-life	14.3 days
Monochromatic beta	1.7 mev
Approximate range in tissue	7 mm

Table 19-3
Radiation Dose to Bone Marrow from
^{32}P*

Contribution from:	Rads/mCi
Marrow	13
Trabecular bone	10
Cortical bone	1
Total	24

*Data adapted from ref. 10.

alkylating agents, the most commonly used chemotherapeutic agents are busulfan (Myleran®), chlorambucil (Leukeran®), and melphalan (Alkeran® or L-phenyl-alanine mustard). Drug treatment in general is more difficult to manage than radio-active phosphorus therapy.

Radiation Therapy

Radiation therapy in polycythemia vera has been tried in two different ways: external radiation and radiation with ^{32}P. ^{32}P-therapy has several advantages, and time has shown that this form of therapy has gained exclusive popularity over the external radiation therapy.

RADIOACTIVE PHOSPHORUS (^{32}P) THERAPY

Physical properties of ^{32}P are shown in Table 19-2. ^{32}P has been used success-fully in the therapy for polycythemia vera for about 35 years. An initial dose of 2 to 5 mCi, by oral or intravenous route, was used in the past. Since absorption through the gastrointestinal tract is not complete and varies from patient to patient and within the same patient at different times, it is advisable that all ^{32}P therapy be given intravenously. The chemical form is ionic phosphate, usually in the form of orthophosphate. In the past, therapeutic dose schedules varied widely in different centers. Now the Polycythemia Vera Study Group recommends an initial dose of 2.3 mCi/m² body surface and not to exceed 5 mCi. This is usually sufficient to produce a remission. But if a remission does not occur in 3 months, the dose should be increased by 25 percent. Another increase by 25 percent, but not ex-ceeding 7 mCi, may be tried as a third dose after a period of another 3 months. Retreatment is usually restricted for 6 months thereafter. These are rather arbi-trary criteria set forth by the Study Group based on past experience of several physicians. Variability in the therapeutic efficacy and dose schedule of ^{32}P in different centers is understandable. After intravenous administration of ^{32}P in ionic form, the isotope selectivity concentrates in the mitotically active cells of the bone marrow and in the trabecular and cortical bone. The endosteal accumulation of ^{32}P causes further radiation to the marrow. Total radiation to the marrow is somewhat variable as it depends on the marrow and bone uptake as well as on its retention time in these sites. In this regard, it is analogous to the factors considered in ^{131}I therapy in hyperthyroidism, namely, the gland size, its uptake of ^{131}I, and retention time within the gland. Unfortunately, unlike the thyroid situation, it is extremely difficult to assess marrow mass, ^{32}P uptake, and its residence time within the marrow and bone. Several authors assessed the radiation dose to the marrow to be between 20 and 50 rads per millicuries.[8] One study showed the radiation dose to be 15 rads/mCi on the basis of 20 percent skeleton uptake and 14.1 days effective half-life.[9] A recent calculation[10] appearing to be more methodical showed the radiation dose to be 24 rads/mCi (Table 19-3). Anyway, the variations in marrow and bone mass, ^{32}P uptake, and its effective half-life make it impossible to predict the accurate radiation dose in each individual patient. Moreover, the radiation sensitivity is another variable in the patient population.

Even with these variations, usually in 80 percent of the cases the blood picture returns to normal in 1 to 2 months following the initial therapy. The response is usually predictably good without any major toxicity, and a smooth remission may be maintained for many months or years, when a repeat therapy may be necessary. It is desirable to treat polycythemia vera conservatively with ^{32}P and, if necessary, to repeat it a few times rather than to cause an overkilling, and thereby inducing a rapid hypofunction of the marrow. The Study Group's dose schedule with an initial radiation dose of roughly 100 rads to the marrow appears to be quite conservative and reasonable.

SURVIVAL OF POLYCYTHEMIA VERA PATIENTS WITH DIFFERENT THERAPEUTIC REGIMENS

The optimum therapy for polycythemia vera has been controversial. Signs and symptoms of this relatively rare disease vary tremendously. It is indeed difficult in many instances to differentiate polycythemia vera from other conditions of erythrocytosis. Some consider polycythemia vera to be a chronic benign condition and prefer to treat the disease symptomatically. As this group relate the morbidity and mortality of the disease mainly to hyperviscosity, vascular distension, and tissue anoxia, phlebotomy remains, to them, the main therapeutic choice. Additional treatment of excess urate production with allopurinol and pruritis with cholestyramine or cyproheptadine (Periactin®) is recommended. Very little attention is given to increased leukocytotic and thrombocytotic activity.

A more dynamic picture is held by others who consider polycythemia vera to be a progressive clonal disease with increased and continued activity of the multipotent stem cells with increased intra- and extramedullary hemopoiesis, hepatosplenomegaly with metaplastic foci, and gradually changing to myeloid metaplasia and myelofibrosis leading to severe anemia and recurrent splenic infarction. This group tend to prevent the hemorrhagic and thrombotic episodes by myelosuppressive therapy. There is belief that phlebotomy alone may activate the hemostatic mechanism leading to thrombohemorrhagic conditions. Among the possible mechanisms of origin of polycythemia vera most commonly suggested are (1) abnormal, unregulated, "neoplastic" proliferation of marrow cells,[11] (2) proliferation of normal stem cells in response to an abnormal myeloproliferative factor,[12] and (3) increased sensitivity of marrow cells to erythropoietin, resulting in erythroid hyperplasia.[13] A recent observation in two polycythemia vera cases virtually excluded the later two possibilities as primary mechanisms.[14] In contrast to unaffected tissue, such as skin fibroblasts, which consisted of both B and A types, the glucose-6-phosphate dehydrogenase of these patients' RBCs, WBCs, and platelets was only of type A. These results provide direct evidence for the stem cell nature of polycythemia vera and strongly imply a clonal origin for this disease.

It has long been shown that the ^{32}P therapy indeed prolonged life much more than that with phlebotomy alone.[15,16] Thus, an average survival of 8 years after the detection of polycythemia vera has been extended to approximately 16 years with the help of ^{32}P therapy. Increased incidence of leukemia in polycythemia vera has been partly attributed, by these authors, to the longer survival of patients treated with ^{32}P, compared to those not so treated.

In a recent article, Landaw[17] has analyzed data from 18 different series or subseries on survival in polycythemia vera patients in relation to age at onset and treatment regimen. The duration of survival in any series of patients treated with ^{32}P depends on the average age of the patients at the onset of disease. Patient survival varies among the available published series, and some of the differences in mean survival may be explained by the variation in average age at the onset of the disease. Thus, it has been shown that the earlier the age at onset of the disease, the longer the survival time of the patient (Fig. 19-3). When a straight line is drawn to represent a least-square best-fit through 14 points representing series with ^{32}P therapy, a remarkable lack of scatter ($r - 0.92$) occurs. Indeed, this graph seems to indicate that the prime factor determining survival of polycythemia vera patients treated with ^{32}P is the age at onset of this disease. Survival of these patients treated with ^{32}P can be fitted to the formula:[17]

Mean survival (years) = 29.4 − (0.3l3) × [age at onset of PV (years)].

The mean survival in these 14 groups of patients treated with ^{32}P was 12 years with the average age of onset of the disease being 57 years.

The average survival in two other series, as analyzed by Osgood[18] and Landaw,[17] for patients with polycythemia vera treated with phlebotomy alone falls below the line drawn in Figure 19-3 (squares). Mean ages of onset of polycythemia vera in these two groups were 56.6 and 60, respectively, but mean survivals were 8.4 and 7.6 years, respectively. These limited data suggest that the survival of polycythemia vera patients treated with phlebotomy alone is somewhat less than for those treated with ^{32}P.

A total of 32 cases (triangles in Fig. 19-3) treated with phlebotomy-supplemented chemotherapy and dying of acute leukemia also fell below the line. These patients had an average survival of 7 years, and the average age of onset of polycythemia vera was 53.8 years. The average age at death for these two groups is far less than that for patients treated with ^{32}P and dying of acute leukemia.

It has been observed recently that with new drugs and improved medical care, survival of the phlebotomized patients without any myelosuppressive therapy has also improved.[19] In some instances it has approached that of the

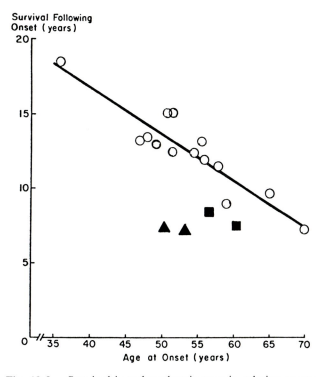

Fig. 19-3. Survival in polycythemia vera in relation to age of onset. Circles represent ^{32}P-treated series or subseries of patients published between 1955 and 1976. Squares represent phlebotomized groups and triangles represent chemotherapeutic groups. (Reprinted with permission from Landaw S. A. Semin. Hemat. 13:33, 1976.)

^{32}P-treated group. But it must be remembered that the complication of thrombotic episodes is greater in the phlebotomized group. It is also noticeable that unlike the result with ^{32}P, control of pancythemia is difficult with phlebotomy and chemotherapy because tolerance is exceeded before the disease is controlled.

LEUKEMOGENIC EFFECT OF ^{32}P AND OTHER CHEMOTHERAPEUTIC AGENTS

Many polycythemia vera cases terminate into acute leukemia following ^{32}P therapy. Appropriate questions have been raised as to the cause of leukemia in these patients. Is this the effect of ^{32}P or is this the natural course of the disease or both?

It is now widely accepted that the incidence of radiation-induced leukemia is much higher than that occurring in a normal population. This is based on the data obtained from the literature dealing with experimental mice, occupational exposure to radiation, chromosome abnormalities in therapeutically irradiated patients, increased rates of leukemia in atom bomb survivors, and incidence of leukemia and chromosome abnormalities in patients receiving diagnostic or therapeutic radiation.

Modan and Lilienfield's survey[21] showed that 10 percent of questionable or correctly diagnosed polycythemia vera patients ultimately developed leukemia. Lawrence, Winchell, and Donald[22] showed in their series that 14 percent of their patients receiving ^{32}P developed terminal acute leukemia. The incidence of acute leukemia in this series was 20 to 40 times that expected due to radiation exposure alone. Osgood[18] has pointed out that the incidence of acute leukemia was not really total radiation dose dependent alone. These findings simply point out that either acute leukemia is a terminal event of polycythemia vera or the polycythemia vera patients are highly susceptible to radiation-induced acute leukemia.

This proves that Lawrence's contention[15,16] of acute leukemia being the natural history of polycythemia vera is at least partially correct. Acute leukemia occurred significantly more often in patients treated with ^{32}P than in those not so treated. This may be in part a real radiation effect and in part because in the past ^{32}P-treated groups outlived the other groups, thereby being more vulnerable to the end stage of the disease, namely, acute leukemic state. There were at least 32 patients terminating into acute leukemia following chemotherapy and never receiving ^{32}P or any other form of radiation.[17] The total number of cases of acute leukemia reported in the world literature is much more in the ^{32}P groups than in the phlebotomy or chemotherapy groups. The main reason for this is that more patients were treated with ^{32}P therapy during the last four decades. It had been difficult to calculate the rate of occurrence of acute leukemia in each group due to the following reasons: (1) not enough records were kept to determine the number of cases in each group; (2) many patients received combined forms of therapy; and (3) follow-up of the group receiving chemotherapy alone has not been complete in many instances since this mode of therapy was started only recently.

Here again, the role of the Polycythemia Vera Study Group will be of immense value. Although we need to wait patiently for more complete data, there is some indication at this stage that myelosuppressive drugs, in general, may not prolong the life of polycythemia vera patients any more than what can be achieved with ^{32}P therapy. Moreover, occurrence of leukemia in the group treated with chemotherapy is no less than that with ^{32}P therapy. It may turn out that the incidence of acute leukemia is more in chemotherapy-treated groups than in the ^{32}P-treated group.

Occurrence of acute leukemia in other diseases where the patients received chemotherapy had been shown to be enormous. Multiple myeloma patients receiving melphalan developed acute leukemia in epidemic proportion.[23,24] There is a report of secondary polycythemia developing acute leukemia following TEM and naphthyl-chloroethylamine.[25] Hodgkin's disease terminating into acute leukemia following multiple chemotherapy in the absence of radiation therapy has also been reported.[26] Similarly, in other forms of malignant and nonmalignant diseases where chemotherapy was used, there is evidence of development of acute leukemia.[27–30]

ROLE OF ^{32}P IN THE TREATMENT OF LEUKEMIA

Although ^{32}P-therapy has been shown to be very effective in polycythemia vera, its role in the treatment of leukemias has not been ideal. Carefully titrated and regularly spaced therapeutic doses of ^{32}P and/or x-ray have been instituted in a large series[31] of patients with chronic lymphocytic leukemia (CLL) and with chronic granulocytic leukemia (CGL). [32]P has been preferred because doses above 25 rads of x-ray have produced nausea, which has never been encountered with [32]P. A few patients originally in x-ray therapy had to be transferred to the ^{32}P regimen because of radiation sickness.

Of the 212 patients with CLL, 63 have lived more than 10 years since onset and 32 more than 10 years after first treatment; 93 have attained the age of 70. Of the 114 patients with CGL, 11 have lived more than 10 years since onset, 5 have lived more than 10 years since first therapy, and 23 have attained the age of 70 years. Five-year survival in these two groups together was 42 percent (52 percent in CLL and 25 percent in CGL). Granulocytic cases reported in this series were later found to be undertreated, as it was shown[32] that the threshold dose of ^{32}P in CGL was much higher than that in CLL. Threshold dose in CGL, to control the WBC count of 15,000 was 10.6 mCi and that in CLL was 6.3 mCi. Median maintenance doses were 17.0 and 7.5 mCi, respectively.

It has been shown[31] that "[32]P is at least as good as Colcemide in CGL and far superior to Mylern, and that it is at least as good as either TEM or Leukeran in the CLL and is much easier to titrate than any of the other agents and less expensive for the patients since it requires far fewer visits and seems much less likely to cause toxic complications."

As mentioned earlier, with the investigational trials of combination drug therapy, the use of ^{32}P in the treatment of leukemia has been minimal during the past two decades. A recent article[33] has emphasized that after the first year of therapy, the annual death rate in the chemotherapeutic group is slightly lower than that of the radiation therapy group. Unfortunately, the comparison is made between very recent series of studies in the chemotherapy group (mostly published in the seventies) and the relatively older series of patients with radiation therapy (studied in the twenties, thirties, and forties). In the latter group, the mode of radiation therapy was mainly x-ray and not [32]P.

It is well recognized that irrespective of basic therapeutic modality in chronic leukemia, management of complications in these patients has been improved during this period of time. One may argue whether the minimal apparent improvement in the survival of these leukemic patients is a reflection of (1) chemotherapeutic drug therapy; (2) supportive care such as cortisone, antibiotics, treatment of anemia, gamma globulin, germ-free chambers, and improved laboratory tests and technology; or (3) greater knowledge of the disease pathophysiology, which would reflect earlier diagnosis and earlier recognition and treatment of complications. It is necessary that a comparison study with ^{32}P be done to determine if any improvement is actually documented with chemotherapy. To be included in the comparison would be the quality of life.

It is understandable at the same time that neither ^{32}P therapy nor other forms of existing chemotherapy are the answer for the treatment of chronic leukemia.

Consequently, search for any better form of therapy or combination of therapy will continue in the foreseeable future.

SUMMARY

^{32}P therapy in polycythemia vera has been shown to achieve normal or near normal survival. Only a few cases can be continued on phlebotomy, and the majority require myelosuppressive therapy. Of the myelosuppressive therapeutics, ^{32}P therapy has been shown to be of more advantage than the chemotherapeutics in terms of patient survival, quality of life, ease to control, and patient expenses. Ten to eighteen percent of ^{32}P-treated patients develop end-stage acute leukemia, but this does not lessen the overall survival rate or quality of life. Recent data indicate that at least the same number of patients in the chemotherapeutic regimen terminate to end-state acute leukemia.

Even though remissions can be achieved in the majority of chronic leukemic patients with any of several chemotherapeutic agents, relatively little improvement in survival has been recorded. In the final analysis, none of these chemotherapeutics have been proven to be of any added advantage over ^{32}P therapy. The results with any therapeutic modality, including ^{32}P, are far from ideal. Hence the search for any better leukemic therapy will be continuing during the foreseeable future.

REFERENCES

1. Pollycove, M., Winchell, H. S., Lawrence, J. H.: Classification and evolution of patterns of erythropoiesis in polycythemia vera as studied by iron kinetics. Blood 28:807–829, 1966.
2. Van Dyke, D. C., Lawrence, J. H., Anger, H. O.: Whole body marrow distribution studies in polycythemia vera. In: Myeloproliferative Disorders of Animals and Man. USAEC Div. Tech. Info., CONF-680529, pp. 721–733, 1970.
3. Chaudhuri, T. K., Ehrhardt, J. C., DeGowin, R. L., et al.: ^{59}Fe whole-body scanning. J. Nucl. Med. 15:667–673, 1974.
4. Berlin, N. I.: Diagnosis and classification of the polycythemias. Semin. Hematol. 12:339–351, 1975.
5. Petitt, R. M., Silverstein, M. N.: Polycythemia vera. In: Conn's Current Therapy. Philadelphia, W. B. Saunders Co., pp. 323–326, 1976.
6. Chaudhuri, T. K., Winchell, H. S., Lawrence, J. H.: Platelet aggregation in polycythemia vera: a possible aid in determining need for therapy with ^{32}P or alkylating agents? J. Nucl. Med. 10:392, 1969.
7. Wasserman, L. R.: Polycythemia vera. In: Conn's Current Therapy. Philadelphia, W. B. Saunders Co., pp. 297–301, 1974.
8. International Commission on Radiological Protection: Protection of the Patient in Radionuclide Investigations. ICRP Publication No. 17. Oxford, Pergamon Press, p. 64, 1971.
9. Mays, C. W.: Cancer induction in man from internal radioactivity. Health Physics 25:585–592, 1973.
10. Spiers, F. W., Beddoe, A. H., King, S. D., et al.: The absorbed dose to bone marrow in the treatment of polycythemia vera by ^{32}P. Br. J. Radiol. 49:133–140, 1976.

11. Gurney, C. W.: Polycythemia vera and some possible pathogenetic mechanisms. Annu. Rev. Med. 16:169–186, 1965.
12. Ward, H. P., Vautrin, R., Kurnick, J.: Presence of myeloproliferative factor in patients with polycythemia vera and agnogenic myeloid metaplasia. I. Expansion of the erythropoietin-responsive stem cell compartment. Proc. Soc. Exp. Biol. Med. 147:805–308, 1974.
13. Zanzani, E. D.: Hematopoietic factors in polycythemia vera. Semin. Hematol. 13:1–12, 1976.
14. Adamson, J. W., Fialkow, P. G., Murphy, S., et al.: Polycythemia vera: stem-cell and probable clonal origin of the disease. N. Engl. J. Med. 295:913–916, 1976.
15. Lawrence, J. H.: Polycythemia, Physiology, Diagnosis and Treatment Based on 303 Cases. New York, Grune and Stratton, 1955, pp. 69–76.
16. Lawrence, J. H., Berlin, N. I., Huff, R. L.: The nature and treatment of polycythemia. Medicine (Baltimore) 32:323–388, 1953.
17. Landaw, S. A.: Acute leukemia in polycythemia vera. Semin. Hematol. 13:33–48, 1976.
18. Osgood, E. E.: Polycythemia vera: age relationship and survival. Blood 26:243–256, 1965.
19. Wasserman, L. R.: The treatment of polycythemia vera. Semin. Hemat. 13:57–78, 1976.
20. Modan, B.: An epidemiological study of polycythemia vera. Blood 26:657–667, 1965.
21. Modan, B., Lilienfield, A. M.: Polycythemia vera and leukemia—the role of radiation treatment: a study of 1,222 patients. Medicine (Baltimore) 44:305–344, 1965.
22. Lawrence, J. H., Winchell, H. S., Donald, W. G.: Leukemia in polycythemia vera. Ann. Intern. Med. 70:763–777, 1969.
23. Holland, J. F.: Editorial: Epidemic acute leukemia. N. Engl. J. Med. 283:1165–1166, 1970.
24. Rosner, F., Grünwald, H.: Multiple myeloma terminating in acute leukemia: report of 12 cases and review of the literature. Am. J. Med. 57:927–939, 1974.
25. Perkins, J., Israëls, M. C. G., Wilkinson, J. F.: Polycythemia vera: clinical studies on a series of 127 patients managed without radiation therapy. Q. J. Med. 33:499–518, 1964.
26. Rosner, F., Grünwald, H.: Hodgkin's disease and acute leukemia. Report of 8 cases and review of the literature. Am. J. Med. 58:339–353, 1975.
27. Allan, W. S. A.: Acute myeloid leukemia after treatment with cytostatic agents. Lancet 2:775, 1970.
28. Garfield, D. H.: Acute erythromegakaryocytic leukemia after treatment with cytostatic agents. Lancet 2:1037, 1970.
29. Schein, P. S., Winokur, S. H.: Immunosuppressive and cytotoxic chemotherapy; longterm complications. Ann. Intern. Med. 82:84–95, 1975.
30. Sypken, S., Smit, C. G., Meyler, L.: Acute myeloid leukemia after treatment with cytostatic agents. Lancet 2:671–672, 1970.
31. Osgood, E. E.: Treatment of chronic leukemias. J. Nucl. Med. 5:139–153, 1964.
32. Osgood, E. E.: The threshold dose of ^{32}P for leukemic cells of the lymphocytic and granulocytic series. Blood 16:1104–1121, 1960.
33. Sokal, J. E.: Evaluation of survival data for chronic myelocytic leukemia. Am. J. Hematol. 1:493–500, 1976.

Ervin Kaplan

20

Historical Development of ^{32}P in Bone Therapy

Therapy for malignant lesions of bone with radionuclides has been the subject of historical treatment. Marshall Brucer in his inimicable, whimsical style has devoted four of his *Vignettes in Nuclear Medicine*[1] to the history of bone scanning and incidently to the history of radionuclide therapy for bone malignancy. The author has summarized radioisotope therapy for malignancy in bone, and in particular, the use of phosphorus 32.[2] Storaasli[3] commented on the use of radiotherapy and phosphorus 32 in metastatic bone disease.

A prologue to treatment of bone malignancy with ^{32}P is found in the pioneering work which defined bone-seeking radionuclides. Bone as a tissue capable of rapid dynamic exchange of its mineral content was characterized by employment of radionuclide tracer experiments. Chiewitz in collaboration with George Hevesy[4] in 1935 demonstrated the rapid incorporation of ^{32}P-phosphate into bone salts and established a kinetic concept of regeneration of the mineral content of the skeleton. Early studies by Hamilton[5] identified the bone-seeking radionuclides. Prominent among these isotopes was the calcium analogue strontium 89. Charles Pecher[6,7] working at the University of California demonstrated by autoradiography the concentration of ^{32}P-phosphate and ^{89}Sr in normal bone. The enhanced localization of ^{89}Sr in reactive bone growth in osteogenic sarcoma was also confirmed by autoradiography (Fig. 20-1). In addition, calcium 45 was, as expected, shown to rapidly accumulate in bone. In 1941 Pecher employed ^{89}Sr-lactate in the treatment of metastatic carcinoma of prostate to bone in a single patient. Treatment of several additional patients with skeletal metastasis from metastatic carcinoma of the prostate followed. Pecher's early and promising work was interrupted by World War II and his untimely death.

The selective localization of ^{89}Sr in the osteoblastic areas surrounding osteogenic and Ewing's sarcoma was confirmed in six patients using direct tissue examination by Low-Beer et al.

The observation of gallium 72 by Dudley et al.[8] from 1948 to 1950 identified it as a bone seeker with high concentration in bone tumors. The subsequent detailed studies by Brucer and Bruner[9] in 1953 led to the application of this radionuclide to

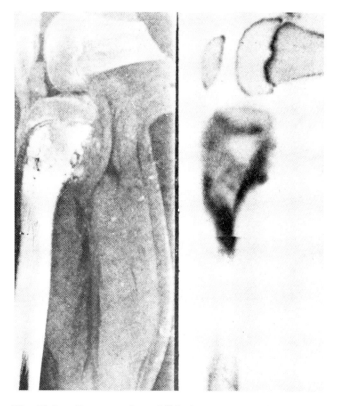

Fig. 20-1. Concentration of ^{89}Sr in an osteogenic sarcoma was demonstrated by Charles Pecher[7] in 1942 using autoradiography in the photograph on the right. The specimen, a human limb in longitudinal section, is seen on the left. (Reproduced with permission from Heller D. A., Adv. Biol. Med. Phys. 2:141, 1951.)

therapy for bone tumors. One-fourth of the patients with a variety of malignant bone tumors had subjective decrease in bone pain. Hematopoietic depression and gallium toxicity as well as the high gamma energy, 2.5 mev, discouraged its further application.

From 1942 to 1948 Friedell with Low-Beer and Lawrence observed a patient with metastatic carcinoma of the breast to bone who was treated with ^{32}P-orthophosphate. This patient responded dramatically to this therapy and inspired Friedell and Storaasli[10] to evaluate treatment of 12 additional patients with skeletal metastasis from breast carcinoma using [32]P. This work published in 1950 initiated a series of clinical trials over the following 20 years.

CLINICAL TRIALS

The treatment of metastatic carcinoma of the breast to bone with ^{32}P-orthophosphate by Friedell and Storaasli[10] resulted in subjective relief of pain in

Table 20-1
Results of Orthophosphate Therapy for Metastatic Carcinoma in Bone*

	No. of Published Reports† (ref. no.)	No. of Patients	No. of Patients with Subjective Pain Relief	% Patients with Pain Relief	No. of Patients with Objective X-Rays of Bone Regeneration	% Patients with Bone Regeneration
Carcinoma of breast	4 (10, 11, 16, 18)	213	186	87	81	39
Carcinoma of prostate	9 (11, 12, 17, 19–24)	113	97	86	25	22
Total	13	326	283	87	106	33

*From ref. 2.
†Papers are limited to those in which subjective and objective evidence was quantitatively reported.

83 percent of 12 patients and 16 percent objective regeneration of bone. The total series of clinical trials reviewed by the author reporting ^{32}P-orthophosphate therapy for skeletal metastasis from breast and prostate are summarized in Table 20-1. Only those papers are included in which subjective evidence of pain relief and objective evidence of bone regeneration by x-ray are quantitatively reported. A total of 328 patients were treated, 87 percent experienced pain relief, and 33 percent had evidence of bone regeneration. Adverse side effects in carcinoma of the breast were largely limited to hematopoietic depression. In addition, patients with prostatic skeletal metastasis experienced enhanced bone pain during pre-treatment with testosterone when given.

The largest clinical series, 137 patients with carcinoma of the breast and 47 with carcinoma of the prostate, were reported in 1958 by the Maxfield's[11] and in 1959 by Vermooten and the Maxfields.[12] Maxfield presented the rationale for the use of testosterone to suppress the breast lesions in bone and to stimulate and render more reactive the prostatic bone lesions. The claim was made in these studies that the prostatic tumor nodule might be concentrating ^{32}P: "It (testosterone) gives significantly large concentration of ^{32}P in the metastases and, therefore, allows adequate irradiation to inhibit the tumor cells.... We concur with Hertz[13] that possibly the testosterone causes a direct increase in the uptake of ^{32}P by the tumor cell itself." It was recommended that "The exact mechanism of this action is not known and investigation should be continued in this phase of the

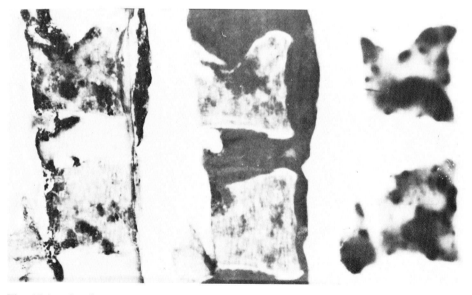

Fig. 20-2. Sections of human lumbar vertebrae in 3-mm section obtained post mortem from a patient who had recently received ^{32}P-orthophosphate therapy following pretreatment with testosterone. The vertebrae show marked metastatic involvement. From left to right, the reproduction is a photograph, a radiograph, and an autoradiograph. The areas of tumor involvement are radiolucent and the uptake of radioactivity is in trabecular bone spicules and not in tumor nodules. (Reproduced with permission from Kaplan E., Miree J., Hirsh E., et al., Int. J. Appl. Radiat. Isot. 5:94–98, 1969.)

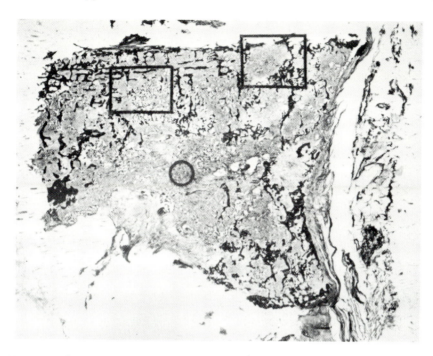

Fig. 20-3. A microsection of the upper vertebrae in Fig. 20-2. The radionecrotic tumor is adjacent to the bone spicules. The rectangle to the left shows total necrosis. The rectangle to the right shows some viable tumor in the center beyond the penetration of the beta emission from the spicules. The center of the large tumor nodule (*circled*) far removed from spicules reveals viable tumor. (Reproduced with permission from Kaplan E., Miree, J., Hirsh, E., et al., Int. J. Appl. Radiat. Isot. 5:94–98, 1969.)

problem.''[11] This aspect of the problem was resolved by the author and his colleagues in 1959.[14] A terminal patient with widespread skeletal involvement from carcinoma of the breast was treated with the Maxfield regimen, and detailed studies were made of gross sections of involved bone by photography, radiography, and autoradiography. The localization of ^{32}P was definitively concentrated in bone spicules. Microscopic sections of identical vertebral specimens revealed radionecrosis of tumor cells within the range of penetration of ^{32}P beta emission from trabecular bone spicules and viable tumor beyond this range (Figs. 20-2, 20-3). The combination of pretherapy with testosterone followed by ^{32}P-orthophosphate continued until the last reported series by Morales et al.[15] in 1970. Other investigators also reported on therapy for metastatic breast and prostate carcinoma.[16–24]

^{32}P - Orthophosphate Following Adrenalectomy

Skeletal metastases of carcinoma of the breast were treated without pretherapy with testosterone by Storaasli et al.[25] in 1961. They studied a series of 42 patients using ^{32}P-orthophosphate only with hematopoietic depression as the endpoint. Subjective results were not recorded, but good evidence of bone regeneration was noted in 11 of 42 patients. In an additional group of 22 patients, ^{32}P-orthophosphate was employed 10 to 14 days post-adrenalectomy. Of these patients, 15 showed objective improvement with bone regeneration and enhanced survival compared with ^{32}P alone. The 68 percent objective improvement is significantly superior to that seen with ^{32}P following testosterone. No other publications are available using ^{32}P following adrenalectomy.

[32]P - Orthophosphate Following Parathormone

The stimulation of reactive bone in metastatic carcinoma of the breast and lung by initial demineralization with parathormone for 1 week prior to ^{32}P-orthophosphate therapy was initially reported in eight patients by Tong and Rubenfeld in 1967.[26] Evidence of bone regeneration occurred in one patient. Bone marrow depression was produced as an adverse side effect. Tong[27] used this therapy for carcinoma of the prostate metastatic to bone in 1971. Pain relief was noted in eight of eight patients. Objectively, three patients showed significant bone regeneration. A drop in elevated acid and alkaline phosphatase was seen. Bone marrow depression did occur.

Pinck and Alexander[28] in 1973 reported a series of 32 patients with prostatic skeletal metastases treated by this method. Bone pain was dramatically relieved in 22 patients and partial relief was noted in 4 additional subjects. Six patients showed improved appetite, weight gain, and increased strength. Eight of ten bedfast patients became ambulatory. Bone regeneration was seen in nine patients. Relief of bone pain was confirmed by Merrin and Bakshi[29] in 1974 using [32]P. Following parathormone, seven of eight patients experienced fair to excellent response. No x-ray evidence of bone regeneration was seen. Editorial comments on this combined therapy have been made by Rubenfeld.[30]

[32]P - Polyphosphate

Polyphosphate as a carrier of technetium-99m is widely known as a bone scanning agent. The biologic activity of this polyelectrolyte was related to its capacity to bind cations and specifically calcium, which led to its widespread commercial use as a water softener and a detergent additive. An additional property, the hydrolysis of this substance by mammalian phosphatase, was described by Kitastato[31,32] in 1928. Fels et al.[33] in 1959 evaluated the ^{32}P-labeled preparation prepared by the method of Jones[34] as an improved agent for therapy for malignancy in bone. This study verified that trimetaphosphate and polyphosphate localized more specifically in bone than orthophosphate. The ^{32}P concentration in bone as compared to the average concentration in soft tissue when administered to mice favored polyphosphate. Orthophosphate was 3.5, trimetaphosphate 5, and polyphosphate 8.2 times concentrated over soft tissue levels. Polyphosphate in addition to having a superior bone to soft tissue ratio actually localized in normal mouse bone in greater total quantity than orthophosphate. Localization showed the identical qualitative distribution as orthophosphate by autoradiograph.

Unpublished studies by Veatch and Kaplan indicated that the whole-body retention of ^{32}P-orthophosphate was approximately eight times the retention of

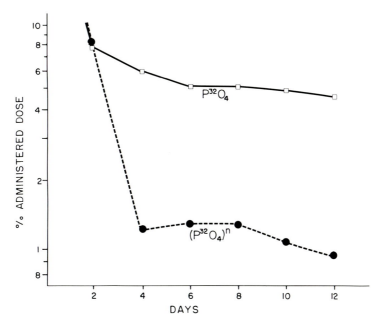

Fig. 20-4. The fractional retention of orthophosphate and polyphosphate in normal mice over 12 days. The polyphosphate was largely confined to bone, whereas orthphosphate was widely distributed in soft tissue as well as bone.

[32]P-polyphosphate (Fig. 20-4). The assumption was made that a significantly greater dosage of radioactivity could be safely delivered to bone with polyphosphate than by using orthophosphate. This was verified in the determination of the minimum lethal dose with 50 percent survival (MLD_{50}) which permitted a 7.2 μCi/g dosage for polyphosphate and a 4.4 μCi/g dosage for orthophosphate in mice (Fig. 20-5). This figure was estimated to be higher for larger mammals, considering the relationship of beta penetration in the small bone marrow–bone compartment in mice.

The first clinical study by the author and his coworkers[35] using ^{32}P-polyphosphate therapy in metastatic prostate cancer to bone appeared in the first issue of the new *Journal of Nuclear Medicine*. Of eight patients treated, seven had relief of bone pain, and several who were bedfast became ambulatory. The bone x-rays showed an initial sclerosis of bone followed by reversion to a trabecular pattern in two patients. Acid and alkaline phosphatase levels dropped.

An additional five patients were treated with combination ^{32}P-polyphosphate and estrogen therapy. All showed rapid complete disappearance of bone pain; weight gain and reversal of paraplegia occurred in two of the five patients. The clinical and laboratory evaluation of these two patients is seen in Figures 20-6 and 20-7. The extensive involvement of the lumbar vertebrae and the subsequent return to normal appearance of the lumbar vertebrae are demonstrated in the second patient (Fig. 20-7), who had a reversal of paraplegia after 120 days. The serial x-rays of this subject are seen in Figure 20-8.

A number of patients were treated by the author and other clinical groups

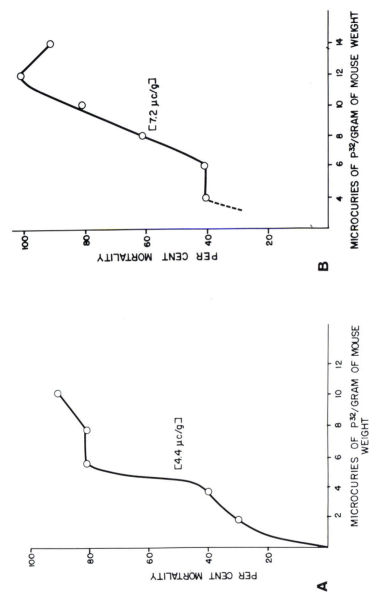

Fig. 20-5. The minimum lethal dose of orthophosphate and polyphosphate in normal mice. (**A**): Fifty percent mortality was produced by 4.4. μCi/g with ^{32}P orthophosphate. (**B**): Fifty percent mortality required nearly double the dosage (7.2 μCi/g) when ^{32}P polyphosphate was used.

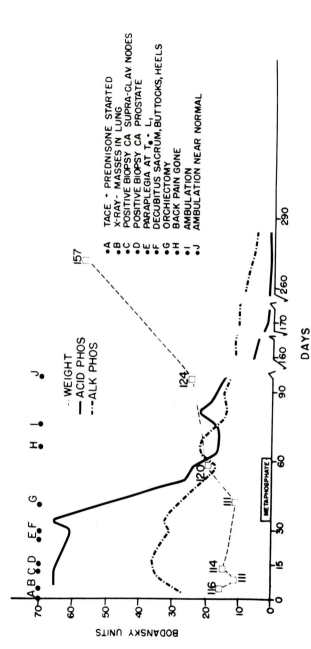

Fig. 20-6. The clinical course of a terminal patient with metastatic carcinoma of the prostate to bone showing response to combined ^{32}P-polyphosphate and hormonal therapy.

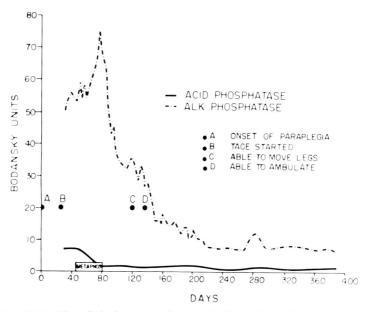

Fig. 20-7. The clinical course of a paraplegic patient with metastatic carcinoma of the prostate demonstrating return of the alkaline and acid phosphatase to normal, reversal of paraplegia, and the return of ability to walk on combined estrogen ^{32}P=polyphosphate therapy.

while the preparation remained commercially available. Only one known study using ^{32}P-polyphosphate was published following the author's work. Corwin et al.[36] studied 20 patients. Eight patients received combination estrogen therapy, which resulted in pain relief in six. Another group of 12 patients received combination testosterone therapy, and 10 of these patients experienced pain relief. X-ray evaluation following therapy was not adequately reported. Hall et al.[37] evaluated ^{32}P-diphosphonate as a potential therapeutic agent in 1975.

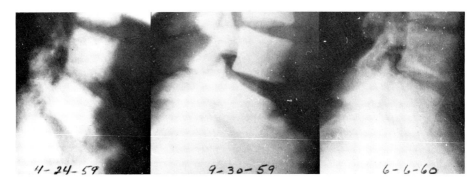

Fig. 20-8. The lumbar vertebrae of the patient in Fig. 20-7 at indicated intervals show transition from marked metastatic involvement to hypermineralization to return of normal trabecular bone pattern.

HISTORICAL CONCLUSION

Specific conclusions can be made based on 30 years of clinical experience using ^{32}P and documentation in more than 20 publications by a variety of investigators in more than 300 patients.

1. Relief of pain occurred in 87 percent of the patients treated for bone metastases.
2. The experience was almost exclusively determined with patients having carcinoma of the prostate and breast.
3. The significant adverse side effect of ^{32}P therapy in any form or with any supportive modality was bone marrow depression.

Tentative conclusions can be made concerning the following:

1. A variety of ancillary hormonal therapies may enhance therapeutic benefit by ^{32}P-orthophosphate. These include treatment with testosterone, estrogen, and parathormone, as well as orchiectomy and adrenalectomy. Hormonal therapy may produce adverse side effects.
2. The use of ^{32}P-polyphosphate may enhance the delivery of radiation dosage to reactive bone surrounding metastatic lesions by increasing the concentration in proportion to the severity of the lesion, while sparing radiation dosage to soft tissue and the whole body.

Specific suggestions can be made from the historical experience described.

1. ^{32}P therapy appears to have a useful role in the palliative therapy for skeletal metastases from prostate and breast and should probably be more widely applied.
2. Whole-body bone scanning with technetium-labeled polyphosphate, diphosphonate, and pyrophosphate should be used as an indicator of severity of disease and perhaps of response to therapy. These bone-seeking agents made with therapeutic quantities of ^{32}P should be evaluated in adequate prospective clinical trials for possible superior palliation.
3. Combination therapy by pretreatment with testosterone, estrogen, and parathormone should be evaluated with polyphosphate, diphosphonate, and pyrophosphate. Pretreatment with agents capable of enhancing immune response to tumor in bone and enhancing reactivity and bone mineralization about metastatic lesions should also be evaluated.
4. Simultaneous therapy with the radioactive phosphate bone seekers should be studied using combination therapy with chemotherapeutic agents and specific hormonal agents such as estrogen in prostatic carcinoma in bone.
5. Such combination therapy should be used in early metastatic disease to bone identified by bone scanning and preceded by vigorous surgical obliteration of the primary lesion in prostatic cancer. The long-term prognosis of early or minimal bone lesions may be altered by such intensive therapy.

^{32}P may yet have a significant role in therapy for metastatic bone disease.

REFERENCES

1. Brucer, M.: Vignettes in Nuclear Medicine, Nos. 80–83. St. Louis, Mallinckrodt, 1975, 1976.
2. Kaplan, E.: Hand-Book Series in Clinical Laboratory Science, D. Seligson and R. P. Spencer (eds.). Cleveland, CRC Press, pp. 476–483, 1977.
3. Storaasli, J.: The role of radiotherapy and radioactive phosphorus (^{32}P). J.A.M.A. 210:1077–1078, 1969.
4. Chiewitz, O., Hevesy, G.: Radioactive indicators in study of phosphorus metabolism in rats. Nature 163:754–755, 1935.
5. Hamilton, J. G.: The metabolism of the fission products and the heaviest elements. Radiology 49:325–343, 1947.
6. Pecher, C.: Biological investigations with radioactive calcium and strontium. Proc. Soc. Exp. Biol. Med., 46:86–91, 1941.
7. Pecher, C.: Biological investigations with radioactive calcium and strontium: preliminary report on the use of radioactive strontium in treatment of metastatic bone cancer. University of California, Publications in Pharmacology 11:117–149, 1942.
8. Dudley, H. C., Munn, J. I., Henry, K. E.: Studies of the metabolism of gallium II. J. Pharm. Exp. Ther. 98:105–110, 1950.
9. Brucer, M., Bruner, H. D.: Physics and radiation characteristics of gallium. Radiology 61:537–543, 1953.
10. Friedell, H. L., Storaasli, J. P.: The use of radioactive phosphorus in the treatment of carcinoma of the breast wtih widespread metastasis to bone. Am. J. Roentgenol. 64:559–575, 1950.
11. Maxfield, J. R., Jr., Maxfield, J. G. S., Maxfield, W. S.: The use of radioactive phosphorus and testosterone in metastatic bone lesions from breast and prostate. South. Med. J. 51:320–327, 1958.
12. Vermooten, V., Maxfield, J. R., Jr., Maxfield, J. G.: The use of radioactive phosphorus in the management of advanced carcinoma of the prostate. West. J. Surg. 67:245–249, 1959.
13. Hertz, S.: Modifying effect of steroid hormone therapy of human neoplastic disease as judged by radioactive phosphorus studies. J. Clin. Invest. 29:821, 1950.
14. Kaplan, E., Miree, J., Hirsh, E., et al.: Autoradiographic localization of P^{32} phosphate in metastatic carcinoma of the breast to bone. Int. J. Appl. Radiat. Isot. 5:94–98, 1959.
15. Morales, A., Connally, J. G., Burr, R. C., et al.: The use of radioactive phosphorus to treat bone pain in metastatic carcinoma of the prostate. Can. Med. Assoc. J. 103:372–373, 1970.
16. Taber, K. W.: Current status of breast cancer treatment including radiophosphorus (P^{32}). W. Va. Med. J. 51:171–174, 1955.
17. Wildermuth, O., Parker, V., Archambeau, J. O., et al.: The management of diffuse metastasis from carcinoma of the prostate. J.A.M.A. 172:1607–1116, 1960.
18. Mandel, P. R., Chiot, H.: Radioactive phosphorus for carcinoma of the breast with diffuse metastatic bone disease. N.Y.J. Med. 62:1970–1976, 1962.
19. Parsons, R. L.: Experience with P-32 in treatment of metastatic carcinoma of prostate: a preliminary report. J. Urol. 85:342–344, 1961.
20. Parsons, R. L., Campbell, J. L., Thomley, M. W.: Experiences with P-32 in the treatment of metastatic carcinoma of the prostate: a follow-up report. J. Urol. 88:812–813, 1962.
21. Smart, J. G.: The use of P-32 in the treatment of severe pain from bone metastases in carcinoma of the prostate. Br. J. Urol. 37:139–147, 1965.
22. Joshi, D. P., Seery, W. H., Goldberg, L. G., et al.: Evaluation of phosphorus 32 for

intractable pain secondary to prostatic carcinoma metastatis. J.A.M.A. 193:621–623, 1965.

23. Dontai, R. M., Ellis, H., Gallagher, N. I.: Testosterone potentiated ^{32}P therapy in prostatic carcinoma. Cancer 19:1088–1090, 1966.
24. Morin, L. J., Stevens, J. C.: Radioactive phosphorus in the treatment of metastasis to bone from carcinoma of the prostate. J. Urol. 97:130–132, 1967.
25. Storaasli, J. P., King, R. L., Krieger, H., et al.: Palliation of osseous metastases from breast carcinoma with radioactive phosphorus alone and in combination with adrenalectomy. Radiology 76:422–430, 1961.
26. Tong, E. C. K., Rubenfeld, S.: The treatment of bone metastasis with parathormone followed by radiophosphorus. Am. J. Roentgenol. 99:422–434, 1967.
27. Tong, E. C. K.: Parathormone and P-32 therapy in prostatic cancer with bone metastases. Radiology 98:343–351, 1971.
28. Pinck, B. D., Alexander, S.: Parathormone. Potentiated radiophosphorus therapy in prostatic carcinoma. Urology 1:201–204, 1973.
29. Merrin, C., Bakshi, S.: Treatment of metastatic carcinoma of the prostate to bone with parathormone and radioactive phosphorus. J. Surg. Oncol. 6:67–72, 1974.
30. Rubenfeld, S.: Editorial: Treatment of bone metastasis from carcinoma of prostate with parathyroid hormone and radioactive phosphorus. Urology 1:268–269, 1973.
31. Kitasato, T.: Uber Meta-phosphatase. Biochem. Zeit, 197:257–258, 1928.
32. Kitasato, T.: Weitere Untersuchungan Uber die Meta-phosphatase. Biochem. Z. 201:206–211, 1928.
33. Fels, I. G., Kaplan, E., Greco, J., et al.: Incorporation in vivo of P^{32} from condensed phosphates. Proc. Soc. Exp. Biol. Med. 100:53–55, 1959.
34. Jones, L. T.: Seminars on pyro-, meta-, and polyphosphate in the presence of one another. Indust. Eng. Chem. Anal. 14:536–542, 1942.
35. Kaplan, E., Fels, I. G., Kotlowski, B. R., et al.: Therapy of carcinoma of the prostate metastic to bone with P^{32} labeled condensed phosphate. J. Nucl. Med. 1:1–13, 1960.
36. Corwin, S. H., Malament, M., Sonall, M., et al.: Experience with P-32 in advanced carcinoma of the prostate. J. Urol. 104:745–748, 1970.
37. Hall, J. N., Tokars, R. P. O'Mara, R. E.: P-32 diphosphonate: a potential therapeutic agent. J. Nucl. Med. 16:532, 1975.

Thomas P. Haynie and Douglas E. Johnson

21

Androgen-Parathormone Primed Phosphorus 32 for Intractable Pain in Carcinoma of the Prostrate

INTRODUCTION

The management of advanced carcinoma of the prostrate often involves the alleviation of severe pain caused by extensive osseous metastases. When hormonal manipulation fails to control symptoms and the extent of disease precludes palliative external radiotherapy, treatment with radioactive phosphorus has been recommended.[1-19]

There is disagreement concerning the best method of administering this therapy. In 1950 Hertz[19] demonstrated that the uptake of phosphorus in new bone formation could be increased 15 to 20 times by the concomitant administration of testosterone. Tong and coworkers,[13,15] however, observed the intensification of bone pain that frequently accompanied the use of testosterone, and proposed an alternate drug regimen that included parathormone administration. Tong hypothesized that there would be an increase in the deposition of radiophosphorus in bone and tumor upon withdrawal of parathormone.

We previously reported a review of our experience with testosterone-^{32}P therapy at M. D. Anderson Hospital.[16] Since testosterone and parathormone presumably involve different mechanisms for enhancing ^{32}P uptake, we reasoned that combining the two might produce an even greater effect, and therefore began treating a series of patients with testosterone and parathormone ^{32}P.

MATERIALS AND METHODS

Patient Selection

Nine patients with histologically verified prostatic carcinoma who were treated at M. D. Anderson Hospital and Tumor Institute from June 1973 to July 1976 were included in the study. The patients ranged in age from 55 to 72 years, with an average age of 63.4 years. Six patients had been treated with orchidectomy and prlonged estrogen administration. In addition to orchidectomy and estrogen therapy, one patient had received chemotherapy with 5-fluorouracil, cyclophosphamide, and streptozotocin. Two patients had received palliative radiotherapy prior to ^{32}P therapy. Widespread metastases were demonstrated scintiphotographically and radiographically in all patients; in each case a ^{99m}Tc-polyphosphate or pyrophosphate bone scan showed abnormal uptake in the metastatic areas. All patients had severe bone pain that was incompletely controlled with large amounts of analgesics and narcotics. Many patients had also received external irradiation in an attempt to control metastatic bone pain.

Treatment Method

All patients were admitted to the hospital and estrogen therapy was discontinued. Testosterone was given intramuscularly in the form of testosterone cypionate, 100 mg daily for 15 days. Intramuscular injections of 100 IU parathormone were administered three times daily for 5 days. Twenty-four hours after the last parathormone injection, intravenous injections of 5 mCi radioactive sodium phosphate-^{32}P were given on each of two consecutive days. Estrogen therapy was resumed after the last injection of testosterone.

Assessment of Treatment Effect

Patients responses were arbitrarily defined as: (1) the patient had complete alleviation of pain and was able to resume usual activities without analgesics or narcotics; (2) the patient resumed normal activities with minimal discomfort that was relieved by the infrequent use of analgesics; (3) pain was reduced, but the frequent use of analgesics or narcotics was required; (4) there was no improvement in the patient's symptoms or the symptoms progressed during and immediately following therapy.

RESULTS

Clinical Observation

Pertinent clinical observations are shown in Table 21-1. For patients who responded to treatment, a noticeable reduction in the severity of pain was experienced between the third and fifth days after completion of intravenous injections of ^{32}P. The duration of response varied from 2 to 6 months, with maximal relief lasting approximately 3 months. One patient (case 4) received a second reduced dose of 6.5 mCi ^{32}P four months after the first and achieved a fair response. Two patients received palliative external radiotherapy following ^{32}P therapy.

Laboratory Observations

Follow-up x-ray and laboratory studies were obtained for six patients, and the results are shown in Table 21-2. Varying degrees of thrombocytopenia developed in every case, usually becoming apparent 4 to 6 weeks after the therapy and in

Table 21-1
Clinical Observations in Patients Receiving ^{32}P for Prostate Carcinoma

Case No.	Age	Previous Therapy	Scintiphotographic Findings	Response to Therapy	Survival after Therapy (Months)
1	72	Orchidectomy and estrogens	Abnormal foci skull, shoulder girdles, ribs, spine, pelvis, femora	Good	3
2	62	Orchidectomy and estrogens	Abnormal diffusely throughout axial skeleton	Excellent	4
3	55	Orchidectomy and estrogens	Abnormal diffusely throughout axial skeleton	Good	6
4	54	XRT to lumbosacral spine	Abnormal foci spine, ribs, pelvis	Good	6
5	69	Orchidectomy and estrogens	Abnormal diffusely throughout axial skeleton	Excellent	9
6	70	Orchidectomy and estrogens	Abnormal foci skull, spine, ribs, pelvis, humeri, femora	Fair	3
7	69	Estrogens	Abnormal diffusely in axial skeleton	Fair	3
8	55	Orchidectomy, estrogens, and chemotherapy	Abnormal diffusely and focally in axial skeleton	Fair	3*
9	65	XRT to neck and right hip; estrogens	Abnormal foci skull, chest, spine, pelvis, femora	Poor	3*

*Lost to follow-up.

253

Table 21-2
Laboratory Observations in Patients Receiving ^{32}P for Prostate Carcinoma

Case No.	Change in Radiography	Alkaline Phosphatase (m-IU/ml) Before/After	% Change	Prostatic Acid Phosphatase (IU/L) Before/After	% Change
2	Progression of multiple metastases	313/248	−21	0.77/0.21	−73
3	Progression of metastatic disease in spine, ribs, pelvis	350/350	0	14.5/53.1	+73
4	Progression of metastatic disease in axial skeleton	255/184	−28	0.92/1.01	+9
5	Progression of metastatic disease in spine & ribs	350/230	−34	0.61/0.16	−73
7	Progression of metastatic disease	350/350	0	0.86/3.2	+73
8	Progression of metastatic disease	350/192	−45	72.8/38.2	−48

several instances persisting until death. In no case, however, was this complication the direct cause of death. All patients displayed progression of metastatic disease on x-ray films obtained after therapy. New bone formation may account for changes in the x-ray films, for it is paradoxical that symptoms appeared to be improving at the same time that the x-ray films showed disease progression. Follow-up scintigrams were not obtained.

Hemoglobin and white blood cell and platelet counts generally decreased after therapy; and most patients required blood transfusions at one time or another. No major complications were associated with these changes.

Phosphatase levels either declined moderately or did not change; however, in one patient (case 3) the prostatic acid phosphatase level increased strikingly within 2 months after therapy at the same time that the patient was showing a good response to therapy.

Other Observations

Two patients (cases 2 and 3) developed evidence of spinal cord compression after therapy. Whether this was related to therapy cannot be determined. Because of previous experience indicating a worsening of neurological symptoms associated with testosterone therapy, patients with premonitory symptoms were excluded from the study.

DISCUSSION

Relief of pain has been obtained in approximately 86 percent of the patients who received testosterone-potentiated ^{32}P therapy. In this series, which combined parathormone rebound and androgen, the response rate was not greatly different from that expected with androgen priming alone. The expectation that a combined preparation would produce a greater therapeutic effect was apparently correct for bone marrow but not for tumor. This series of patients differed from those treated with testosterone alone in that thrombocytopenia, leukopenia, and anemia developed in many patients. This bone marrow depression has been noted by others who have combined testosterone and parathormone priming.[17]

The failure to achieve complete relief from pain in these patients was not unexpected and does not detract from the benefits derived from ^{32}P therapy. Selected patients were in the terminal stage of their disease. In addition to widespread skeletal metastases, visceral and soft tissue metastases may have been present. Currently, androgen priming alone appears to be the simplest and most effective priming method for sodium phosphate ^{32}P therapy in the control of intractable pain due to extensive osseous metastases from prostatic carcinoma. We look forward to evaluating the newer radionuclides and radioactive compounds currently under development for this form of therapy.

REFERENCES

1. Maxfield, J. R., Jr., Maxfield, J. G. S., Maxfield, W. S.: The use of radioactive phosphorus and testosterone in metastatic bone lesions from breast and prostate. South. Med. J. 51:320–327, 1958.
2. Vermooten, V., Maxfield, J. R., Jr., Maxfield, J. G. S.: The use of radioactive phosphorus in the management of advanced carcinoma of the prostrate. West. J. Surg. 67:245–249, 1959.
3. Kaplan, E., Fels, I. G., Kotlowski, B. R., et al.: Therapy of carcinoma of the prostate metastatic to bone with ^{32}P labeled condensed phosphate. J. Nucl. Med. 1:1–3, 1960.
4. Wildermuth, O., Parker, D., Archambeau, J. O., et al.: Management of diffuse metastasis from carcinoma of the prostate. J.A.M.A. 172:1607–1611, 1960.
5. Parsons, R. L.: Experiences with ^{32}P in treatment of metastatic carcinoma of prostate: A preliminary report. J. Urol. 85:342–344, 1961.
6. Parsons, R. L., Campbell, J. H., Thomley, M. W.: Experiences with P[32] in the treatment of metastatic carcinoma of the prostate. A followup report. J. Urol. 88:812–813, 1962.
7. Smart, J. G., Lond, M. B.: Radioactive phosphorus treatment of bone-metastatic carcinoma of the prostate. Lancet 2:882–883, 1964.
8. Smart, J. G.: The use of P[32] in the treatment of severe pain from bone metastases of carcinoma of the prostate. Br. J. Urol. 37:139–147, 1965.
9. Joshi, D. P., Seery, W. H., Goldberg, L. G., et al.: Evaluation of phosphorus-32 for intractable pain secondary to prostatic carcinoma metastases. J.A.M.A. 193:621–623, 1965.
10. Walton, R. J.: Palliative treatment of osseous metastases from carcinoma of the breast and carcinoma of the prostate with radioactive phosphorus and testosterone. J. Can. Assoc. Radiol. 16:213–216, 1965.

11. Donati, R. M., Ellis, H., Gallagher, N. I.: Testosterone potentiated ^{32}P therapy in prostatic carcinoma. Cancer 19:1088–1090, 1966.
12. Morin, L. J., Stevens, J. C.: Radioactive phosphorus in the treatment of metastasis to bone from carcinoma of the prostate. J. Urol. 97:130–132, 1967.
13. Tong, E. C. K., Rubenfeld, S.: The treatment of bone metastases with parathormone followed by radiophosphorus. Am. J. Roentgenol. 99:422–434, 1967.
14. Corwin, S. H., Malament, M., Small, M., et al.: Experiences with P-32 in advanced carcinoma of the prostate. J. Urol. 104:745–748, 1970.
15. Tong, E. C. K.: Parathormone and ^{32}P therapy in prostatic cancer with bone metastases. Radiology 98:343–351, 1971.
16. Johnson, D. E., Haynie, T. P.: Phosphorus-32 for intractable pain in carcinoma of the prostate. Tex. Med. 67:57–59, 1971.
17. Rodriguez-Antunez, A., Cook, S. A., Jelden, G. L., et al.: Management of primary and metastatic carcinoma of the prostate by the radiotherapist. Am. J. Roentgenol. 118:876–880, 1973.
18. Edland, R. W.: Testosterone potentiated radiophosphorus therapy of osseous metastases in prostatic cancer. Am. J. Roentgenol. 120:678–683, 1974.
19. Hertz, S.: Modifying effect of steroid hormone therapy of human neoplastic disease as judged by radioactive phosphorus (P-32) studies. J. Clin. Invest. 29:821, 1950.

Robert E. O'Mara

22
New ^{32}P Compounds in Therapy
for Bone Lesions

Treatment of patients suffering from advanced metastatic carcinoma to bone resulting in intractable bone pain presents a very difficult clinical problem, despite
many reports of at least palliative success in trials with ^{32}P-orthophosphate. This
use of radiophosphorus in the treatment of metastatic carcinoma has never gained
wide acceptance. Lawrence and coworkers[1] in the 1940s investigated the treatment of leukemias and lymphomas with ^{32}P. Friedell and Storaasli[2] in 1950 published their experience for the treatment of osseous metastatic carcinoma of the
breast using testosterone in combination with ^{32}P. This therapy resulted in calcifica-
tion and control of the lesions for periods as long as 6 years. Hertz[3] noted in 1950
that exogenous androgens resulted in increased deposition of radiophosphorus in
newly developed bone. Maxfield and coworkers[4] in 1958 suggested the combination of radiophosphorus with androgens in the management of osseous metastatic
breast neoplasm.

More recently, studies by Tong and Rubenfeld[5,6] have demonstrated the beneficial effects of pretreatment with parathormone followed by radiophosphorus for
the treatment of diffuse bony metastatic bone lesions from prostatic and breast
carcinoma. The theory behind this is that the rebound effect caused when
parathormone is withdrawn results in an increased uptake of ^{32}P in bone and
osseous metastatic tumors.

All of these attempts at treatment with orthophosphate take advantage of the
fact that the radiation dose from the ^{32}P will destroy neoplastic tissue. Maxfield's
group demonstrated that ^{32}P uptake in bone neoplasm is greater than that in the
same neoplasm in soft tissue and also greater than that in normal bone. However,
the isotopic uptake differential between neoplastic and normal osseous tissue is not
great enough to allow cancerocidal doses to be administered without significant
damage to surrounding normal tissue, including bone marrow. Testosterone and
parathormone have been utilized in attempts to allow augmentation of the uptake
of ^{32}P in neoplastic bony areas. Unfortunately, testosterone, which apparently
stimulates new bone formation, also results in an exacerbation of bone pain. The
use of testosterone does appear to reduce the severity of unwanted marrow response to ^{32}P.

The use of parathormone for enhancement of ^{32}P uptake as described by Tong and Rubenfeld is based on the fact that the parathormone desaturates calcium and phosphorus from the matrix of bone and increases urinary phosphate excretion. When parathormone is withdrawn, a rebound effect occurs resulting in high phosphorus accumulation in bone. One advantage that the parathormone treatment appears to offer is that the initial increase in bone pain that accompanies testosterone administration is not seen.[7] The disadvantages are the need to maintain adequate hydration in the patient in order to prevent the formation of renal calculi and the inability to apply this process with parathormone in patients suffering from preexisting renal disease.

Treatment with ^{32}P following either of these preadministration techniques is such that most people now prefer to use 1 to 2 mCi of ^{32}P intravenously over a 7- to 12-day period with a total dose of 10 to 12 mCi. The radioactive material may also be given orally. Most groups report substantial palliative effects, but deleterious hematopoietic effects of the standard ^{32}P-orthophosphate administration are frequently seen as noted in the preceding chapter.[4,5,7-10] The platelet count is prominently decreased, usually between 4 to 8 weeks following therapy. The hematopoietic effects appear to be less severe in patients pretreated with testosterone rather than parathormone.

Because of the difficulties with standard forms of treatment, other forms of ^{32}P have been evaluated. Kaplan et al.[11] reported their results utilizing a ^{32}P-labeled polymetaphosphate ("condensed phosphate") without pretreatment regimens in 1960. In eight patients with metastatic prostatic neoplasms, they achieved good relief of symptoms in four, minor relief in three, and no change in one. They also experienced a transient leukocyte drop and decreased alkaline and acid phosphatase serum levels as well as radiographic evidence of healing. In addition, they suggest that a combined estrogen and polymetaphosphate treatment regimen may produce a synergistic palliative effect.

Hall and coworkers[12] proposed in 1975 that ^{32}P-labeled diphosphonate be utilized. They demonstrated that in Fischer-344 rats, the bone marrow ratio for ^{32}P-diphosphonate was similar to that of ^{32}P-orthophosphate at 24 hours postintravenous administration but approximately double at 5 to 7 days. Diphosphonates have been shown to inhibit hydroxyapatite dissolution in vitro and bone resorption and tissue culture in vivo.[13] They inhibit bone resorption induced by parathyroid extract in mouse calvaria. Oral administration of diphosphonate has been used in the treatment of Paget's disease and myositis ossificans resulting in a decrease of the alkaline phosphatase in plasma and hydroxyproline in plasma and urine.[14,15] This decrease usually reaches half of the initial value after 2 to 3 months of therapy. This suggested that the diphosphonate may reduce excessive bone turnover in conditions such as Paget's disease. Clinical trials by Ferman et al.[15,16] demonstrate improvement in clinical symptoms and bone scans in such patients. Cessation of therapy results in return of biochemical and clinical evidence of the disease.

In 1976 Francis and coworkers[17] reported on the distribution and effect of ^{32}P-labeled EHDP (ethane-1-hydroxy-1, 1-diphosphonate) both in dogs that were normal and in those carrying osteogenic sarcoma. They demonstrated palliative effects in the tumor-bearing animals and suggested that this agent might represent a reasonable choice for treatment of osseous neoplastic disease. This group also studied the use of [32]P- and ^{33}P-radiolabeled EHDP in comparison to ^{32}P-pyrophosphate and ^{32}P-orthophosphate in rats.[18] They noted markedly increased bone to muscle and bone to bone marrow retention rates for the labeled EHDP in comparison to the others and felt that this indicated that the EHDP would give significantly lower total radiation exposure to the patient despite adequate treatment doses. In addition, they suggested that the use of ^{33}P, with its lower energy beta particle, would also further reduce patient and marrow exposure. Bigler et al.[19] suggested that ^{32}P-EHDP may be of value as an adjuvant to present methods of managing osteogenic sarcoma patients as a result of the high uptakes and similar patterns of distribution between this compound and ^{99m}Tc-labeled diphosphonates in patients with osteogenic sarcoma.

Potsaid et al.[20] also reported in 1976 on a group of five patients with stage IV prostatic carcinoma treated with ^{32}P-EHDP. Within this group, two received 3 mCi of ^{32}P-EHDP a week apart and three patients received a single 3-mCi dose. In the 9-mCi total dose pair, one patient underwent a drop in peripheral white count and platelets but made a good recovery from his bone marrow depression and had relief of pain. No change was noted in the other. Two of the patients given the single-dose regimen had no change in any parameters monitored as well as no relief of bone pain. Their work would suggest that despite the highly specific bone activity, marrow competence must be assessed prior to attempted palliation even with the diphosphonates.

McCormack (*unpublished observations*) followed a group of 40 patients with osseous metastatic cancer whom he treated with 2 to 2.5 mCi of ^{32}P-EHDP every day for four to five doses. No pretreatments were given, but any prior estrogen therapy was stopped 3 to 5 days commencing the regimen. He reports a good palliative response in 60 percent of these patients with periods of relief lasting 6 months or longer. However, in his experience, there has been no effect on patient longevity and marrow depression remains a problem.

Despite the repeated success many investigators have had with ^{32}P treatment of widespread osseous metastatic disease, this treatment has failed to gain wide acceptance. I feel that the one reason for this is the marked complexity involved in the use of pretreatment agents, such as testosterone and/or parathormone. The early investigative work with ^{32}P-labeled EHDP offers promise of a mechanism to increase localized bone radiation dose while decreasing or holding constant the marrow and total-body dose as well as avoiding complicated therapeutic regimens. However, a basic concept remains important, even with possibly improved agents. Patient evaluation is necessary in a preselection mode. Patients to be selected should (1) have evidence of widespread metastatic disease to bone, (2) be in pain, and (3) demonstrate adequate marrow function and reserve. This last item is most important, since most patients to be considered for this type of therapy will also have undergone or be involved in a therapeutic regime utilizing marrow-depressing chemotherapeutic agents or radiotherapy. Further investigative and clinical work is necessary to fully assess the practicality of applying the organic diphosphonate as a more simplified mechanism of treatment for patients suffering from this condition. Such work should be a correlated effort with standardized patient evaluations, dosage regimens, and follow-up in order to avoid the hodgepodge approach currently available in the literature. Only then can we expect to be able to offer patients a reasonable hope of palliation with a simple treatment program involving the use of radiophosphorus as a treatment in osseous metastatic neoplasm.

REFERENCES

1. Lawrence, J. H., Tuttle, L. W., Scott, K. G. et al.: Studies on neoplasms with the aid of radioactive phosphorus. 1. The total phosphorus metabolism of normal and leukemic mice. J. Clin. Invest. 19:267–271, 1940.
2. Friedell, H. L., Storaasli, J. P.: Use of radioactive phosphorus in treatment of carcinoma of the breast with widespread metastases to bone. Am. J. Roentgenol. 64:559–575, 1950.
3. Hertz, S.: Modifying effect of steroid hormone therapy of human neoplastic disease as judged by radioactive phosphorus (P-32) studies. J. Clin. Invest. 29:821, 1950.
4. Maxfield, J. R., Jr., Maxfield, J. G., Maxfield, W. S.: Use of radioactive phosphorus and testosterone in metastatic bone lesions from breast and prostate. South. Med. J. 51:320–327, 1958.
5. Tong, E. C. K., Rubenfeld, S.: The treatment of bone metastases with parathormone followed by radiophosphorus. Am. J. Roentgenol. 99:422–434, 1967.
6. Tong, E. C. K.: Parathormone and ^{32}P therapy in prostatic cancer with bone metastases. Radiology 98:343–351, 1971.
7. Pinck, B. D., Alexander, S.: Parathormone-potentiated radiophosphorus therapy in prostatic carcinoma. Urology 1:201–204, 1973.
8. Morin, L. J., Stevens, J. C.: Radioactive phosphorus in the treatment of metastasis to bone from carcinoma of the prostate. J. Urol. 97:130–132, 1967.
9. Morales, A., Burr, R. C., Bruce, A. W.: The use of radioactive phosphorus to treat bone pain in metastatic carcinoma in the prostate. Can. Med. Assoc. J. 103:372–373, 1970.
10. Donati, R. M., Ellis, H., Gallagher, N. I.: Testosterone potentiated ^{32}P therapy in prostatic carcinoma. Cancer 19:1088–1090, 1966.
11. Kaplan, E., Fels, I. G., Kotlowski, B. R., et al.: Therapy of carcinoma of the prostate metastatic to bone with P^{32} labeled condensed phosphate. J. Nucl. Med. 1:1–13, 1960.
12. Hall, J. N., Tokars, R. P., O'Mara, R. E.: P-32 diphosphonate: a potential therapeutic agent. J. Nucl. Med. 16:532, 1975 (Abst.).
13. Fleisch, H., Russell, R. G. G., Francis, M. D.: Diphosphonates inhibit hydroxyapatite dissolution in vitro and bone resorption in tissue culture and in vivo. Science 165:1262–1264, 1969.
14. Smith, R., Russell, R. G. G., Bishop, M.: Diphosphonates and Paget's disease of bone. Lancet 1:945–947, 1971.
15. Weiss, I. W., Fisher, L., Phang, J. M.: Diphosphonate therapy in a patient with mysitis ossificans progressiva. Ann. Intern. Med. 74:933–936, 1971.
16. Finerman, G. A. M., Gonick, H. C., Smith, R. K., et al.: Diphosphonate treatment of Paget's disease. Clin. Orthop. 120:115–124, 1976.
17. Francis, M. D., Slouth, C. L., Tofe, A. J.: Distribution and effect of P-32 EHDP in normal and bone tumor bearing dogs. J. Nucl. Med. 17:548, 1976 (Abst.).
18. Tofe, A. J., Francis, M. D., Slough, C. L., et al.: P-33 EHDP and P-32 (EHDP, PPi, and Pi) tissue distribution in considerations of palliative treatment for osseous neoplasms. J. Nucl. Med. 17:548, 1976 (Abst.).
19. Bigler, R. E., Rosen, G., Tofe, A. J., et al.: Comparative distribution of P-32 and Tc-99m diphosphonates in patients with osteogenic sarcoma. J. Nucl. Med. 17:548, 1976 (Abst.).
20. Potsaid, M., Irwin, R., Castronovo, F., et al.: Phosphorus-32 EHDP clinical study of patients with prostate carcinoma bone metastases. J. Nucl. Med. 17:548–549, 1976 (Abst.).

Savita Puri and Richard P. Spencer

23
Intralesional Therapy

By intralesional therapy we mean deposition of the chemotherapeutic or radioactive material directly into the lesion. That is, it is introduced into the region of interest without passing through systemic pathways. There are several ways in which this can be accomplished; these can be divided into two major categories:

1. Direct approach: By injecting the therapeutic agent directly into the lesion.
   a. Skin lesion.
   b. Ocular lesion—injecting under microscopic control.
   c. Internal lesion—introducing the agent via injection guided by scan, radiograph, or other modality.
2. Indirect approach: Delivery of the therapeutic agent into the lesion by routes other than direct injection.
   a. Transbronchial—treating lesions connected with the bronchial tree.
   b. Intrapleural injection.
   c. Endoarterial injection—i.e., into the vessel feeding the tumor.
   d. Endolymphatic injection—i.e., into the lymphatics by selective catheterization.

Before dwelling on this, we must inquire as to the rationale of such therapy. If we institute a different means of therapy, do the benefits far outweigh the risks? There are several advantages to intralesional therapy.

1. A small benefit, but one which may have great psychological significance for the patient, is that some skin lesions can be made to regress by direct injection. The patient's elation at observing the regression of a tumor, no matter how small, cannot be neglected.
2. The destruction of a skin metastatic tumor prevents it from serving as a focus for further spread of the neoplasm. Hence, not only is there local benefit, but additional spread may be slowed.

Supported by U.S. Public Health Service Grant CA 17802 from the National Cancer Institute.

3. The radiation dose delivered to a tumor by intralesional therapy with radionuclides can be very high. If alpha or beta ray emitters are utilized, the radiation exposure of surrounding tissue is negligible. Hence, additional radiation via external sources can be used if necessary. In a way this is like delivering a massive radiation dose to the center of a tumor and a much smaller dose elsewhere. The combination of intralesional therapy and then external irradiation requires much additional study.

4. As tumor tissue is destroyed, various products are discharged into the bloodstream. Some of these are tumor-related antigens. Apparently, antibody production occurs or there are other abscopal effects. That is, the destruction of local tumor is often associated with the regression of tumor elsewhere.

5. Several tumors are unresectable because of their extent or location, such as tumors situated in the vital organs or in their close proximity. These lesions could conceivably be treated by intraarterial injection of highly energetic particles by selective catheterization of the major tumor-feeding blood vessel. Under such circumstances an invasive procedure such as catheterization is less of a life threat than surgery, and yet might have hope for tumor regression.

6. It has been shown that certain tumors (e.g., malignant melanoma) are radiosensitive in vitro but radioresistant in vivo. This radioresistance to external radiation therapy is partly attributed to low oxygen tension in the tumor. In such situations where external radiotherapy fails, intralesional therapy with radioisotopes might have some promise. High-energy particles deposited directly into the lesion will have a better chance to kill the cells.

7. Prophylactic radiation of the lymphatic system via endolymphatic injection of radiocolloids, before detectable metastases occur, may be needed if we are treating the patients for cure.

The basis for trying one type of intralesional therapy, immunotherapy, was that the chemically induced sarcomas in animals were shown to be antigenic.[1,2] The host could thus potentially be made to develop an immune response against its tumor. At the turn of the century, Calmette and Guerin had developed an attenuated strain of *Myocobacterium bovis* which became known as the bacillus Calmette-Guerin, or BCG. During studies of the immune response to tuberculosis, after administration of BCG, it was noted that immunity to other apparently antigenically unrelated bacteria was also increased. This led to the concept of a heightened immune response, and the use of BCG in attempted immunotherapy of tumors. For example, Zbar and coworkers[3] used direct injection of a modified BCG into intradermal transplants of a guinea pig tumor. Not only did the tumors regress, but the animals failed to show lymph node metastases. Further, many of these guinea pigs rejected later transplants of the tumor, suggesting systemic tumor immunity. Attempts to modify the immune response of the body have also proceeded by intradermal injection of BCG,[4] by use of PPD and components of the immune system,[5] and by a variety of other techniques.[6]

The criteria for successful use of BCG in tumor immunotherapy, by direct intratumor injection, can be listed as follows:[7]

1. The animal host must be immunologically competent.
2. A sufficient number of the BCG bacteria have to be injected.

3. The response is more favorable by direct injection into tumor within the skin; tumor in lymph nodes or muscle responds less completely.
4. The tumor burden must be small.

The last point leads directly to the intralesional use of chemotherapeutic agents or radionuclides. *If the tumor burden can be reduced, then immunotherapy or chemotherapy has a better chance of success.* Direct intralesional therapy with chemotherapeutic agents has been tried. Bast and coworkers[8] studied intradermal hepatoma cells in guinea pigs. These animals with intradermal tumors were not helped by intraperitoneal injection of drugs. However, cures were obtained with several intralesional injections of actinomycin D, 1-3-bis (2-chloroethyl)-1-nitrosourea, adriamycin, mitomycin D, or melphalan. The intradermal cures were obtained even when tumor cells were in the lymph nodes draining the area. The immune nature of the cure was shown by the later rejection, by these guinea pigs, of freshly injected tumor cells. An interesting variant was described by Takahashi and associates.[9] These workers prepared an emulsion of bleomycin, which they tested in animals and in eight patients by intralesional injection. Six of the eight patients with skin squamous cell carcinoma or recurrent adenocarcinoma of the breast responded to the intralesional therapy as shown by tumor regression.

If we are to attempt direct intralesional placement of radionuclides, what approaches are available? Table 23-1 lists some of the possibilities. The placement of removable sources of radiation into a tumor, such as wires or sutures, is being increasingly employed in the treatment of carcinoma of the breast.[10] This has been an area of interest to the radiation therapist, and it forms a bridge to the following discussion of direct introduction of nonremoveable radionuclides. By analogy to the use of chemotherapeutic agents in emulsion, radionuclides could be given in emulsion form. This has the potential of treating not only the tumor locally, but also the draining lymph nodes, as the drainage occurs into the regional lymph nodes. The number of radiopharmaceuticals capable of being emulsified is presently limited, but the number will increase in the future as lipid carriers such as liposomes are investigated.

Table 23-1
Possible Techniques of Intralesional Therapy with Radionuclides

Technique	Reference
1. Interstitial radiation with removable wire or sutures.	10
2. Local radionuclide injection in form of emulsion (by analogy to administration of anticancer agents).	9
3. Possible local application, by analogy to Moh's chemosurgery.	11
4. Direct introduction with uptake by an organ-specific function (radioiodide injection into thyroid?).	
5. Radiation via deposited nonremovable radionuclides, such as radiocolloids.	This chapter
6. Endoarterial injection.	12
7. Endolymphatic injection.	13

Another approach is provided by examining the Mohs technique of "chemosurgery."[11] Here a keratinolytic agent is applied to the tumor and a fixative is used so that a small piece of the tumor can be excised. The procedure is repeated until the final specimen reveals no tumor. The radionuclide equivalent would be one in which the radioactive agent diffused through all or part of a tumor. If a gamma ray emitting radionuclide were used, it might be possible to image the distribution and, hence, to delineate the boundaries of the tumor. If a pure beta ray emitter were utilized, application might be by "stages" to distribute the material throughout the tumor. A variant of this is theoretically possible and is shown as number 4 in Table 23-1. In selected cases, the directly introduced radionuclide might incorporate into a metabolic function of the tumor, thus limiting itself to the neoplasm. A conceptual example would be the direct injection of small quantities of radioiodide into the thyroid, with trapping within the gland.

The fifth approach noted in Table 23-1 is direct intratumor injection of non-removable radionuclides such as a radiocolloid. This provided the starting point for a number of studies in our laboratory. Obviously, some radioactivity will be lost as the tumor regresses.

Mouse sarcoma 180 was grown in the flank subcutaneously, and the tumor was allowed to attain a diameter of 1.2 cm. In 11 experimental tumors 0.08 ml (0.4 mCi) of ^{32}P-chromic phosphate was injected intralesionally, and in 5 control tumors 0.08 ml of saline was injected intralesionally. The tumors were measured daily in two dimensions. At the time of sacrifice the tumor, liver, and carcass were counted for ^{32}P.

Control tumors grew from 1.24 to 2.86 cm in diameter between days 8 and 24 ($\Delta = 2.86 - 1.24 = 1.62$ cm). The experimental tumors grew from 1.18 to 1.85 cm in diameter between days 8 and 24 ($\Delta = 1.85 - 1.18 = 0.67$ cm). Hence, the intralesional ^{32}P-chromic phosphate inhibited tumor growth.

Some ^{32}P escaped as shown by activity in the liver and carcass. Variants being pursued are multiple injections and use of agents to retard escape from the local site. Direct intralesional injection of cis-Pt(NH$_3$)$_2$ Cl$_2$ at 15 mg/kg in B16 melanoma resulted in melanoma regression but renal toxicity suggested escape from the local sites.

In summary, then, the activity of radiopharmaceuticals alone, in emulsion form or in combination with chemotherapeutic agents by direct or indirect route, will be of value in reducing the tumor burden, minimizing the systemic side effects, and treating unresectable tumors. Prophylactic irradiation of lymphomas by endolymphatic injection of radiocolloids may prove to be one useful variant of this mode of therapy.

REFERENCES

1. Foley, E. J.: Antigenic properties of methylcholanthrene-induced tumors of the strain of origin. Cancer Res. 13:835–837, 1953.
2. Prehn, R. T., Main, J. M.: Immunity to methylcholanthrene-induced sarcomas. J. Natl. Cancer Inst. 18:769–778, 1957.
3. Zbar, B., Ribi, E., Meyer, T.: Immunotherapy of cancer: regression of established

intradermal tumors after intralesional injection of mycobacterium cell wall attached to oil droplets. J. Natl. Cancer Inst. 52:1571–1577, 1974.

4. Eilber, F. R., Morton, D. L., Holmes, E. C., et al.: Adjuvant immunotherapy with BCG in treatment of regional-lymph node metastases from malignant melanoma. Engl. J. Med. 294:237–240, 1976.

5. Klein, E., Holtermann, O., Milgrom, H., et al.: Immunotherapy for accessible tumors utilizing delayed hypersensitivity reaction and separated components of the immune system. Med. Clin. North Am. 60:389–418, 1976.

6. Carter, S. K.: Immunotherapy of cancer in man. Am. Sci. 64:418–423, 1976.

7. Pliskin, M. E., Mastrangelo, M. J., Bellet, R., et al.: BCG immunotherapy of a mucous membrane malignant melanoma. Oral Surg. 42:73–79, 1976.

8. Bast, R. C., Jr., Segerling, M., Ohanian, S. H., et al.: Regression of established tumors and induction of tumor immunity by intratumor chemotherapy. J. Natl. Cancer Inst. 56:829–832, 1976.

9. Takahashi, T., Veda, S., Kono, K., et al.: Attempt at local administration of anti-cancer agents in the form of fat emulsion. Cancer 38:1507–1514, 1976.

10. Scott, W. P.: Surgical radiation therapy with vicryl-^{125}I absorbable sutures. Surg. Gynecol. Obstet. 142:667–670, 1976.

11. Olshansky, K., Robins, P.: Moh's chemosurgery and skin cancer. South. Med. J. 69:1126–1127, 1976.

12. Dogliotti, A. M., Caldersola, L., Badellino, F., et al.: Regional injection of radioisotopes in the treatment of malignant tumors. Int. J. Appl. Radiat. 17:51, 1968.

13. Lienen, E. J.: An appraisal of radioactive therapeutics lymphography. Am. J. Roentgenol. 93:110, 1965.

I. Ross McDougall, June K. Dunnick,
and Joseph P. Kriss

24
Therapeutic Implications of
Radiolabeled Vesicles

INTRODUCTION

The therapeutic uses of radionuclides and radiopharmaceuticals depend on their active localization in disease sites. If active uptake occurs, it is usually due to an alteration in physiology, such as an increase in blood supply, rather than to specific properties of the tumor actively concentrating the radiolabeled drug. This applies even in the treatment of functioning thyroid cancer, where it is necessary to ablate normal thyroid tissue before the neoplastic thyroid tissue will concentrate sufficient radioiodine for a therapeutic effect.

   The purpose of this chapter is to discuss a novel technique, in which packages of therapeutic (or diagnostic) agents are entrapped in minute lipid spheroids (vesicles) to be delivered to target sites. The communication describes the structure of vesicles, their method of production, and how they are loaded with radioactive materials. Techniques for altering the rate of release of the entrapped materials are described, and finally methods of directing the radiolabeled vesicles to target sites are discussed.

STRUCTURE AND PRODUCTION OF VESICLES

   Phospholipids, such as lecithin, form a monolayer when they are applied to an air-water interface. This is because the polar head group of the molecule is hydrophilic (mixes with water), whereas the nonpolar fatty acid chains are hydrophobic (do not mix with water) (Fig. 24-1). If the phospholipids are agitated and thoroughly mixed in an excess of water, the molecules form closed envelopes of lipids, each envelope consisting of a bilayer with a structure as shown in Figure 24-2. In this spherical structure the hydrophilic segments of the phospholipid molecules are in contact with the aqueous medium, whereas the hydrophobic segments are in contact with each other. At this stage the spherules consist of

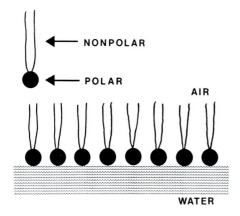

Fig. 24-1. The upper part of the figure shows diagrammatically the structure of a phospholipid molecule. The lower half of the diagram shows the orientation of phospholipid molecules at an air-water interphase. The hydrophilic segments (*circular parts*) are miscible in water, whereas the fatty acids (*linear parts*) are not.

multiple concentric phospholipid bilayers, separated from one another by aqueous layers. The multicompartmental onionlike structure is called a *liposome.*

Liposomes are an inhomogeneous collection of lipid spherules varying greatly in size from 500 Å to 1 to 2 μm in diameter. If the liposomal solution is subjected to ultrasonic irradiation by a probe or in a bath sonicator, progressively smaller envelopes are formed until a homogeneous population of single-compartment spheres surrounded by a single phospholipid bilayer is produced. The lipid composition of vesicles is not critical; lecithin, gangliosides, phosphatidic acid, and cholesterol are used most frequently. The exact composition and quantities used by several groups of investigators are to be found in references 1, 2, and 3. We have used 44 μmoles phosphatidylcholine (lecithin), 4 μmoles gangliosides as the standard constituents of artificial vesicles.

Since the membrane structure of the vesicle wall is similar to the lipid bilayer of biological membranes, these tiny spherules have been adopted by membranologists as research tools. They have provided valuable information about bilayer permeability, physical characteristics of phospholipids, phospholipid-protein interactions, and the effect of drugs and anesthetics on lipid bilayers.[4-7]

Recently, Dunnick and Kriss[8] have made vesicles by sonicating whole plasma from animals. These vesicles contain both lipids and protein, and provisional

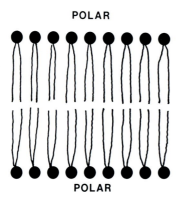

Fig. 24-2. Segment of vesicle membrane illustrating how the phospholipid molecules are orientated when there is an aqueous medium on both sides of the membrane.

analysis of human plasma vesicles indicates that they are composed of lecithin, cholesterol, cholesterol esters, and β globulins, probably lipoproteins.

LOADING OF VESICLES WITH RADIONUCLIDES

Provided the radionuclide (or drug) is water soluble, it can be entrapped within the central cavity of vesicles, or the multiple aqueous compartments of liposomes. The radioactive marker is dissolved in the aqueous medium to which the phospholipids are added. As the liposomes form, a proportion of buffer solution, and radioactivity, is enclosed by lipid bilayers. Sonication of liposomes causes fragmentation and reforming of the phospholipids until single compartmental vesicles are formed, the central cavity containing a proportion of the buffer and radioactive marker. The "labeled" liposomes or sonicated vesicles can be separated from the nonentrapped label by Sephadex or Sepharose gel filtration. Some investigators have purified labeled liposomes by ultracentrifugation; however, small single-compartmental vesicles do not centrifuge reliably.[9,10] In the experiments described below, we have used ^{99m}Tc (as pertechnetate TcO$_4^-$) as the radioactive marker, but we recognize that this would not be of therapeutic value. It is possible to entrap nonradioactive molecules such as proteins, hormones like insulin, and antitumor drugs which could have value in therapy.[2]

An alternative method of placing radioactivity within the central cavity of vesicles has been described by Gregoriadis et al.[1] who enclosed albumin in liposomes and iodinated the albumin with ^{125}I using the monochloride method. Similarly, transferrin has been entrapped and subsequently labeled within indium. All of these methods place the label within the central cavity of the vesicle. In addition, there are methods of introducing radiomarkers by incorporation into the membrane structure, or by chemical combination with active groups on the periphery of the vesicle. Phospholipids or cholesterol (^{3}H or ^{14}C labeled) are incorporated into vesicle membranes, and lipid-soluble drugs are positioned similarly. We have attached proteins, including labeled antibodies, to the outside of preformed vesicles by the carbodiimide reaction.[11] Possible sites of labeling vesicles are shown in Figure 24-3.

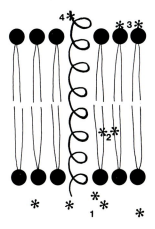

Fig. 24-3. Asterisks show potential site for labeling vesicles with radionuclides: (1) in central cavity; (2) in fatty acid chains; (3) to polar head groups; (4) to molecules incorporated into, or onto, the vesicle membrane.

CONTROL OF RATE OF RELEASE OF ENTRAPPED AGENT

It would be a great disadvantage if all of the therapeutic package escaped from the carrier system before reaching the desired target. It would also be a disadvantage if the entrapped agent, a drug that acts on a specific intracellular organelle, could not escape across the limiting membrane of the vesicle. There is now considerable knowledge of how the lipid constituents of the phospholipid bilayer, the method of production of vesicles, and the properties of the enclosed marker such as size and electrical charge affect the rate of transfer of the trapped marker across the membrane. Vesicle membranes fashioned from lecithin alone are relatively permeable to small molecules but can be made progressively less so by the addition of gangliosides, cholesterol, or both.[3] Phospholipids whose fatty acids are saturated and of long chain length make impermeable membranes, whereas increasing degrees of unsaturation or shortening in fatty acid chain length increase permeability. This has been demonstrated by many workers in vitro and in our laboratory in vitro and in vivo.[3] Liposomes or vesicles containing identical lipid constituents are made progressively impermeable for entrapped molecules as the length of sonication increases. The addition of protein to vesicles has variable effects on the membrane permeability. We found incorporation of polyamino acid chains of tyrosine and phenylalanine reduced it, whereas polylysine increased it.[11]

DISTRIBUTION OF VESICLES IN VIVO

Vesicles prepared and loaded with radiopharmaceuticals in vitro have been injected intravenously into rats and mice. The animals showed no ill effects, and mice (weight 25 to 30 grams) survived injections of 0.5 to 0.8 ml of vesicles. In control experiments, small volumes of vegetable oils (0.1 ml) injected intravenously caused almost instantaneous death; thus lipid vesicles, unlike lipid emulsions, cause no acute or short-term demise to mice.

A significant proportion (20 to 80 %) of the vesicle-entrapped radioactivity is found in the liver and spleen after intravenous injection. This can be shown by killing mice at timed intervals after injection or by computer analysis of gamma camera images of rats. In spite of this it has been possible, using a nonradioactive spin label, to demonstrate intact vesicles in the circulation for as long as 3 hours.

The uptake of vesicles in the liver and spleen presents a major problem, since in most clinical situations the desired treatment site would be neither of these organs. Because of this, there has been considerable effort to define the factors which promote or reduce hepatic and splenic clearance of vesicles. Factors which augment hepatic clearance are (1) addition of cholesterol to the constituent lipids and (2) increasing the time of sonication. Therefore, a mutually unresolvable problem arises: those alterations to the membrane which prevent leakage of the entrapped marker are also the factors which cause vesicles to be rapidly cleared from the circulation by the liver and spleen. There is indisputable evidence that circulating vesicles are not cleared from the circulation as quickly as colloidal particles.[3] In spite of this, there is controversy about which liver cells are more important in causing uptake. The weight of evidence indicates that the reticuloendothelial (Kupffer) cells are the more important.[12] Nevertheless, electronmicroscopic studies have demonstrated liposomes within hepatocytes.[13] Therefore, treatment of diseases of hepatocytes might be possible. Unfortunately, few diseases are seldom restricted to hepatocytes, but there are a variety of viral and autoimmune conditions and inborn errors of metabolism which affect these cells predominantly and might be amenable to treatment. Drugs used to treat viral hepatitis and chronic active hepatitis include glucocorticosteroids and immunosuppressive drugs, but the systemic doses of these drugs necessary to alter the course of the diseases usually, perhaps inevitably, cause toxic effects. However, if the therapeutic dose could be delivered specifically to the hepatocytes, side effects might be averted.

Nevertheless, in the majority of patients diseases are not restricted to the liver. Thus, in most cases rapid hepatic uptake of vesicles would be a great disadvantage, and detailed studies will be required to define those conditions which minimize hepatic clearance. One possible solution to this problem could well be the use of vesicles prepared from native plasma ingredients.[8] Labeled plasma vesicles remain intact in the circulation of experimental animals for many hours and are slowly cleared by the liver. Analysis of the constituents of human plasma vesicles could well provide us with a formula for artificial vesicles which would not be extracted rapidly by the liver. Plasma vesicles made from each patient might be the simplest vehicle.

METHODS OF DIRECTING VESICLES TO TARGET SITES

Although it is possible to alter the distribution of vesicles in vivo by changing the lipids which make up the limiting membrane, in most instances it will be necessary to introduce a homing mechanism to produce specific localization. Dunnick et al.[11,14] and Gregoriadis and Neerunjun[15] approached this problem by using antibodies to produce specificity in vitro. Liposomes associated with anti-cell IgG increased liposome uptake by the specific cell,[15] and antibody to thyroglobulin complexed to vesicles augments vesicle attachment to thyroglobulin.[14] Weissmann et al.[16] demonstrated augmented uptake of liposomes by dogfish phagocytes when the liposomes were coated with IgM. The latter example appears to be a nonspecific phenomenon and probably would not help in dictating exact tissue localization.

Gregoriadis and Neerunjun[15] showed that incorporation of the protein fetuin into liposomes increased hepatic uptake. However, it has been our experience that hepatic uptake can be increased by addition of cholesterol to the constituent lipids and the problem is to diminish, not to increase, localization to the liver.

There has been a growing knowledge of protein-lipid interactions in liposomes and vesicles. Proteins such as rhodopsin,[17] spectrin,[18] and ATPase[19] have all been incorporated into the lipid bilayers and shown to function. These specific proteins might not be of value as localizing agents, but the expertise and methodology obtained are of importance and should be applicable to the utilization of other homing mechanisms.

Provided the probe does in fact direct the radiolabeled vesicle to the target site, there are still difficulties to be resolved. The intact vesicle must be able to leave the circulation, and there is some evidence from electron microscopic studies showing intact vesicles inside cells that can do so. Investigations of the distribution of radiolabeled vesicles injected subcutaneously show a pattern similar to intravenous injection.[20] This is probably due to the vesicles gaining access to lymphatic channels and then entering the systemic circulation, but indicates that they can cross one endothelial barrier and gain access to the bloodstream. If the vesicle has the ability to cross capillaries and come in contact with target cells, several outcomes are possible and have been described.

1. There may be no interaction.
2. The vesicle wall can fuse with the cell membrane and rupture. This could result in the intracavitary contents of the vesicle being injected into the cytoplasm of the cell; alternatively, the contents might be lost in the extracellular fluids.
3. There may be complete endocytosis of vesicles.
4. It has been shown that lipids of vesicle membranes and those of tumor cell membranes can interchange in vitro.[21,22] When stearylamine is a constituent of the vesicle wall, this phospholipid transfers to the tumor membrane and slows tumor growth. This mechanism could be of value as a therapeutic adjuvant.

SUMMARY

Vesicles and liposomes can entrap packages of water-soluble radiolabeled drugs (or hormones, enzymes). The rate of release of the entrapped drug can be altered in vitro by changing the constituents of the vesicle membrane or by altering the conditions of preparation. The distribution of the drug in an experimental animal can be altered substantially by entrapping the drug in vesicles, and the new distribution is dictated by the properties of the carrier system. This system of delivery is still in infancy, and the major problem to be answered is the one of specific direction to target sites. There is still work to be done!

REFERENCES

1. Gregoriadis, S., Swain, C. P., Wills, E. J., et al.: Drug-carrier potential of liposomes in cancer chemotherapy. Lancet 1:1313–1316, 1974.
2. Gregoriadis, G.: Carrier potential of liposomes in biology and medicine. N. Engl. J. Med. 295:704–710, 1976.
3. McDougall, I. R., Dunnick, J. K., McNamee, M., et al.: Distribution and fate of synthetic vesicles in the mouse. A combined radionuclide and spin label study. Proc. Natl. Acad. Sci. U.S.A. 71:3487–3491, 1974.
4. Boggs, J. M., Hsia, J. C.: Effect of cholesterol and water on the rigidity and order of phosphatidylcholine bilayers. Biochim. Biophys. Acta 290:32–42, 1972.
5. Hsia, J. C., Long, R. A., Hruska, F. E., et al.: Steroid-phosphatidylcholine interactions in oriented multibilayers—a spin label study. Biochim. Biophys. Acta 290:22–31, 1972.
6. Papahadjopoulos, D., Nir, S., Ohki, S.: Permeability properties of phospholipid membranes: effect of cholesterol and temperature. Biochim. Biophys. Acta 266:561–583, 1972.
7. Phillips, M. C., Finer, E. G., Hauser, H.: Differences between conformations of

lecithin and phosphatidylethanolamine polar groups and their effects on interactions of phospholipid bilayer membranes. Biochim. Biophys. Acta 290:397–402, 1972.

8. Dunnick, J. K., Kriss, J. P.: Studies of radiopharmaceuticals enclosing lipid-protein vesicles formed from native plasma components. J. Nucl. Med. (in press).

9. Johnson, S. M.: The inability of macrophages to digest liposomes containing a high proportion of cholesterol. Biochem. Soc. Trans. 3:160–161, 1975.

10. Roseman, M., Litman, B. J., Thompson, T. E.: Transbilayer exchange of phosphatidylethanolamine for phosphatidylcholine and N-acetimidoylphosphatidylethanolamine in single-walled bilayer vesicles. Biochemistry 14:4826–4830, 1975.

11. Dunnick, J. K., McDougall, I. R., Aragon, S., et al.: Vesicle interation with polyamino acids and antibody. *In vivo* and *in vitro* studies. J. Nucl. Med. 16:483–487, 1975.

12. Segal, A. W., Gregoriadis, G., Black, C. D. V.: Liposomes as vehicles for the local release of drugs. Clin. Sci. Mol. Med. 49:99–106, 1975.

13. Segal, A. W., Gregoriadis, G., Lavender, J. P., et al.: Tissue and hepatic subcellular distribution of liposomes containing bleomycin after intravenous administration to patients with neoplasms. Clin. Sci. Mol. Med. 51:421–425, 1976.

14. Dunnick, J. K., Badger, R. S., Takeda, Y., et al.: Vesicle interactions with antibody and peptide hormone. Role of vesicle composition. J. Nucl. Med. 17:1073–1076, 1976.

15. Gregoriadis, G., Neerunjun, D. E.: Control of the rate of hepatic uptake and catabolism of liposome-entrapped proteins injected into rats. Possible therapeutic applications. Eur. J. Biochem. 47:179–185, 1974.

16. Weissmann, G., Bloomgarden, D., Kaplan, R., et al.: A general method for the introduction of enzymes, by means of immunoglobulin-coated liposomes, into lysosomes of deficient cells. Proc. Natl. Acad. Sci. U.S.A. 72:88–92, 1975.

17. Montal, M., Korenbrot, J. I.: Incorporation of rhodopsin proteolipid into bilayer membranes. Nature 246:219–221, 1973.

18. Juliano, R. L., Stamp, D.: The effect of particle size and charge on the clearance rates of liposome and liposome encapsulated drugs. Biochem. Biophys. Res. Commun. 63:651–658, 1975.

19. Jilka, R. R., Martonosi, A. N., Tillack, T. W.: Effect of purified $(Mg^{2+} + Ca^{2+})$ activated ATPase of sarcoplastic reticulum upon the passive Ca^{2+} permeability and ultrastructure of phospholipid vesicles. J. Biol. Chem. 250:7511–7524, 1975.

20. McDougall, I. R., Dunnick, J. K., Goris, M. L., et al.: *In vivo* distribution of vesicles loaded with radiopharmaceuticals: a study of different routes of administration. J. Nucl. Med. 16:488–491, 1975.

21. Dunnick, J. K., Kallman, R. F., Kriss, J. P.: Alteration of growth and lipid composition of EMT-6 tumor cells after exposure to lipid vesicles. Biochem. Biophys. Res. Commun. 73:619–624, 1976.

22. Pagano, R. E., Huang, L.: Interaction of phospholipid vesicles with mammalian cells. J. Cell Biol. 67:49–60, 1975.

23. Dapergolas, G., Neerunjun, D. E., Gregoriadis, G.: Penetration of target areas in the rat by liposome associated bleomycin, glucose oxidase and insulin. FEBS Lett. 63:235–239, 1976.

Larry A. Spitznagle

25

Use of ³H- and ¹⁴C-Labeled Compounds in the Therapy for Specific Metabolic Pathways

The use of radioactive molecules for therapeutic purposes began shortly after the discovery of radioactive decay. The most common use of a radioactive drug for therapeutic purposes, the use of sodium iodide-¹³¹I for treatment of hyperthyroidism, is an excellent example of therapy for a specific metabolic pathway. Before discussing the use of ³H- and ¹⁴C-labeled compounds in therapy, let us review the properties which a therapeutic radiopharmaceutical should possess. Figure 25-1 lists some important properties of a therapeutic radiopharmaceutical.

A therapeutic radiopharmaceutical should possess tissue specificity. The radiopharmaceutical should accumulate, hopefully rapidly, in the target tissue and should be cleared rapidly from nontarget tissues and excreted from the body. In addition, high specific activity is often important to prevent toxicity to nontarget tissues.

A therapeutic radiopharmaceutical should have a long effective half-life in the target tissue and at the same time have a short effective half-life in nontarget tissue. In the ideal case the radiopharmaceutical would be bound to the target tissue.

Therapeutic radiopharmaceuticals must deliver a high radiation dose to the target tissue and at the same time should not produce high radiation doses to nontarget tissues. Therefore, the radionuclides incorporated into therapeutic radiopharmaceuticals should emit nonpenetrating radiation.

Advances in radiopharmaceutical development often result from serendipitous discoveries; however, the design of radiopharmaceuticals is usually based on the principles of biochemistry and pharmacology. Those principles led to the proposal of organic compounds containing carbon, hydrogen, oxygen, and often nitrogen and sometimes sulfur as pharmaceuticals. For imaging purposes we know that there really are no useful radionuclides of any of these elements.

It has been suggested that ³H and ¹⁴C might prove useful for therapy if they were incorporated into the appropriate molecule (R. P. Spencer, *personal communication*). These radionuclides have long been used in biochemical research because of the ease with which they can be incorporated into biologically interest-

1. Tissue specificity
   Accumulation
   Clearance
   Specific activity

2. Effective half-life
   Long physical half-life
   Long biological half-life

3. Nonpenetrating radiation

Fig. 25-1.   Properties of a therapeutic radiopharmaceutical.

ing compounds. In fact, much of what we know about biosynthesis and metabolism has come from studies utilizing ^{3}H- and ^{14}C-labeled compounds.

Many of the chemical and physical properties of ^{3}H and ^{14}C suggest that they may be useful for incorporation into specific therapeutic radiopharmaceuticals. Tritium may be produced by a ^{6}Li(n,α)^{3}H reaction, whereas ^{14}C may be produced by a ^{14}N(n,p)^{14}C reaction. Both reactions result in relatively inexpensive, high specific activity, carrier-free sources of radionuclide. Figure 25-2 lists a few of the wide range of chemical forms of these two radionuclides available from radiochemical manufacturers. Figure 25-3 lists some physical information concerning these radionuclides and the radiation resulting from their decay.

The half-lives of ^{3}H and ^{14}C are long enough for both nuclides to be useful therapeutically. Both radionuclides are pure beta emitters and thus all the radiation will be absorbed in the vicinity of the decaying atoms rather than elsewhere in the body. It should be noted that the beta particles from ^{14}C are almost 10 times more energetic than those from ^{3}H. It is also important to note that the maximum range of the beta particles from ^{3}H is less than the diameter of the average cell.

The short range of the beta particles from ^{3}H has led to speculation about the radiation hazards from ^{3}H-labeled compounds and their potential as therapeutic agents.[1] As a result of this interest, several investigators have discussed the microdosimetry of tritium. Tagder and Scheuermann[2] presented the results of microdosimetry calculations made by themselves and by other investigators, each

Compound	Specific Activity	Cost
T_2	Carrier free 2.6 Ci/cc at STP	$42 + 3/Ci
HTO	20 Ci/g	$45/Ci
Testosterone-7-T	10–25 Ci/mM	$103/mCi
$^{14}CO_2$	1–60 mCi/mM	$48/mCi
$Ba^{14}CO_2$	40–60 mCi/mM	$28/mCi
Testosterone-4-^{14}C	50–60 mCi/mM	$150/0.1 mCi

Fig. 25-2.   Some common chemical forms of ^{3}H and ^{14}C.

Property	³H	¹⁴C
Half-life (years)	12.2	5700
Radiation emitted	β	β
E_{max} (kev)	18	156
E_{ave} (kev)	5.5	50
*Range ave (μm)	0.6	35
*Range max (μm)	6	250

*Range in tissue equivalent material.

Fig. 25-3. Some physical properties of ³H and ¹⁴C.

using different assumptions. They also made similar calculations for ¹⁴C. The results of their calculations are summarized in Figure 25-4. One important conclusion evident from their paper is that once the diameter of the cell nucleus or target cell reaches the maximum range of the beta particle, the dose rate levels out. In addition, none of the methods used gave results differing by more than 20 percent; therefore, as a first approximation, any of the methods will suffice. What the calculations do not consider, which is particularly important for ¹⁴C, is that the cell is not suspended in a vacuum and is most likely being irradiated by beta particles originating from surrounding cells. Therefore, all the energy from the decay of ¹⁴C will be rather uniformly distributed in the target tissue.

Figure 25-5 gives a simple view of when microdosimetry calculations might be useful for ³H-labeled compounds. If, as in part A, tritium were localized only in the nucleus, then the dose to the genetic material would be much higher than that calculated, assuming a uniform distribution of ³H within the cell. However, even with ³H-labeled nucleic acids much of the ³H is metabolized and ends up as THO and irradiates the whole cell rather than just the nucleus. If, as in part B, ³H were localized only in the cytoplasm, then the genetic material would receive less radiation dose than from a uniform distribution of ³H. If, as in part C, ³H were

Cell Diameter (μm)	Radiation Disintegration/μm³ ³H	¹⁴C
1	25–50	—
2	45–70	—
3	55–75	—
4	60–85	—
5	65–85	50–80
10	68–85	100–150
20	70–85	175–250
40	''	300–400
100	''	500–600

Fig. 25-4. Summary of microdosimetry calculations.

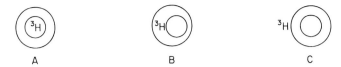

Fig. 25-5. Microdosimetry of tritium.

localized in the extracellular fluid or on the cell membrane, then the nucleus would receive very little radiation. Such microdosimetry calculations are of little value for ^{14}C since even if ^{14}C were located only on the surface of the cell, the cell would be rather uniformly irradiated.

A term which can be useful for comparing various potential radionuclides for possible use in therapeutic radiopharmaceuticals is the reciprocal of the *specific dose constant* as used by MIRD committee. This new term gives the concentration in microcuries per gram which would produce 1 rad for every hour that the concentration is maintained. Figure 25-6 gives the results for ^3H and ^{14}C.

From the above discussion it becomes apparent that ^3H and ^{14}C may be useful as components in therapeutic radiopharmaceuticals, provided that the compounds concentrate in the target tissue. Figure 25-7 lists several factors concerned with the incorporation of a compound into a specific metabolic pathway.

Other contributors to this volume discuss the effects of mode of administration on delivery of a therapeutic radiopharmaceutical to a tumor. Under circulation effects, a factor which can sometimes be controlled is the size of the circulating pool of the precursor. If the pool is large, little of the administered radiopharmaceutical will reach the target tissue. It may be possible to reduce the size of the circulating pool of precursor pharmacologically by administration of enzyme inhibitors or blocking agents. Cellular factors influencing the incorporation of agents into metabolic pathways can seldom be altered but must not be ignored when considering the therapeutic potential of various pathways.

Most specific metabolic pathways have a low capacity. Therefore, one must use high specific activity materials, otherwise specific carrier or uptake mechanisms will become saturated and nonspecific mechanisms will predominate.

The obvious extension of the above discussion is to consider which metabolic pathways might lend themselves to therapeutic applications of radiopharmaceuticals. Attention has been drawn to tissues and tumors containing high concentrations of certain metabolic products. It is known, for example, that the adrenal glands contain high concentrations of ascorbic acid,[3] DOPA,[4] dopamine,[4] and cholesterol.[5] Several types of tumors utilize tyrosine or one of its metabolic products, i.e., neuroblastomas,[6,7] pheochromocytomas,[8] and melanomas.[9] I have purposely not included nucleic acids since such pathways are general and found in all cell types.

^3H $1/\Delta = 82.6 \dfrac{\mu\text{Ci-hr}}{\text{g-rad}}$

^{14}C $1/\Delta = 9.5 \dfrac{\mu\text{Ci-hr}}{\text{g-rad}}$ **Fig. 25-6.** Theoretical maximum dose from *MIRD*.

Administration	Circulation	Cellular Incorporation
Intravenous	Entrance into circulation	Cellular pool of precursor
Intraarterial	Hemodynamics	Metabolic renewal
Intraperitoneal	Vascularization of target tissue	Biological half-life
Ingestion	Circulating pool of precursor	Reutilization

Fig. 25-7. Some factors influencing incorporation of metabolic precursors.

Even though we have information concerning the concentration or utilization of a metabolic product in certain tissue types, the information necessary to evaluate the therapeutic potential of radioactive derivatives is lacking. Information such as the fate and time course of exogenously administered materials or the percentage of the administered dose taken up by target and non-target tissues is seldom available even for common metabolic precursors. Where such information has been obtained, such as with nucleic acids, one often finds that the target tissue receives only a small fraction of the injected dose while nontarget tissue receives a large part of the dose.

For the purposes of this chapter I will consider one metabolic pathway in which ^{3}H or ^{14}C might be incorporated for therapeutic purposes. It is known that cholesterol is taken up by the adrenal cortex and stored as an esterified derivative.[10] Other metabolic modifications of the steroid nucleus take place in the adrenal cortex leading to steroids with other target organs.[5] These metabolic products are subsequently cleared from the body rapidly.[5]

Figure 25-8 illustrates dosimetry calculations of a model ^{3}H-labeled radiopharmaceutical based on cholesterol. Three different uptakes were used—

		Dose Administered to Produce:	
Ave. Exposure Time (1.44 × B½) Hr	Ave. % Uptake (% Dose/g)	1 rad μCi	5000 rads mCi
24	0.5	688	3441
1728	0.5	9	48
3456	0.5	5	24
24	1.0	344	1720
1728	1.0	5	24
3456	1.0	2	12
24	2.0	172	860
1728	2.0	2	12
3456	2.0	1	6

Fig. 25-8. Dosimetry for a model ^{3}H-labeled radiopharmaceutical in the adrenal glands.

		Dose Administered to Produce:	
Ave. Exposure Time (1.44 × B½) Hr	Ave. % Uptake (% Dose/g)	1 rad μCi	5000 rads mCi
24	0.5	79	395
1728	0.5	1	6
3456	0.5	0.6	2.75
24	1.0	39	198
1728	1.0	0.6	2.75
3456	1.0	0.3	1.4
24	2.0	20	99
1728	2.0	0.3	1.4
3456	2.0	0.1	0.7

Fig. 25-9. Dosimetry for a model ^{14}C-labeled radiopharmaceutical in the adrenal glands.

0.5, 1, and 2 percent of dose per gram of target tissue—each with three different average exposure times—1, 72, and 108 days. Two values were calculated, the total dose which must be administered to produce 1 rad in the adrenals of a 70-kg human and the dose required to produce 5000 rads. Figure 25-9 gives the results of similar calculations for a ^{14}C-labeled radiopharmaceutical.

An approximation of the whole-body dosimetry for these model radiopharmaceuticals was made with the following assumption:

The adrenals weighed 16 grams and contained 32 percent of the dose; the remainder of the dose was distributed over 70 kg; the biological half-life was 75 days. Using these assumptions, one could calculate that 6 mCi of ^{3}H-labeled steroid would produce a whole-body dose of approximately 1.4 rads, and 0.7 mCi of ^{14}C-labeled radiopharmaceutical would produce a whole-body dose of approximately 2.5 rads.

The figure of merit for these two model radiopharmaceuticals as therapeutic agents appears to be very high; however, ^{3}H- and ^{14}C-labeled compounds are not used routinely for therapy. Other features must be responsible for this situation. One factor may be lability of the label. Tritium is easily removed from most organic molecules either by exchange or by metabolic transformations. In addition, ^{14}C is certainly labile in the positions of a molecule in which it is easily introduced. Furthermore, the ^{14}C available has a low specific activity which is particularly important when only one carbon of a compound containing 20 to 30 carbon atoms is being labeled. Another reason ^{3}H and ^{14}C compounds are not widely used as therapeutic radiopharmaceuticals may be the cost of doing research with them. For instance, at current market prices, the ^{3}H-labeled steroid necessary to produce a 5000-rad dose to one patient would cost approximately $600, and the ^{14}C steroid would cost approximately $1050.

In conclusion, ^{3}H and ^{14}C are not likely to find use in radiotherapeutic agents until more tissue-specific radiopharmaceuticals have been developed. Even then, radionuclides with higher specific dose constants than ^{3}H and ^{14}C such as ^{32}P and ^{131}I should be considered first.

REFERENCES

1. Feinendegen, L.: Tritium Labeled Molecules in Biology and Medicine. New York, Academic Press, 1967.
2. Tagder, K., Scheuermann, W.: Estimation of absorbed doses in the cell nucleus after incorporation of ^{3}H and ^{14}C-labeled thymidine. Radiat. Res. 41:202–216, 1970.
3. Yovarsky, M., Almaden, P., King, C. G.: The vitamin C content of human tissues. J. Biol. Chem. 106:525, 1934.
4. Morales, J. O., Beierwaltes, W. H., Counsell, R. E., et al.: The concentration of radioactivity from labeled epinephrine and its precursors in the dog adrenal medulla. J. Nucl. Med. 8:800–809, 1967.
5. Appelgren, L. E.: Sites of steroid hormone formation. Acta Physiol. Scand. [Suppl 71] 301:1–108, 1967.
6. VonStudnitz, W., Kaser, H., Sjoerdsma, A.: Spectrum of catecholamine biochemistry in patients with neuroblastoma. N. Engl. J. Med. 269:232, 1963.
7. Lieberman, L. M., Beierwaltes, W. H., Varma, V. M., et al.: Labeled dopamine concentrations in human adrenal medulla and in neuroblastoma. J. Nucl. Med. 10:93–97, 1969.
8. Anderson, B. G., Beierwaltes, W. H., Harrison, T. S., et al.: Labeled dopamine concentration in pheochromocytomas. J. Nucl Med. 14:781–784, 1973.
9. Meier, D. A., Beierwaltes, W. H., Counsell, R. E.: Radioactivity from labeled precursors of melanin in mice and hamsters with melanomas. Cancer Res. 27:1354–1359, 1967.
10. Kirschner, A. S., Ice, R. D., Beierwaltes, W. H.: Radiation dosimetry of ^{131}I-19-iodocholesterol. J. Nucl. Med. 14:713–717, 1973.

H. Donald Burns

26

Relationship Between the Development of Radioactive and Nonradioactive Pharmaceuticals

The goal of this chapter is to encourage increased cooperation between researchers working on the development of radioactive pharmaceuticals and those concerned with the development of stable pharmaceuticals. Although there has been some cooperation in the past, it is likely that additional interaction between the two groups will be very beneficial to both fields. The term "radiopharmaceutical" has been used to identify several types of radioactive compounds: (1) radioactive compounds administered to a patient to elicit a therapeutic effect, (2) radioactive compounds administered to a patient to obtain diagnostic information about the patient, (3) radioactive compounds administered to a patient to obtain information concerning the fate of the compound in vivo (e.g., drug distribution and metabolism studies), and (4) radioactive compounds used in vitro to aid in analyzing for the chemical concentration of various substances in samples of body fluids or tissues obtained from the patient. The concepts used in designing each of these types of radiopharmaceuticals are quite similar; however, there are some important differences. Because of these differences, it is essential to emphasize that this discussion is concerned only with those radiopharmaceuticals which are administered to patients to obtain diagnostic information about the patient (by means of external detection of radiation being emitted from within the patient) and those used for therapy.

There are two important differences between diagnostic and therapeutic radiopharmaceuticals; the first concerns the choice of the radionuclide to be used, and the second concerns the need for specificity. When one chooses a radionuclide for use in a diagnostic radiopharmaceutical, the ideal is to maximize the externally detectable photon yield, while minimizing the radiation absorbed dose to the patient. To accomplish this, a radionuclide which emits either gamma or x-radiation is preferred. Ideally, no particulate radiation should be emitted, and any gamma or x-radiation should be at least 30 kev and preferably higher. For a therapeutic radiopharmaceutical, the opposite is true. The radiation emitted should be absorbed by the tissue. In this case, nuclides which emit nonpenetrating, particulate radiation are preferred. Beta emitters have been the most widely used, although interest in the use of alpha emitting nuclides is increasing.

The need for specificity is important for both types of radiopharmaceuticals, with the requirements for therapeutic pharmaceuticals greater than those for diagnostic radiopharmaceuticals. For imaging purposes, it is only necessary to achieve regional specificity. For example, a radiopharmaceutical which localized in brain tumors would be useful for diagnosis, even if the majority of the radioactivity administered to the patient were concentrated in the kidney, since kidney activity would not interfere with the resulting brain scan. On the other hand, when considering therapeutic radiopharmaceuticals, it is important that the major concentration of the radiopharmaceutical be in the target tissue, i.e., whole-body specificity must be achieved. The need for this greater degree of specificity is a consequence of the fact that the degree of damage to any given tissue by the nonpenetrating radiation is directly related to the concentration of the radiopharmaceutical in that tissue. (Some tissues are more radiosensitive than others; however, in some cases this is a disadvantage.) Thus, a radiopharmaceutical for the treatment of brain tumors would not be very useful if it delivered a high radiation dose to a nontarget organ such as the kidney. Apart from the higher degree of specificity required for therapeutic radiopharmaceuticals and the fact that different radionuclides are used, the characteristics of therapeutic radiopharmaceuticals are essentially the same as those of diagnostic radiopharmaceuticals. The concepts used to design and the methods used to develop both types of radiopharmaceuticals are very similar. These concepts and methods are also similar to those used for the development of stable pharmaceuticals. In an attempt to point out some of these similarities, we will discuss the methods of developing stable pharmaceuticals. An attempt will be made to demonstrate that the same general approaches are used, and some examples of instances where each field has benefited from work done in the other will be given.

There are several systems for classifying the methods used for the development of stable pharmaceuticals. One of the most widely accepted (and the one preferred by the author) is the following:

1. Empirical approach
2. Serendipity
3. Exploration of side effects
4. Molecular modification of biologically active compounds
5. Rational design

EMPIRICAL APPROACH

The empirical approach to radiopharmaceutical development can be defined as that approach based solely on experiment and observation rather than on deliberate design. This approach is similar to the random screening of organic compounds for the development of stable drugs. Since many radioactive compounds can be eliminated on the basis of unsuitable physical properties (radiations, half-life, etc.), this method of radiopharmaceutical development should more correctly be compared to the directed random screening or organic compounds for the development of stable drugs. Much of our current understanding of the relationship between molecular structure and biodistribution resulted from the random evaluation of the biodistribution of various compounds of radionuclides which were considered to have desirable physical properties for incorporation into radiopharmaceuticals.

Studies such as those conducted by Durbin[1] in the 1950s led to a partial understanding of the properties of an element which dictate the biological distribution and excretion of the element. The major benefit derived from this type of study was a wealth of information from which conclusions can be drawn about the factors which determine the biological distribution of various substances. Many of our currently used stable drugs resulted from random screening programs similar to the study by Durbin. However, Korolkovas and Burckhalter[2] have estimated that for a new anticonvulsant to be discovered by such a screening process, it might be necessary to evaluate 500,000 compounds. Although the problems associated with the development of a radiopharmaceutical are somewhat different than those involved with the development of an anticonvulsant, it is likely that random screening of radiolabeled compounds will be less productive in the future than it has been in the past. More deliberate approaches to radiopharmaceutical design such as some of those discussed below are likely to be the source of most new radiopharmceuticals.

Even though a deliberate approach is now preferred, one should not underestimate the value of random screening. In the late 1950s, a group headed by Dudley[3] at Oak Ridge National Laboratories conducted an investigation which involved the study of the biodistribution of various radionuclides. During this investigation, they discovered that gallium (Ga^{3+}) accumulated in bone. They suggested at that time that radioisotopes of gallium be used to study bone metabolism, thus, a radiopharmaceutical of potential use for bone imaging was discovered by an empirical approach.

SERENDIPITY

Serendipity is defined as the discovery of something useful—by accident. In 1969 Edwards and Hayes[4] were evaluating the use of ^{67}Ga-citrate for the study of bone metabolism (as suggested by Dudley) when they discovered that this radionuclide localized in lymph nodes of a patient suffering from Hodgkin's disease. Since that time, ^{67}Ga-citrate has been found to localize in a wide variety of neoplastic lesions and has become the most widely used tumor localizing radiopharmaceutical today. This discovery of a very useful tumor imaging agent is clearly an example of serendipity. Even today, almost 20 years later, there is still no clear understanding of the mechanism responsible for the tumor localization of gallium.

The finding that Ga^{3+} accumulates in tumors has been very useful to those interested in the diagnosis of cancer. It has also been useful to those interested in cancer chemotherapy. Based on this tumor-seeking property of gallium, a group at the National Cancer Institute[5] decided to test gallium nitrate (nonradioactive) for antineoplastic activity. They found that the compound possessed significant activity against several types of tumors. This activity was significant enough to warrant phase I clinical trials in patients which are currently in progress. Thus, this is an example of an instance where people interested in the development of stable pharmaceuticals benefited from work done by radiopharmaceutical researchers.

A more recent example of a serendipitous discovery of a radiopharmaceutical is the development of the hepatobiliary agent ^{99m}Tc-HIDA by Loberg and coworkers[6] at the University of Maryland. The radiopharmaceutical was originally designed as an analogue of the local anesthetic lidocaine in hopes of obtaining a myocardial imaging agent (based on the finding that ^{14}C-lidocaine showed as high as a 5:1 heart to blood ratio in experimental animals). Although ^{99m}Tc-HIDA did not accumulate in the myocardium as desired, it was rapidly removed from the circulation by the liver and was excreted in the bile. This behavior suggested that ^{99m}Tc-HIDA might be useful as a radiopharmaceutical for the evaluation of hepatobiliary function. Additional animal and patient studies with this radiopharmaceutical have supported this expectation, and ^{99m}Tc-HIDA appears to be the most promising of the hepatobiliary agents currently under investigation. Although serendipity may be considered an accidental discovery of something useful, it requires an alert investigator who is able to recognize the value of some unexpected behavior of the system under investigation.

EXPLORATION OF SIDE EFFECTS

Somewhat similar to serendipity is the exploration of side effects as a method of developing radiopharmaceuticals. This method of developing stable pharmaceuticals has been very productive and is discussed in detail by Korolkovas and Burckhalter; however, it has not been used to any great extent for the development of radiopharmaceuticals. Perhaps the best example of this approach applied to radiopharmaceuticals is the recent development of in vivo red cell labeling procedures.

At the 1975 Society of Nuclear Medicine Meeting, there were three reports of delayed blood clearance of ^{99m}Tc when [99m]TcO$_4^-$ was used for brain scans.[7-9] All of these reports involved brain scans which were performed within several days after a bone scan with a stannous-containing bone agent. The investigators were able to show that the delayed blood clearance was a consequence of binding of ^{99m}Tc to circulating red cells. Since these observations were made, several investigators have attempted to develop an in vivo red cell labeling procedure which would involve injection of a small quantity of stannous complex, followed by an injection of TcO$_4^-$ a short time later.[10] Although all of the problems have not yet been solved, initial results appear quite promising. A procedure such as this is very attractive since it does not involve the removal, in vitro labeling, and reinfusion of each individual's red cells.

MOLECULAR MODIFICATION

It has long been known that polyphosphate, pyrophosphate, and other phosphate-containing compounds accumulated in the bone.[11] Based on this information, Subramanian and McAfee[12] attempted to label pyrophosphate with ^{99m}Tc in order to combine the desirable physical characteristics of ^{99m}Tc with the bone-seeking properties of polyphosphate. They found that the ^{99m}Tc complex did in fact localize in the bone. The complexation of ^{99m}Tc to polyphosphate may be loosely regarded as an example of molecular modification of the polyphosphate ion to form a useful radiopharmaceutical. Although calling the developing of ^{99m}Tc-polyphosphate an example of molecular modification may be somewhat tenuous, the development of subsequent ^{99m}Tc bone-seeking radiopharmaceuticals definitely is an example of this approach. Since the finding by Subramanian that ^{99m}Tc-polyphosphate localized in bone, many other bone agents have been discovered. The binding of Tc to the polyphosphate molecule involves the coordination of the phosphate oxygens to Tc (Fig. 26-1). Because of this, other phosphate-type compounds were evaluated. Most of these compounds fit into the general structure shown in Figure 26-1 with the only modification being the identify of X. This is clearly an example of the use of molecular modification to develop new radiopharmaceuticals. The molecular modification of biologically important molecules for the development of new *stable* drugs is currently the most productive source of new drugs. Often the discovery of a new class of drugs is serendipitous, such as the discovery of the central nervous system activity of the benzodiazapines; molecular modification of this lead compound has led to many new drugs with similar activity. The discovery of radiopharmaceuticals by molecular modification is also quite productive and probably the source of most of the currently used radiopharmaceuticals.

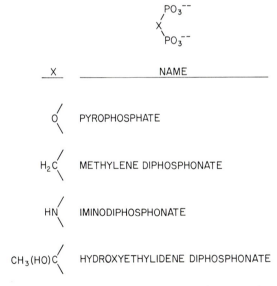

Fig. 26-1. Structure of compounds used to complex technetium in the preparation of ^{99m}Tc-bone imaging radiopharmaceuticals.

RATIONAL DESIGN

The most satisfying method of developing stable pharmaceuticals is the rational design of new drugs. Unfortunately, this method has not been very productive in the past due to the complicated nature of the relationship of structure to biological activity of medicinal agents. The development of radiopharmaceuticals by rational design has been considerably more productive, due in part to a relatively good understanding of the relationship of molecular structure to biodistribution. Radiopharmaceuticals such as particles for lung perfusion and colloids for imaging the reticuloendothelial system are rationally designed radiopharmaceuticals. Of the simpler organic compounds (more closely related to the types of compounds used as stable drugs), one of the best examples of a rationally designed radiopharmaceutical is the adrenal imaging agent 19-iodocholesterol (Fig. 26-2).[13]

The design of the pancreas imaging agent ^{75}Se-selenomethionine by Blau and Bender in 1962 relied on the high requirement by the pancreas for amino acids and on the well-known principle of bioisosterism,[2] which is often utilized in the development of nonradioactive drugs. Another example of the application of the principle of bioisosterism in the design of radiopharmaceuticals is the development of ^{125}I-5-iododeoxyuridine (Fig. 26-3).[14]

As mentioned earlier, one of the important characteristics of radiopharmaceuticals (both diagnostic and therapeutic) is the need for specificity. In the case of radiopharmaceuticals, this specificity is achieved as a result of a selective localization of the radiopharmaceutical in the target tissue. With nonradioactive drugs, specificity is also important; however, in this case it is the parmacological action caused by the drug that must be selective. There is generally no requirement that the drug accumulate in the target tissue. In many cases the drug's activity is a consequence of the drug binding to a highly specific receptor. The action occurs, therefore, only in tissues that possess the receptor. There is no effect in tissues that do not possess the receptor. Furthermore, Butler[15] has pointed out that, "With most drugs, only a very small portion of the total amount in the body is at any time in direct interaction with the receptors producing the pharmacological action. Usually a very high proportion of the total drug in the

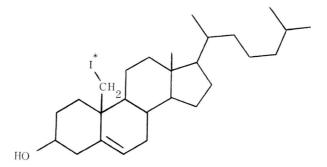

Fig. 26-2. Structure of the adrenal imaging agent 19-iodocholesterol.

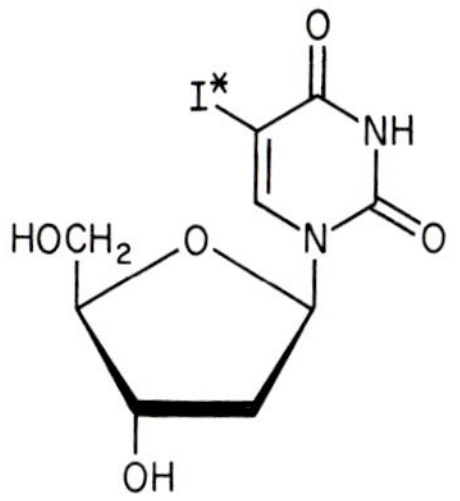

Fig. 26-3.   The structure of 5-iodo-2'-deoxyuridine.

body is localized in parts of the body remote from the site of action.'' Although most nonradioactive drugs do not need to selectively accumulate in the target tissue, such selectivity is important for one group of drugs—the antineoplastic chemotherapeutic agents.

Antineoplastic drugs are generally toxic compounds which interfere with cell growth and replication. Unfortunately, these drugs are often toxic to normal cells as well as tumor cells. Because of this toxicity to normal tissue, much effort is currently being expended by medicinal chemists to design specificity into their toxic compounds in an attempt to develop antineoplastic drugs which retain their cancericidal activity but are free of the many unpleasant and harmful side effects normally associated with cancer chemotherapy. One way of achieving this specificity of action is to develop toxic compounds which selectively concentrate in tumor tissue. In this general area of investigation, additional cooperation between medicinal chemists and radiopharmaceutical chemists might be fruitful. The remainder of this discussion is concerned with several examples of what medicinal chemists are currently doing to achieve selective localization of antineoplastic drugs in cancerous tissue.

Generally, two methods can be used to increase selective localization of antineoplastic compounds in tumor cells. The first involves the use of carrier groups, such as metabolic substrates or tumor-specific antibodies, and the second involves a mechanistic approach. A good example of the use of metabolic substrates as a carrier group is the development of l-phenylalanine mustard (Fig. 26-4).[16] The toxic portion of this molecule is the bis-(2-chloroethyl)amino-group enclosed in the circle. In this case, the phenylalanine molecule serves as a carrier

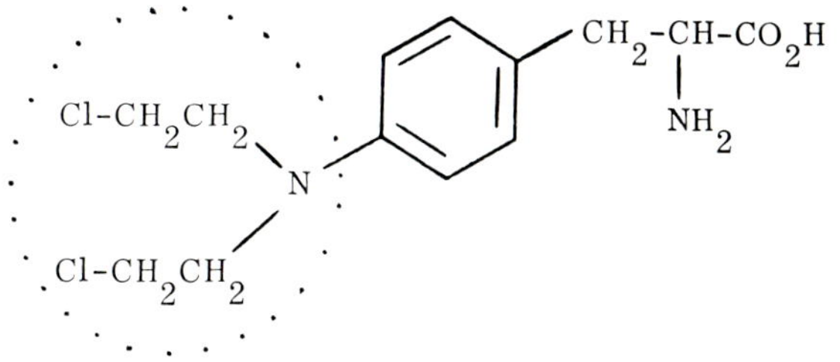

Fig. 26-4.   Structure of l-phenylalanine mustard. The phenyl-alanine portion of the molecule serves as a carrier for the nitrogen mustard function (group enclosed in dotted circle).

group for the toxic nitrogen mustard functionality, assuming that active transport of the phenylalanine will assure an elevated concentration of the chemotherapeutic agent intracellularly, where it can exert its toxic effect. The fact that the L-isomer of phenylalanine mustard shows marked superiority over the D-isomer suggests that active transport indeed occurs. Such use of metabolic substrates as carrier groups has proven useful for the development of radiopharmaceuticals as well as nonradioactive pharmaceuticals; examples are ^{75}Se-selenomethionine, ^{123}I-iodohexadecanoic acid,[17] and ^{18}F-glucose.[18] Cooperation at this level will permit researchers from both fields to better predict which metabolic substrates are useful and in which part of the molecule significant structural modifications can be made without destroying the compound's ability to participate in its normal metabolic reactions.

An interesting example of the use of a "metabolic" substrate" as a carrier to increase the tumor specificity of an antineoplastic drug has recently been reported by Trouet and coworkers.[19] Adriamycin and daunomycin (Fig. 26-5) are two new antitumor agents whose mechanism of action involves inhibition of nucleic acid synthesis as a result of intercalation between base pairs in nuclear DNA. Both drugs have displayed significant antileukemic activity as well as activity against a broad spectrum of solid tumors.[20] Both of these compounds display many toxic side effects common to most antitumor agents. The most serious side effect is a rapidly progressing syndrome of congestive heart failure and cardiopulmonary decompensation. This cardiotoxicity is the side effect most limiting to the use of these drugs at the present time, because treatment must be stopped while the tumor is still responding to the drug.

Trouet attempted to decrease the cardiotoxicity and enhance the antineoplastic activity of adriamycin by altering the biodistribution of the drug in a manner which would decrease the concentration of the drug in the heart and increase its concentration in the tumor. Based on the fact that tumor cells have a higher pinocytosis rate than normal cells, Trouet reasoned that a DNA-adriamycin complex would be selectively taken up by tumor cells. Lysosomal metabolism of the

Fig. 26-5. Adriamycin and daunomycin, two antitumor agents whose mechanism of action involves inhibition of nucleic acid synthesis as a result of intercalation between base pairs in nuclear DNA.

DNA after accumulation in the tumor cell would release the adriamycin intracellularly where it would intercalate with nuclear DNA, thus inhibiting replication. They found that the DNA-adriamycin complex was clearly superior to the free drug at all dose levels. Also, the toxicity of the complex was substantially reduced. This work by Trouet suggests that a radiolabeled adriamycin analogue complexed to DNA may prove to be a useful tumor imaging agent.

A method for increasing the tumor specificity of daunomycin was reported by Hurwitz and coworkers in 1976.[21] They coupled daunomycin to (Fab')₂ fragments to deliver the drug specifically to the tumor. They found that the activity of the complexed drug was greater than the combined activity of the drug and antibody, suggesting that the drug was in fact selectively delivered to the tumor cells. It is not clear how the drug would have reached the nucleus of the tumor cells since it was covalently attached to the (Fab')₂ molecules. Furthermore, there is no actual proof that an increased concentration of the drug in the tumor was attained. Again, a radiolabeled adriamycin might prove useful for determining if an increased concentration of the drug is delivered to the tumor. Such a radiolabeled drug-antibody complex might be useful as a tumor imaging radiopharmaceutical. The concept of labeling antibodies for radiopharmaceutical development is currently being actively pursued by several radiopharmaceutical researchers. These are being evaluated as both therapeutic and diagnostic radiopharmaceuticals. Researchers concerned with using antibodies as carriers for nonradioactive drugs and those using antibodies as carriers for radionuclides can benefit from the methodologies developed by both groups.

The second general method of increasing the tumor specificity of antineoplastic drugs is the mechanistic approach. Probably the most sophisticated example of this approach currently under investigation is the design of "suicide substrates." Suicide substrates are a special type of irreversible enzyme inhibitors which require chemical activation by the target enzyme. Rando[22] has recently reviewed the work which has been done to date on these compounds.

The sequence of events which occur when a substrate interacts with an enzyme can be summarized as follows:

$$S + E \underset{K_s}{\rightleftarrows} ES \underset{K_{cat}}{\rightleftarrows} EP \underset{K_d}{\rightleftarrows} E + P,$$

where S is the substrate, E is the enzyme, K_s is the dissociation constant for the binding of the substrate to the enzyme, K_{cat} is the catalytic constant which is a measure of the probability that substrate molecule bound to the enzyme will be converted to product, and finally K_d is the dissociation constant of the enzyme-product complex.

Irreversible enzyme inhibitors are usually molecules whose structure closely resembles that of the substrate. In addition, they possess a chemically reactive functional group (usually an alkylating agent). Since these compounds are highly reactive, they are not very specific, i.e., they alkylate many functional groups in addition to the active site of the enzyme. In an attempt to increase the selectivity of these alkylating agents for the active site of the enzyme, several investigators have designed compounds which possess "latent" reactive groups that require activation by the enzyme to become highly reactive alkylating groups. Ideally, the enzyme should convert the substrate to such a highly reactive compound that it immediately alkylates the active site before the enzyme-product complex dissociates. The sequence of events which occur can be summarized as follows:

$$S + E \underset{\overline{K}_s}{\rightleftharpoons} ES \underset{\overline{K}_{cat}}{\rightleftharpoons} EP \overset{\nearrow K_a \quad E - P}{\searrow K_d \quad E - P}$$

Again, K_d is the dissociation constant of the enzyme-product complex. K_a is the rate at which the product alkylates the active site of the enzyme leading to irreversible inhibition of the enzyme. The derivation of the term "suicide substrate" should be clear after considering the above sequence. The enzyme converts the nonlethal substrate to the lethal product, essentially "pulling the trigger" on itself to commit suicide. The substrate itself is not an alkylating agent, therefore it does not alkylate any functional groups other than those at the active site of the enzyme.

Robinson and coworkers[23] have recently reported on a suicide substrate for the enzyme Δ^5-3-ketosteroid isomerase. The normal reaction of this enzyme is outlined in Figure 26-6. The enzyme converts Δ^5-3-ketosteroids (I) to Δ^4-3-ketosteroids (II) via the intermediate $\Delta^{3,5}$-dienol (III). The acetylentic steroid analogue (IV, shown in Fig. 26-7) was prepared by Robinson and shown to irreversibly inhibit Δ^5-3-ketosteroid isomerase by the mechanism shown in Figure 26-7. The formation of the highly reactive allenic ketone (V) is catalyzed by the enzyme and is not formed in the absence of the enzyme. Thus, only functional groups located in the close vicinity of the active site of the enzyme will be alkylated.

How can such a mechanistic approach be applied to the design of radiophar-

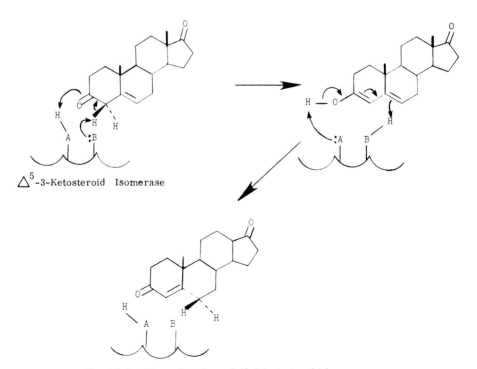

Δ^5-3-Ketosteroid Isomerase

Fig. 26-6.   Normal action of Δ^5-3-ketosteroid isomerase.

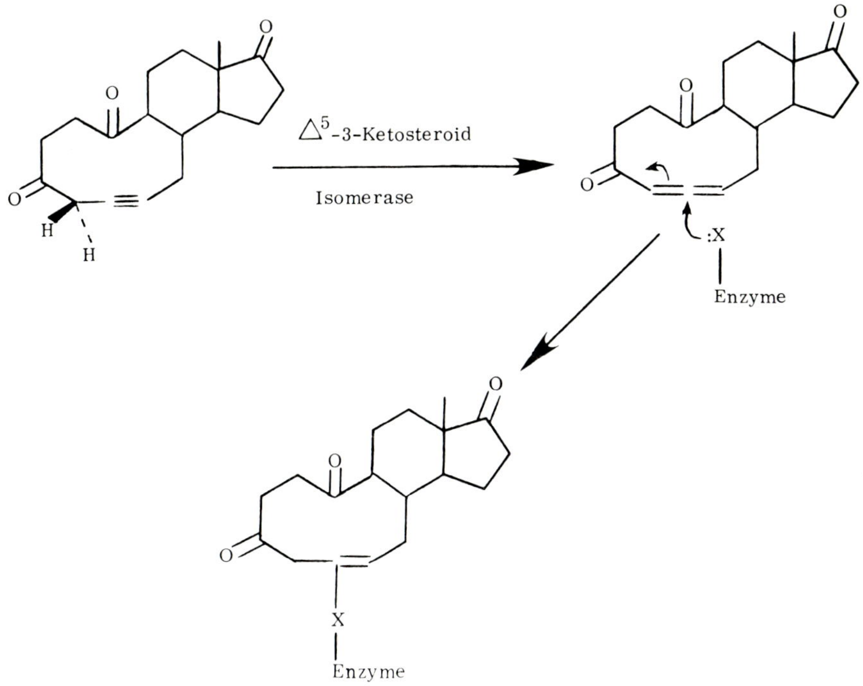

Fig. 26-7. Mechanism of action of Δ^5-3-ketosteroid isomerase "suicide substrate."

maceuticals? Theoretically, the degree of specificity of biodistribution which can be obtained is limited only by the degree of localization of the enzyme. Take, for example, an enzyme which is present only in functionary prostate tissue. A radiolabeled suicide substrate which is specific for this enzyme should concentrate selectively in functioning prostate tissue as a result of alkylating the enzyme's active site.

SUMMARY

An attempt has been made to demonstrate that the concepts used to design nonradioactive and radioactive pharmaceuticals are very similar. Particular emphasis was placed on attempts to design target tissue specificity into nonradioactive pharmaceuticals, especially antineoplastic chemotherapeutic agents. The goal of this discussion has been to encourage readers to more actively pursue cooperation between investigators concerned with the development of nonradioactive pharmaceuticals and those concerned with the development of radioactive pharmaceuticals.

REFERENCES

1. Durbin, P. W.: Metabolic characteristics within a chemical family. Health Phys 2:225, 1960.

2. Korolkovas, A., Burckhalter, J. H.: Essentials of Medicinal Chemistry. New York, John Wiley & Sons, 1976.
3. Dudley, H. C., Maddox, G. E., LuRue, H. C.: Studies on the metabolism of gallium. J. Pharmacol. Exp. Ther. 96:135–138, 1949.
4. Edwards, C. L., Hayes, R. L.: Scanning malignant neoplasms with gallium 67. J.A.M.A. 212:1182, 1970.
5. Symposium on the role of metal complexes and metal salts in cancer chemotherapy. Cancer Chemother. Rep. 59:587, 1975.
6. Harvey, E., Loberg, M., Cooper, M.: Tc-99m-HIDA: A new radiopharmaceutical for hepatobiliary imaging. J. Nucl. Med. 16:533, 1975.
7. Chandler, W.M., Shuck, L.: Abnormal technetium-99m pertechnetate imaging following stannous pyrophosphate bone imaging. J. Nucl. Med. 16:581, 1975.
8. Walker, A. G.: Effect of Tc-99m-Sn bone scan agents on subsequent pertechnetate brain scans. J. Nucl. Med. 16:579, 1975.
9. Khetigan, A., Garrett, M., Lum, D., et al.: Effect of prior administration of Sn (II) complexes used in nuclear medicine on in vivo distribution of subsequently administered Tc-99m-pertechnetate and Tc-99m-compounds. J. Nucl. Med. 16:541, 1975.
10. Zimmer, A. M., Pavel, D. G., Patterson, V. N.: In-vivo red blood cell labeling using consecutive injections of stannous pyrophosphate and technetium-99m-pertechnetate. J. Nucl. Med. 17:566, 1976.
11. Fels, I. G., Kaplan, E., Greco, J., et al.: Incorporation *in vivo* of ^{32}P from condensed phosphates. Proc. Soc. Exp. Biol. Med. 100:53–55, 1959.
12. Subramanian, G., McAfee, J. G.: A new complex of ^{99m}Tc for skeletal imaging. Radiology 99:192–196, 1976.
13. Blair, R. J., Beierwaltes, W. H., Lieberman, L. M., et al.: Radiolabeled cholesterol as an adrenal scanning agent. J. Nucl. Med. 12:176–178, 1971.
14. Eidinoff, M. L., Cheong, L., Rich, M. A.: Incorporation of unnatural pyrimidine bases into deoxyribonucleic acid of mammalian cells. Science 129:1550–1551, 1959.
15. Butler, T.: The distribution of drugs. In: Fundamentals of Drug Metabolism and Drug Disposition. Baltimore, Williams & Wilkins Co., 1971.
16. Bergel, F., Stock, J. A.: Cytoactive amino acid and peptide derivatives. Part I. Substituted phenylalanines. J. Chem. Soc., pp. 2409–2417, 1954.
17. Poe, N. D., Robinsonj G. D., Graham, L. S., et al.: Experimental basis for myocardial imaging with ^{123}I-labeled hexadecanoic acid. J. Nucl. Med. 17:1077–1082, 1976.
18. Straatmann, M. G., Welch, M. J.: ^{18}F-DAST as a reagent in the synthesis of an ^{18}F-sugar. Abstracts of the First International Symposium on Radiopharmaceutical Chemistry. Brookhaven, N.Y., Brookhaven National Laboratories, 1976.
19. Trouet, A., Deprez-de-Campeneere, D., Schmedt-Malengraux, M., et al.: Experimental leukemia chemotherapy with a "lysosomotropic" adriamycin-DNA complex. Eur. J. Cancer 10:405–411, 1974.
20. Henry, D. W.: Adriamycin. In: Cancer Chemotherapy, A. C. Sartorelli (ed.). Washington, D.C., American Chemical Society, 1976.
21. Hurwitz, E., Levy, R., Maron, R., et al.: The covalent binding of daunomycin and adriamycin to antibodies, with retention of both drug and antibody activity. Cancer Res. 35:1175–1181, 1975.
22. Rando, R. R.: Chemistry and enzymology of K_{cat} inhibitors. Science 185:320–324, 1974.
23. Batzold, F. H., Robinson, C. H.: Irreversible inhibition of Δ^5-3-ketosteroid isomerase 5, 10-secosteroids. J. Am. Chem. Soc. 97:2576–2578, 1975.

Robert E. Belliveau and Joseph T. Witek

27
Possible Therapeutic Use
of Radiolabeled Antibodies:
A Review

The further developments in the understanding of the relationships of immunology, cellular and humoral, to cancer has provided a basis for the use of immune mechanisms for the detection and treatment of neoplasms. Reports on the use of immune therapy to supplement present chemo- and radiotherapeutic modalities have been noted and reviewed in patients with different cancers.[1,2]

The effectiveness of action of humoral agents in the body's immune tumor defense has been questioned with major emphasis on cellular mechanisms. In some tumor systems, both in vivo and in vitro, no definitive effect of antibody in neutralizing tumor growth has been noted.[3,4] In others, definite cytostasis followed by tumor cell death has been documented.[5,6] In 1953 Pressman[1] first suggested that radioiodinated antibodies might be used for in vivo localization and therapy. Since then, many studies utilizing radiolabeled antibodies for the detection and treatment of tumors have been conducted in human and nonhuman tumor systems. The present chapter reviews the literature and summarizes the conceptual basis and suggestions for the development of these tagged antibodies in the treatment of neoplasms. The advantages and disadvantages of these systems are discussed.

The normal cell surface consists of many antigens which are continually synthesized and cleared from this membrane. With neoplastic alteration of the cell, the identity of the cell surface becomes altered with the expression of new antigens. Isolation of these tumor antigens and the production of specific antibodies to these have been pursued with varying success. The radioiodination of these same antibodies has been studied in human and nonhuman hosts.

Table 27-1 presents chronological listing of reports dealing with various tumor systems and antibodies. Survival times following in vivo exposure to radiolabeled antibodies were reported in only three of these studies.[12,19,20] Significantly increased survival times were recorded in all of these. The other studies emphasized distribution and concentration of labeled antibody without survival data. In addition to tumor localization, most of these studies reported preferential uptake of the labeled antibody in nontumor tissues, including the lungs, liver, spleen, and kid-

Table 27-1
Tumors and Radiolabeled Antibodies in Human and Nonhuman Tumor Localization and Therapy

Reference (Year) (No.)	Tumor Type	Host	Tumor Site*	Agent (Isotope)	Tumor/Blood Ratio†	Survival‡	Critical Organ Ratio†
Pressman & Korngold (1953) (7)	Wagner osteo-genic sarcoma	Mouse (A km)	S.C.	^{131}I-anti WOS Ig	U	U	Blood < 1.0
Korngold & Pressman (1954) (8)	Lymphosarcoma—Murphy-Strum	Sherman rat	S.C.	^{131}I-antilymphosarcoma Ig	U	U	Spleen > 1.0
Day et al. (1956) (9)	Lymphosarcoma—Murphy-Strum	Wistar rat	S.C.	^{131}I-antitumor Ig	U	U	Liver > 1.0
Spar et al. (1960, 1967) (10, 11)	Various tumors	Human	X	^{131}I-antifibrinogen Ig	U	U	U
Reif (1971) (12)	Myeloma MOPC-21A	Mouse (BALB/c)	S.C.	^{125,131}I-antimyeloma & N Ig	U	+	U
Izzo et al. (1971) (13)	Fischer MC tumor	Buffalo, Fischer rats	S.C.	^{125}I-Fischer transplantation Ig	≈ 3.7	U	Blood ≈ 3.7
Kellen et al. (1973) (14)	Mammary tumors R35, R3230AC	Sprague-Dawley rat	S.C.	^{125}I-antitumor assoc. Ig	U	U	Kidney, liver ≈ 1.7, 2.2
Goldenberg et al. (1974) (15)	Human colonic Cancer GW-39	Hamster	C.P.	^{125}I-anti-CEA & N Ig	5.06 ± 0.74	U	Blood ≈ 5.1
Goldenberg et al. (1974) (15)	Sarcoma HS-1	Syrian hamster	C.P.	^{125}I-anti-CEA & N Ig	U	U	Blood ≈ 0.6

Table 27-1
Continued.

Reference (Year) (No.)	Tumor Type	Host	Tumor Site*	Agent (Isotope)	Tumor/Blood Ratio[†]	Survival[‡]	Critical Organ Ratio[†]
Goldenberg et al. (1974) (15)	Melanoma A. Mel.-3	Syrian hamster	C.P.	^{125}I-anti-CEA & N Ig	U	U	U. Bladder $\simeq 0.6$
Hoffer et al. (1974) (15)	Colonic tumor GW-39	Syrian hamster	S.C.	^{125}I-anti-CEA Ig	0.81	U	Blood 0.81
Reif et al. (1974) (17)	Carcinoma colon	Human	X	^{131}I-anti-CEA Ig	U	U	Liver, lungs
Terman et al. (1975) (18)	Neuroblastoma C-1300	Mouse (A/J)	S.C.	^{125}I-Ig	U	U	U
Ghose et al. (1975, 1976) (19, 20)	Lymphoma EL4	Mouse (C57/BL)	I.P.	^{131}I-anti-EL4 & N Ig	U	+	Heart $\simeq 23.0$
Ghose et al. (1975, 1976) (19, 20)	Ehrlich ascites carcinoma	Mouse (BALB/c)	I.P.	^{131}I-anti-EAC & N Ig	U	+	U
Ghose et al. (1975, 1976) (19, 20)	Various tumors	Human	X	^{131}I-antitumor Ig	U	U	U
Belliveau (1976) (unpublished observations)	Neuroblastoma C-1300	Mouse (A/J)	S.C.	^{125}I-anti-PGE Ig	$\simeq 7.0$	U	Lung $\simeq 0.8$

*Abbreviations for tumor sites: S.C., subcutaneous; X, multiple sites; C.P., cheek pouch; I.P., intraperitoneal.
†Ratio expressed on basis of % injected dose/g tissue studied; U, unknown.
‡Survival abbreviations: U, unknown; +, improved or lengthened.

neys. Organs which demonstrated greatest localization of labeled antibody are listed in Table 27-1 as critical organs. In addition, the ratios of percent injected dose per gram for tumor to critical organ are also expressed. In some instances, more activity was located within nontumor structures than in tumors. Tumor to blood ratios of labeled antibody derived from percent injected dose per gram data showed great variability with many studies not listing this information. Certainly, the ability to detect and treat tumors with radiolabeled antibodies depends on a sufficiently high tumor target localization when compared to other organs and blood levels.

The conceptualized delivery and binding of labeled antibodies to cellular antigens can be considered based on the model outlined in Figure 27-1. Injected and labeled antibodies delivered intravenously distribute themselves in proportion to circulatory perfusion. At the capillary level, immunoglobulins diffuse through endothelial pores and into the extracellular space at the rate of T½ of 18 to 24 hours.[23] Further, tumor sites are associated with neovascular structures which have larger pores facilitating greater transport of labeled immunoglobulins. However, circulating labeled antibodies can combine with circulating tumor antigens, and thereby neutralize the antibody which as a complex is phagocytized by the RE system without reaching the tumor binding sites.[21-23]

Within the extracellular space, the labeled antibody comes in contact with cellular surface antigens. The complex may be bound for a period of time or

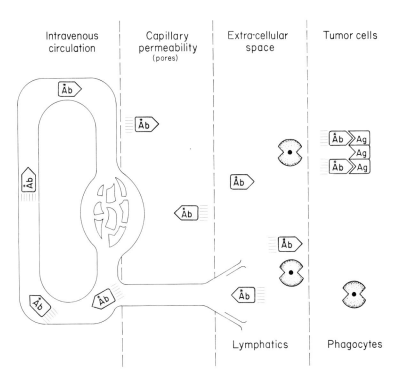

Fig. 27-1.   Schematic representation of distribution of radiolabeled antibody (Ab*) following intravenous administration and desired binding to tumor antigen (Ag).

Table 27-2

Characteristics of Radiolabeled Antibody

---

1. Specificity for tumor antigen without cross reactivity to normal cellular membrane antigens.
2. Capable of binding isotope and maintenance of specificty and biologic activity (with ^{131}I, 2 molecules ^{131}I/molecule Ab).
3. Use of ^{131}I as isotope is capable of delivering therapeutic and cytocidal dose of 500 rads (beta radiation).
4. Combination with tissue-bound antigen and consequent cellular destruction.
5. Preferential localization in tumor with rapid clearance of blood and nontumor levels with time.
6. Short-lived isotopes advantageous since less opportunity for free isotope formation and effects on other tissues (thyroid).

---

liberated through cell destruction and necrosis. In turn, phagocytes distributed locally may engulf these complexes, including labeled antibody. Altered or damaged antibody prior to antigen binding may also be taken up by macrophages and metabolized. During this equilibration, reentry of antibodies into the circulation is occurring. This is achieved through capillary diffusion or entry into both old and newly formed lymphatics. The slow development of lymphatics in zones of tumor growth retards the egress of immunoglobulins.[22,23]

The scheme presented is rather idealized since many of the same cellular phenomena such as capillary changes and local extracellular processes are shared by inflammatory and necrotic sites of tissue reaction. Therefore, localization of labeled antibodies may not be specific to neoplastic processes. The reports listed in Table 27-1 on radiolabeled antibodies and tumor localization have not included comparative measurement of antibody behavior at nontumor sites of tissue reaction, including inflammation.

The production of specific tumor antibody requires extensive investigation before actual use (Tables 27-2, 27-3, and 27-4).[21-23] A pure tumor antigen must be isolated before actual immunization is conducted. Immunization will result in many different antibodies with varying degrees of specificity and titer. The ultimate yield of a specific antibody with minimal cross reactivity with nontumor tissue is quite low. Starting with an immunoglobulin pool from an immunized animal, a tumor-related fraction of 5 to 10 percent is considered sizeable. This

Table 27-3

Characteristics of Tumor Antigens and Corresponding Tumors

---

1. Present along cellular membrane and distinctly different from normal cellular antigens.
2. Tumor antigens must demonstrate a long T½ at the cellular surface.
3. Different antigens with different tumors.
4. Some tumor antigens should be present in circulation at very low or negligible levels.
5. Number of tumor binding sites many times greater than number of radioantibodies needed to deliver tumoricidal dose.
6. Tumor mass limiting factor—circulating tumor cellular elements more responsive than solid tumor.
7. Amenable to storage with retention of immunological activity and subsequent use for immunization.

Table 27-4

Disadvantages and Problems of Labeled Antibodies for Treatment of Neoplasms

1. Antibody purification efficiency is very low (5-10%).
2. Antibody can bind circulating antigens.
3. Complexes of antigen-antibody taken up by RE system leading to high concentrations in liver and spleen.
4. Antibody specificty quite variable with consequent binding to nontumor tissue.
5. Antibody may localize in sites of inflammation.
6. Antigenic sites on tumor cells may be covered by blocking antibodies and thus prevent binding.
7. Antibody administration may blunt host immune responses—immunologic enhancement.
8. Isotope liberated from antibody may interact with other organs (thyroid).
9. Antibodies to other substances, such as brain gangliosides, known to cause epileptiform activity.
10. Xenogenic antisera may cause serum sickness or anaphylaxis upon repeated exposure.

fraction is further reduced following radioiodination since some damage and alteration of the immunoglobulin molecule occurs in the process. [131]I or [133]I has been considered an appropriate isotope for the delivery of adequate tumoricidal dose.[21]

Following intravenous administration to the tumor host, the labeled antibody can be neutralized by the presence of corresponding circulating tumor antigen with resultant complex formation and sequestration within the RE system. Radiolabeled antibody may not combine with tumor antigens as a consequence of blocking antibodies on the surface of the tumor cells.[3,4] However, if there is binding to tumor antigens, then the determinant factor of radiation exposure of the tumor cells depends on the stability and sufficiently long T½ of the cell membrane antigens. Meanwhile, the exposure of nontumor cells to radiation should be minimized.

To date, the primary choice of isotope has been ^{131}I since efficient binding to immunoglobulin and delivery of an adequate radiation dose of 500 rad/cell in the form of beta radiation can be achieved.[21] The number of labeled antibodies needed is far less than the number of binding sites available on the tumor cell surface. The combination of two ^{131}I molecules per antibody molecule can well provide the necessary dose as well as maintain the functional behavior of the antibody. The feasibility of effective antigen and antibody interaction using radiolabeled antibodies has been discussed and mathematically analyzed in great detail by McGaughey.[21] The major determinant of efficacy relates to the adjustment of the appropriate dose of labeled antibody to match the estimated tumor mass. Circulating tumor cells are more amenable to therapy than localized cellular masses.

The literature as reviewed in Table 27-1 revealed tumor localization with the use of different radiolabeled antibodies. However, high concentrations of these were also noted within the blood and other tissues. Some of the greater tumor localization of isotope has been noted in the presence of ^{131}I-fibrinogen antibodies and not in that of tumor-specific antibodies as expected.[10,11] The difficulty in purifying labeled antibody has been advanced as the most significant problem inhibiting success with this modality. Consequently, the effectiveness of radiolabeled antibody would be limited solely by the presence of circulatory antigens or blocking antibodies at the tumor cell surface. The purity of antibodies is most important since serum sickness or anaphylaxis with repeated use may occur. A recent report[24] has noted the ability of antibodies to gangliosides to cause seizures. Therefore, possible impurities of these in human preparations should be evaluated. In addition, further concern about alteration of the body's usual immune reactions is to be considered since the passive administration of antibodies may blunt the host's natural defenses with consequent immunologic enhancement.[3,4]

The utilization of radiolabeled antibodies in humans has been limited to the reports of Ghose et al.,[19,20] Spar et al.,[11] and Reif and coworkers.[17] Ghose's group conducted investigations using xenogenic ^{131}I-radiolabeled antibody in patients having carcinomas of the kidney and lung and malignant melanoma. These patients demonstrated localization of labeled antibody within their tumors as well as in liver, spleen, and lungs. However, assessment of improved survival or cell death in these patients was beyond the scope of the study. The localization of activity was not attributed secondary to fibrinogen antibodies. Spar and his colleagues[11] have noted neoplastic localization of labeled fibrinogen antibodies in 75 percent (129/172) of patients with various tumors. In some instances clinical improvement was documented. However, since their initial reports in the 1960s, there has been no additional information on the use of this agent. In the report of Reif and his group,[17] there was no evidence of localization of ^{131}I-anti-CEA Ig in the metastatic sites of CEA-producing carcinoma of the colon. There was, however, preferential uptake within the liver and lungs showing no evidence of tumor.

The future prospects of developments of radiolabeled antibodies and their impact on diagnostic and therapeutic nuclear medicine should be reviewed with cautious optimism. Table 27-5 lists some of the considerations which should be applied in the assessment of the use and efficacy of radiolabeled antibodies.[25,26] Many more studies using nonhuman tumor models seem indicated before their potential applicability to clinical nuclear medicine can be judged. Further, some standardization of approach and reporting as well as study of nontumor conditions are warranted.

Table 27-5

Suggestions for Future Development and Evaluation of Radiolabeled Antibody

---

1. More complete information of tumor model biochemistry, biophysiology, immunology, and tumor uptake.
2. Development of new tumor models.
3. Standardization of data reporting on tumor localization of radiolabeled antibody.
   a. Use of internal standard such as blood pool agent (^{131}I-serum albumin).
   b. Internal ratios such as liver for uptake comparison.
   c. Uptake standardization (Beierwaltes et al.[26])

$$\text{Percent kg dose/g} = \frac{\mu\text{Ci in organ/g} \times 100}{\mu\text{Ci (dose)/kg body weight}}$$

4. Study of nontumor conditions using the same radiolabeled antibody (inflammation).

REFERENCES

1. McKhann, C. F., Gunnarsson, A.: Approaches to immunotherapy. Cancer 34:1521–1531, 1974.
2. Kramer, S.: Radiation therapy and immunotherapy in research plan for radiation oncology. Cancer 37:2108–2119, 1976.
3. Kaliss, N.: Dynamics of immunologic enhancement. Transplant. Proc. 2:59–67, 1970.
4. Hellström, K. E., Hellström, I.: Immunological enhancement as studied by cell culture techniques. Annu. Rev. Microbiol. 24:373–398, 1970.
5. Shin, H. S., Pasternack, G. R., Economou, J. S., et al. Immunotherapy of cancer with antibody. Science 194:327–328, 1976.
6. Segerling, M., Ohanian, S. H., Borsos, T.: Chemotherapeutic drugs increase killing of tumor cells by antibody and complement. Science 188:55–57, 1975.
7. Pressman, D., Korngold, L.: The in vivo localization of anti-Wagner osteogenic-sarcoma antibodies. Cancer 6:619–622, 1953.
8. Korngold, L., Pressman, D.: The localization of antilymphosarcoma antibodies in the Murphy lymphosarcoma of the rat. Cancer Res. 14:96–99, 1954.
9. Day, E. D., Planinsek, J., Korngold, L., Tumor localizing antibodies purified from antisera against Murphy rat lymphosarcoma. J. Natl. Cancer Inst. 17:517–532, 1956.
10. Spar, I. L., Bale, W. F., Goodland, R. L., et al.: Distribution of injected I^{131}-labeled antibody to dog fibrin in tumor-bearing dogs. Cancer Res. 20:1501–1504, 1960.
11. Spar, I. L., Bale, W. F., Marrock, D., et al.: ^{125}I-labeled antibodies to human fibrinogen. Cancer 20:865–870, 1967.
12. Reif, A. E.: Studies on the localization of radiolabeled antibodies to a mouse myeloma protein. Cancer 27:1433–1439, 1971.
13. Izzo, M. J., Buchshaum, D. J., Bale, W. F.: Localization of an ^{125}I-labeled rat transplantation antibody in tumors carrying the corresponding antigen. Proc. Soc. Exp. Biol. Med. 139:1185–1188, 1972.
14. Kellen, J. A., Lo, J. S.: Localization of I^{125}-labeled antibodies against tumor-associated proteins from experimental rat mammary neoplasms. Res. Commun. Chem. Pathol. Pharmacol. 5:411–420, 1973.
15. Goldenberg, D. M., Preston, D. F., Primus, J. F., et al.: Photoscan localization of GW-39 tumors in hamsters using radio-labeled anticarcinoembryonic antigen immunoglobulin G. Cancer Res. 34:1–9, 1974.
16. Hoffer, P. B., Lathrop, K., Beckerman, C., et al.: Use of ^{131}I-CEA antibody as a tumor scanning agent. J. Nucl. Med. 15:323–327, 1974.
17. Reif, A. E., Curtis, L. E., Duffield, R., et al.: Trial of radio-labeled antibody localization in metastases of a patient with a tumor containg carcinoembryonic antigen (CEA). J. Surg. Oncol. 6:133–147, 1974.
18. Terman, D. S., Stewart, I., Tavel, A., et al.: Localization of neuroblastoma in vivo with tumor-specific antibodies. Cancer Res. 35:1761–1766, 1975.
19. Ghose, T., Tai, J., Guclu, A., et al.: Antibodies as carriers of radionuclides and cytotoxic drugs in the treatment and diagnosis of cancer. Ann. N.Y. Acad. Sci. 277:671–689, 1976.
20. Ghose, T., Guclu, A., Tai, J. et al.: Antibody as carrier of ^{131}I in cancer diagnosis and treatment. Cancer 36:1646–1657, 1975.
21. McGaughey, C.: Feasibility of tumor immunoradio-therapy using radioiodinated antibodies to tumor-specific cell membrane antigens with emphasis on leukemias and early metastases. Oncology 29:302–319, 1974.
22. Spar, I. L.: An immunologic approach to tumor imaging. Semin. Nucl. Med. 6:379–387, 1976.

23. Winchell, H. S.: Mechanisms for localization of radiopharmaceuticals in neoplasms. Semin. Nucl. Med. 6:371–378, 1976.
24. Karpiak, S. E., Graf, L., Rapport, M. M.: Antiserum to brain gangliosides produces recurrent epileptiform activity. Science 194:735–737, 1976.
25. Haynie, T. P., Konikowski, T., Glenn, H. F.: Experimental models for evaluation of radioactive tumor localizing agents. Semin. Nucl. Med. 6:347–369, 1976.
26. Kirschner, A. S., Ice, R. D., Beierwaltes, W. H.: Letter to the editor/Author's reply. J. Nucl. Med. 16:248–249, 1975.

SECTION V

"Limited Access" Use of Radionuclides

Tapan A. Hazra and Robert Howells

28

Uses of Beta Emitters for Intracavitary Therapy

The use of radiocolloids in the treatment of malignant disease was first reported in 1945 by J. H. Muller[1] of Zurich. Not until 1951 was the use of a similar modality of treatment with colloidal gold 198 described by King and his associates in the United States. The primary objective of this form of therapy was the reduction of fluid accumulation in the serosal cavities, and this is still the main application of the method. The types of tumors whosedissemination results in exudation of fluid in serosal cavities are metastatic carcinoma of the lung, and ovary, and disseminated lymphoma and certain cases of gastrointestinal cancer and renal cancer. Parcentesis gives relief, but accumulation may be rapid and frequent tappings are inconvenient for the patient, especially as considerable loss of protein occurs.

There are three colloidal radioisotopes used for intracavitary therapy: namely, gold 198 (^{198}Au), chromic phosphate 32 (^{32}P), and yttrium 90 (^{90}Y). The physical characteristics of the isotopes are as follows:

Isotope	Half-Life (days)	Max. Energy (mev)	Gamma Energy (mev)	Max. Range (cm)	Production
^{198}Au	2.7	0.96	0.412	0.39	Reactor
^{32}P	14.3	1.7	—	0.8	Reactor
^{90}Y	2.68	2.2	—	1.05	Fission

The presence of a penetrating gamma ray component in the decay scheme of gold 198 is a disadvantage. The rationale of radiocolloid therapy is the exploitation of short-range beta particles to give a high dose to tissue surfaces in contact with the isotope. Underlying tissues are spared and hence large volume doses are not given.

In general, the therapeutic end results appear to be the same no matter which isotope is used, provided equivalent doses are delivered. For instance, it is generally accepted that 10 mCi of ^{32}P delivers the equivalent dose as 100 mCi of ^{198}Au. Despite the early enthusiasm for radiogold, radiophosphorus has become the most widely used isotope. Card, Cole, and Henschke[2] in a 10-year review of cases, list their reasons for this:

1. The higher ^{32}P beta energy may be more effective, particularly in the destruction of disseminated cancer cells.
2. The longer half-life of ^{32}P eliminates critical shipping time problems and may allow some advance stocking of the colloid.
3. The abasence of any gamma ray reduces the hazard to personnel considerably, although, of course, spillage of the material is still a hazard. Also, the patient is allowed more mobility as the beta rays are absorbed in the patient, and almost no irradiation sickness (nausea, vomitting, bowel damage, depressed bone marrow or white blood cell count, etc.) is observed.

Hahn[3] reported after gold 198 therapy "a syndrome resembling irradiation sickness." He also noted definite but mild hematological changes which are usually noticeable, but a few patients have developed a persistent leukopenia following large doses. Bone marrow changes were mild.

^{90}Y, while having suitable physical characteristics, requires a stable yttrium carrier in amounts which are close to toxic levels. Hence, it has never been widely used.

Radiogold was commercially available in a suitably prepared medium as a fine colloid with a particle size of 0.05 to 0.1 microns. Radiophosphorus is prepared in the form of chromic phosphate ($Cr^{32}P\ O_4$). It is a coarser colloid than radiogold with a particle size in the range of 0.05 to 1.0 microns and is commercially available as a glucose suspension. It has a tendency to agglutinate more rapidly than gold, particularly in pockets of the peritoneum.

MECHANISM OF ACTION

The pathogenesis of fluid accumulation within the serosal cavities has been ascribed to increased fluid production coupled with a decreased removal rate. There are several theories as to the mechanism by which radiocolloids decrease serosal cavity fluid accumulation:

1. Direct action of radiation on the "free" neoplastic cells in the effusion and on the seedings of tumor present in the serosal surfaces.
2. Radiation fibrosis of the mesothelium and of the small blood vessels of the serosal surfaces which decrease fluid formation.
3. The colloidal particles are engulfed by the phagocytic cells which are present both free in the fluid and on the serosal surface. After being engulfed, the particles are carried to the regional lymph nodes where local irradiation of the nodes is carried out.

Hirabayashi and Graham[4] have made studies that showed malignant peritoneal effusions to be caused by an increased production of fluid by peritoneal surfaces apparently free of tumor. There appears to be a consistent increase in portal pressure in this type of patient.

Coates et al.[5] in a study of 38 patients with ascites caused by neoplasms concluded that "blockage to the normal lymphatic pathways draining the peritoneal cavity may be one of the mechanisms involved in the accumulation of ascites in malignant disease.'' Feldman[6] has demonstrated lymphatic blockage in mice following injection of ascites tumor cells into the peritoneum. He has studied the appearance of rapid inflammatory reactions to the ascitic fluid tumor cells that occlude the conduits connecting the peritoneal cavity to the subdiaphragmatic lymphatic plexus. The inflammation responded to corticoid therapy.

METHOD OF ADMINISTRATION

The administration of radiocolloids should be carried out with full aseptic precautions, and a radiation safety official should be consulted as to the rules governing the handling of unsealed radioisotopes.

The bulk of the fluid is first removed from the serosal cavity by routine paracentesis. This is extremely important, or else the colloid will become greatly diluted, and this dilution will markedly decrease the radiation dose delivered. It is usual to allow some fluid to remain to facilitate rapid and even distribution of the isotope through the serosal cavity. This is much simplified when radiochromic phosphate is used, requiring much less shielding.

In patients receiving colloidal therapy for subclinical disease in early ovarian carcinoma, proper care should be taken to ensure that the tip of the needle is within the peritoneal cavity, and not in the bowel or abdominal wall. Failure to ensure this could result in local necrosis. One method of checking the needle position, other than direct visualization, is by the installation of radiopaque material through the needle, and obtaining a flat plate of the abdomen. Table 28-1 lists the recommended doses of radiocolloids.

After radiocolloids have been given, to ensure uniform bathing of the serosal surfaces the patient is asked to move from side to side as well as to lie prone and supine at intervals for a period of a few hours. Since the heart is in constant motion, it is not necessary to move the patient from one position to the other immediately following the injection of radiocolloid in the pericardium.

MEASUREMENT AND DISTRIBUTION OF RADIATION DOSAGE

It is important to determine the distribution of the radioisotope with the serosal cavity at different times. Local accumulations of the isotope can occur, usually the result of masses or adhesions which cause "pockets" to form. Radiogold is relatively easy to detect because of its gamma rays, and an isoactivity

Table 28-1
Recommended mCi Doses of Radiocolloids

Serosal Cavity	^{32}P	^{198}Au	^{90}Y
Pleura	10–15	75–100	15–20
Peritoneum	15–20	75–150	20–25
Pericardium	5–10	50–75	5–10

map can be measured with a simple detector. The bremsstrahlung from ^{32}P beta rays can be imaged with a 1-inch thick sodium iodide crystal detector, although the scans show only the general distribution of the isotope.

Using ^{99m}Tc-pertechnetate, Vider et al.[7] claim that even peritoneal distribution of the isotope is very difficult to achieve, there being so many peritoneal pockets and cavities where fluid may collect, particularly after surgery. Some unevenness of the distribution is not disastrous, provided that all the serosal surfaces receive an adequate dose. Injection of the isotope into small loculated spaces, however, could result in local "hot spots." Based on autopsy data, an estimate of the dose delivered to various organs, after intraperitoneal administration of 150 mCi of colloidal ^{198}Au in 400 ml of saline has been reported to be about 750 rads from the gamma radiation plus the beta ray component (7,000 rads average for retroperitoneal lymph nodes, 6,000 rads to the omentum, 4,000 rads to the peritoneal serosa, 170 rads to the liver, 150 rads to the spleen, and 30 rads to the kidneys).

The rationale of isotope therapy is that the beta rays will deliver a high surface dose, with very limited penetration of the radiation. If the beta emitting isotope is distributed throughout a simple volume (say a sphere) rather than a plane, then provided that the range of the beta particles is small, the dose throughout most of the volume will be constant. The surface dose will be approximately one-half of the dose within the volume, rising to its maximum at a depth inside the sphere equal to the particle range. Outside the sphere, or other volume, the dose falls away rapidly.

In the therapeutic use of radiocolloids, the isotope plates out onto the serosal surfaces. In the case of radiogold, Walton and Sinclair[8] have shown that the precipitation is slow, most of the dose being given from the colloidal isotope, and that the average dose delivered is dependent on the volume injected. The precipitation rate of radiochromic phosphate is fairly rapid, and the longer half-life of ^{32}P ensures that a large part of the dose is given from the plated out isotope.

Any calculations must be regarded as approximate because of variations in the isotope distribution and uncertainty of the exact contact area of the serosal surfaces.

COMPLICATIONS

Besides the mild radiation sickness as evidenced by nausea, vomiting, and diarrhea, one occasionally sees patients with increasing shortness of breath accompanied by cyanosis and elevation of temperature during intrapleural installation of radiocolloids. Ileus and gastrointestinal complications have also been recorded with intraperitoneal installation of colloids. Gastrointestinal complications have been seen up to 10 years after treatment when the serosa is found to be thickened and fibrosed. Adhesions are formed and the bowel wall is fragile and the damage does not repair easily. These effects are apparent throughout the small intestine. Hematological complications are not common but are seen occasionally.

RESULTS

In patients with malignant disease, survival is a function of the stage of the disease at the time of presentation. Hence, for those patients with diseeminated malignancy presenting with serosal effusion, radiocolloidal therapy does not seem to change the natural outcome. Thus, in most instances such therapy would be considered palliative. Since the advent of chemotherapeutic agents which can be more easily administered, no radiocolloid therapy should be carried out unless the life expectancy of the patient is at least 3 to 6 months. Rapid accumulation of pleural effusion or ascites is a contraindication for colloidal therapy. Colloidal therapy in malignant pericardial effusion often produces very dramatic results.

However, patients with stage I (disease confined to the ovaries) ovarian carcinoma treated with radioactive colloidal solution immediately after surgery have a better 5-year survival rate. Piver[9] found that 94 percent of patients who received colloidal therapy soon after surgery with stage I ovarian carcinoma were alive without evidence of disease compared to 22 percent who had surgery alone. Similar results have also been reported by Hilarisand his associates.[10] At Johns Hopkins Hospital we carried out colloidal therapy in 40 patients soon after surgery for stage I ovarian carcinoma. Our results are also suggestive of a better survival rate when compared to historical controls.

Colloidal gold, yttrium, and arsenic 76 trisulfate have been used in the treatment of superficial bladder cancer. This modality of treatment is unsatisfactory because of the limited dose penetration, which precludes the effective treatment of infiltrating lesions. Moreover, the risk of serious complications—rectal ulceration, bladder contraction, hematuria, urethral insufficiency—is very high. This form of therapy is at present not recommended for bladder carcinoma.

Overton and Shaffell,[11] Trippi et al.,[12] and Young et al.[13] have obtained a marked clinical improvement in patients with inoperable cystic recurrent craniopharyngioma by installation of ^{32}P.

REFERENCES

1. Muller, J. H.: Uber die Verwendung von kunstlichen radioaktiven Isotopen zur Erzielung von lokalisierten biologischen Strahlenwirkungen. Experientia 1:199–200, 1945.
2. Card, R. Y., Cole, D. R., Heschke, U. K.: Summary of ten years of the use of radioactive colloids in intracavitary therapy. J. Nucl. Med. 1:195–198, 1960.
3. Hahn, P. F.: Therapeutic use of artificial isotopes. New York, John Wiley and Sons, 1956.
4. Hirabayashi, K., Graham, J.: Genesis of ascites in ovarian cancer. Am. J. Obstet. Gynecol. 106:492–497, 1970.
5. Coates, G., Bush, R. S., Aspin, N.: A study of ascites using lymphoscintigraphy with Tc-99m sulphur colloid. Radiology 107:577–583, 1973.
6. Feldman, G. B.: Lymphatic obstruction in carcinomatous ascites. Cancer Res. 35:325–332, 1975.

 7. Vider, M., DeLand, F. H., Maruyama, Y.: Loculation as a contraindication to intracavitary ^{32}P chromic phosphate therapy. J. Nucl. Med. 17:150–151, 1976.
 8. Walton, R. J., Sinclair, W. K.: Intracavitary irradiation with radioactive colloidal gold in the palliative treatment of malignant pleural and peritoneal effusions. Brit. Med. Bull. 8:165–171, 1952.
 9. Piver, M. S.: Radioactive colloids in the treatment of stage I-A ovarian cancer. Obstet. Gynecol. 40:42–44, 1972.
10. Hilaris, B. S., Clark, D. G. C.: The value of postoperative intraperitoneal injection of radiocolloids in early cancer of ovary. Am. J. Roentgenol. 112:749–754, 1971.
11. Overton, M. C. III, Sheffel, D. D.: Recurrent cystic formation in craniopharyngioma treated with radioactive chromic phosphate. J. Neurosurg. 20:707–710, 1963.
12. Trippi, A. C., Garner, J. T., Kassabian, J. T., et al.: A new approach to inoperable craniopharyngiomas. Am. J. Surg. 118:307–310, 1969.
13. Young, H. F., Fu, Y. S., Fratkin, M. J.: Organ culture of craniopharyngioma and its cellular effects induced by colloidal chromic phosphate. J. Neuropathol. Exp. Neurol. 35:404–412, 1976.

Irving M. Ariel

29

Lymphography and the Endolymphatic Administration of Radioactive Isotopes for the Treatment of Certain Cancers

Living lymphography (lymphangioadenography) is the roentgenography of the lymphatic channels (lymphangiography) and the lymph nodes (lymphadenography) following the injection or a radiopaque material into a lymphatic vessel. Accordingly, a new dimension is provided in the visualization of the lymphatic dynamic state when cancerous metastases are transferred via a lymphatic vessel to a lymph node, as well as a means for studying the sequence of events that follow such transmission. The administration of a cancerocidal agent, a radioactive isotope, permits the internal irradiation not only of cancerous deposits within a lymph node, but also of in-transit metastases.

Lymphography in the Diagnosis of Malignant Neoplasms

The diagnosis of metastases within the lymph node is dependent on the fact that metastases do not concentrate the injected contrast medium Ethiodol.[1] Normally, the lymph nodes concentrate Ethiodol; when a metastasis of a given size is present, a vacuole remains.

APPEARANCE OF NORMAL LYMPH NODES

The normal lymph node is usually ovoid with a regular contour. However, the normal node may also be of V or J shape, and frequently a small notch in the

---

Grants-in-Aid from the Arnold and Muriel Rosen Cancer Fund, the Harold S. Brady Memorial Cancer Fund, and the Foundation for Clinical Research, New York, New York, are gratefully acknowledged.
[1] E. Fougera & Co., Hicksville, N.Y.

margin known as the hilum is present, which is the point of entry of the lymphatic trunk. The opacified normal lymph node presents a homogeneous and granular appearance. Sometimes a normal lymph node may be partially replaced by fat and/or fibrous tissue lending an appearance similar to that of a cancerous metastasis, and a false-positive diagnosis is made. Fischer and Thornbury[1] call attention to another defect which may create a false-positive diagnosis: when two nodes lie closely adjacent, they give the radiographic appearance of a single node with a small space between, suggesting a metastasis. Special studies and oblique views help to delineate these defects.

APPEARANCE OF METASTASES

Metastases appear as a clear area, or vacuole, in an otherwise homogeneously filled lymph node (Fig. 29-1A). The observed patterns of metastases are numerous and varied. Frequently, lymph nodes containing metastases demonstrate marginal filling defects due to the presence of small metastases in the subcapsular region, presenting a "moth-eaten" appearance. Usually, these nodes are of normal size and do not become enlarged until extensive metastases are present.

Koehler, Wohl, and Schaffer[2] demonstrated that a metastasis must be at least 5 to 10 mm in diameter before it can be visualized roentgenographically. Numer-

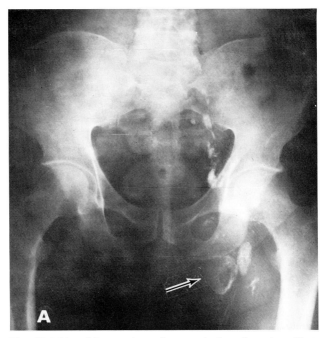

Fig. 29-1(A). Metastatic melanoma in lymph nodes. Note vacuolated appearance (*arrow*). (Reprinted with permission from N.Y. State J. Med. 68:1247, 1968.)

ous examples have been observed of completely normal-appearing lymph nodes which contained microscopic deposits of cancer.

When a lymph node is completely replaced by cancer, the flow of the injected Ethiodol completely circumvents this node, and it is not visualized radiographically. Therefore, the absence of opacification may give the surgeon a false sense of security.

The accuracy of diagnosing lymph node metastases by means of lymphography averages about 30 percent. Errors may be made on two points: from the standpoint of false negatives in which no metastases are observed in a lymph node that appears radiographically normal; and false positives where defects are observed within a node which are not the result of metastases.

RADIOGRAPHIC APPEARANCE OF LYMPHOMA IN LYMPH NODES

Lymphography lends its greatest diagnostic accuracy in the field of lymphomas. In the lymphomas the lymph nodes are markedly enlarged and present a "moth-eaten" appearance throughout. Baum and his colleagues[3] have stressed the fact that lymphography demonstrates even the most minor changes within the lymph nodes due to lymphoma.

The most typical picture seen in lymphosarcoma is a mottled appearance in

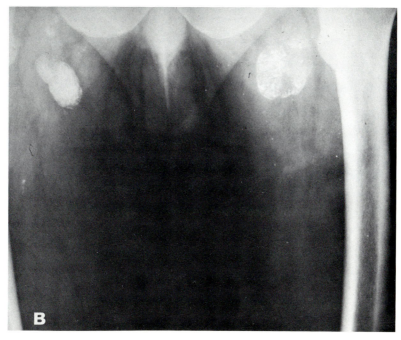

Fig. 29-1(B). Lymphosarcoma in lymph nodes. Note lymphadenopathy and moth-eaten appearance. (Reprinted with permission from N.Y. State J. Med. 68:1247, 1968.)

an enlarged lymph node, defined as producing a "salt and pepper" effect (Fig. 29-1B). Giant follicular lymphoblastoma gives a similar picture; however, the lymph nodes are markedly enlarged and present the salt and pepper effect. In reticulum cell sarcoma, in addition to the lymphadenopathy and the salt and pepper effect, there are "blotchy" areas caused by incomplete filling. This blotchy appearance is noted to a greater degree in Hodgkin's disease (Fig. 29-1C). In lymphatic leukemia and in certain instances of myelogenous leukemia a picture similar to that of lymphosarcoma may be observed. Occasionally, the lymph nodes of metastatic seminoma and sarcoidosis may simulate lymphosarcoma in appearance. Rarely does lymphadenitis of a nonspecific nature mimic the appearance of the lymph nodes as produced by the lymphomas.

Lymphography is a valuable adjunct, not only as an aid in diagnosis, but also in the assessment of the extent of the malignant neoplastic involvement. Recently, a patient was referred to us for therapy with a diagnosis of Hodgkin's disease made histologically. A lymphogram was interpreted as lymphadenitis; review of

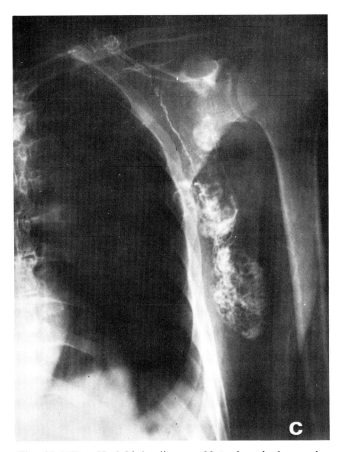

Fig. 29-1(C). Hodgkin's disease. Note lymphadenopathy and blotchy appearance of lymph nodes. (Reproduced with permission from *Progress in Cancer,* N.Y. State J. Med. 68:1247, 1968.)

the biopsy slide confirmed this diagnosis. The benefit accorded this patient by lymphography needs no further comment.

Since the increased use of lymphography in the lymphomas, it has been observed that from 30 to 40 percent of patients with stage I or stage II lymphosarcoma or Hodgkin's disease will have evidence of involvement of their retroperitoneal lymph nodes.

OTHER USES OF LYMPHOGRAPHY

Additional benefits may be derived from lymphography:

1. It permits the oncologist to study both normal and abnormal lymphatic dynamics, and to learn more about cancer spread.
2. Since the lymph nodes will retain the radiopaque medium for from 6 to 9 months, any change within the lymph node can be observed, such as either a response to therapy or an increase in size due to cancerous growth.
3. It offers the radiotherapist a landmark for the placement of radiotherapeutic portals.
4. One can study the response to x-ray therapy by observing any change in the size of the lymph node, particularly a decrease in size.
5. A repeat lymphogram, especially in patients with lymphoma who must be followed for prolonged periods, will provide an assessment of the status of the malignant process.

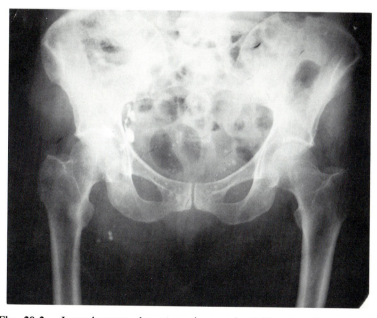

Fig. 29-2. Lymphogram demonstrating retained iliac lymph nodes after superficial groin dissection. Metastases produced painful edematous extremity; symptomatic improvement after isotopic lymphogram. (Reprinted with permission from N.Y. State J. Med. 68:1247, 1968.)

6. When chlorophyll is combined with Ethiodol, all the opacified lymph nodes are stained light green. Therefore, preoperative lymphography aids the surgeon, especially the surgical resident, in the visualization of the lymph nodes during the performance of a lymphadenectomy for cancer. (The Federal Drug Administration now prohibits the use of chlorophyll in this instance.)

7. Lymphography demonstrates to the surgeon the adequacy of his lymph node dissection. A preoperative lymphogram is performed, and upon completion of a lymphadenectomy a repeat roentgenogram taken on the operating table will demonstrate the presence of any retained lymph nodes (Fig. 29-2). It must be borne in mind that a lymph node completely replaced by cancer (unopacified) will not be exhibited on x-ray. However, such cancerous nodes are usually markedly enlarged and are readily visible to the surgeon at the time of operation.

8. Lymphography demonstrates abnormalities of the mediastinum by any alteration in the anatomy of the thoracic duct.

COMPLICATIONS

Fischer and Thornbury,[1] in a review of 100 consecutive lymphograms performed, cite a minimum of complications; none serious.

In our series of 325 lymphograms, no complications were encountered. Ten patients complained of a transient sense of ill feeling which they could not pinpoint; five of these patients complained of transient mild nausea. The only reaction we have observed was slow healing of the incision at the injection site. Inasmuch as many of our patients received radioactive isotopes endolymphatically administered with the Ethiodol, we believe the slow healing to be, in all probability, the result of leakage at the site of incision. The simple procedure of pouring 1 liter of normal saline solution over the wound before it is suture closed has obviated this difficulty.

Spillage of the contrast medium into the lung parenchyma via the thoracic duct is inherent in the technique. As a result, although symptoms are not produced in a patient with normal pulmonary function, a few serious sequelae have been described in patients with extensive pulmonary disease, and two fatal fat embolizations have been reported.[4,5] This complication has been averted in our patients by means of limiting the amount of contrast medium injected. We do not inject more than 10 ml into each lower extremity lymphatic vessel, and a maximum of 5 ml into each upper extremity lymphatic vessel.

LYMPHATIC DYNAMICS

A knowledge of the normal lymphatic anatomy and physiology provides us with a better understanding of the changes that may occur as a result of metastases, those changes that may occur following the performance of certain surgical and radiological procedures, and will illuminate our understanding as to the best possible course of treatment to be followed.

NORMAL LYMPHATIC DYNAMICS

Normally, when Ethiodol is injected into a lymphatic vessel, the medium will be transported throughout the lymphatic network with only a slight delay before deposition in the lymph nodes draining the region. The radiopaque material remains within the lymphatic vessels for a period varying from 3 to 6 hours, and will drain within 24 hours in almost every instance. In contrast to blood flow, lymphatic flow is either extremely slow or stagnant when the extremity is in the dependent position. With the patient in a horizontal position, it may take from 5 minutes to 2 hours to inject 10 ml of Ethiodol using a pressure pump. Accordingly, following the intralymphatic injection of Ethiodol, serial roentgenograms will provide an index of the lymphatic distribution pattern.

Lower Extremity Lymphatic Vessels

The lymphatic trunks of the lower extremity usually follow the course of the greater saphenous vein (saphena magna system). The lymphatic vessels vary from 0.25 to 1.0 ml in diameter, usually retaining their caliber as they ascend toward the inguinal region and usually following a straight course to end abruptly (Fig. 29-

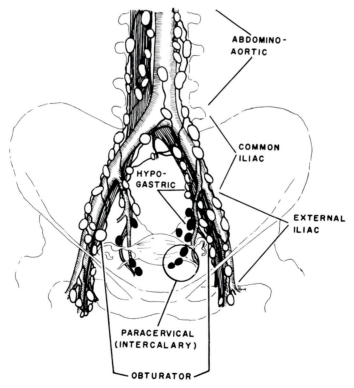

Fig. 29-3(A). Anatomy of lower abdominal lymph nodes. (Reprinted with permission from Arch. Surg. 94:117, 1967.)

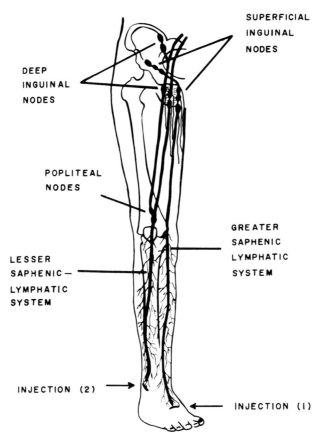

Fig. 29-3(B). Lymphatic vessels of lower extremity. Injection site 1, on dorsum of foot, drains into greater saphenous lymphatic system. Injection site 2, lateral aspect of ankle, drains into lesser sephenous system, into popliteal nodes, and then to inguinal lymph nodes. (Reproduced with permission from Arch. Surg. 94:117, 1967.)

3A). When a contrast medium is injected into a lymphatic vessel on the dorsum of the foot (injection site 1, Fig. 29-3B), the lymphatic vessels are visualized as one or more trunks coursing proximally along the anteromedial aspect of the leg, converging toward the knee, then ascending and branching into 12 to 16 divisions as they enter the superficial inguinal lymph nodes. If the opaque material is injected into a lymphatic vessel along the lateral aspect of the foot (injection site 2, Fig. 29-3B), the lymphatic vessels are seen to course proximally toward the popliteal fossa (saphena parva system), where one or two popliteal nodes are usually found; the latter are found routinely in dogs, whereas in the human they are absent in a significant number of patients (Fig. 29-4). The lymphatic vessels continue to course proximally to the deep lymphatic chain and terminate in the superficial inguinal vessels which course to the thigh and extend medially to enter the groin in juxtaposition to the femoral vessels. Somewhere along the course of the lymphatic vessels, valves are usually found which tend to prevent backflow. The lymph

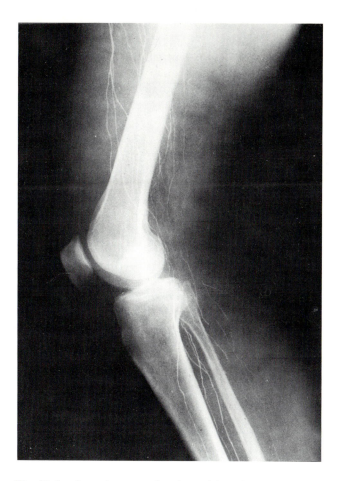

Fig. 29-4. Lymphogram of patient with melanoma, demonstrating well-developed chain of lymphatic vessels coursing
through the popliteal space; no lymph nodes present. Dissection revealed one popliteal lymph node completely replaced
by fat. (Reprinted with permission from Arch. Surg. 94:117,
1967.)

nodes of the saphena parva system (draining the back of the leg and following the
course of the lesser saphenous vein) are said to lie deeper and more craniad than
those draining the trunk of the greater saphenous system.

Inguinal and Iliac Lymph Nodes

There are from 4 to 10 inguinal nodes normally, both superficial and deep,
presenting a variable pattern. Efforts to divide this group into subgroups based on
a relationship to the greater saphenous vein are believed to be of no practical use
in clinical radiographic diagnoses.

As originally described by Rouvier,[6] the efferent lymphatic vessels from the
inguinal nodes continue proximally to the external iliac chain of nodes to divide

into three chains: a lateral chain located lateral to the external iliac artery (one to four nodes), a middle group which lies on the posterior surface of the external iliac vein (two to four nodes), and a medial group (three to four nodes) posterior to the external iliac vein usually in juxtaposition to the lateral pelvic wall. The obturator node is considered a part of the medial group of the external iliac chain of nodes and is found radiographically related; it may either lie in direct continuity with the remainder of the medial chain, or it may be somewhat distant as a solitary node within the obturator fossa usually between the external iliac vein and the obturator nerve and vessels.

Continuing proximally, the common iliac chain (4 to 12 nodes lying in close relationship to the common iliac artery and vein) subdivides into the hypogastric nodes (two to eight in number), and courses along the hypogastric artery; from the common iliac nodes, several trunks course craniad along the aorta and inferior vena cava to form the abdominoaortic lymph node group (25 to 45 nodes). The abdominoaortic nodes are divided into four groups: (1) right lateral aortic, (2) left lateral aortic, (3) preaortic, and (4) retroaortic. Efferent lymphatic vessels from the abdominoaortic chain empty into the cisterna chyli usually at the level of the second lumbar vertebra. Rarely can lymph nodes be visualized in the posterior mediastinum, but not infrequently supraclavicular nodes may be seen in the region of the termination of the thoracic duct.

Upper Extremity Lymphatics

There are usually two groups of lymphatic vessels in the upper extremity, a lateral and medial, which join above the elbow and usually follow the basilic vein along the inner aspect of the arm to the axillary chain of lymph nodes (Fig. 29-5). The axillary nodes vary in number, are interconnected by many trunks, and their efferents may drain either directly into the subclavian vein, or may lead to the supraclavicular nodes and then empty into the subclavian vein. Inconsistently, one to two small lymph nodes may be visualized in the epitrochlear region along the medial aspect.

Lymphatic-Vascular Communications

A communication normally exists between the lymphatic and venous systems. Rusznyak, Foldi, and Szabo[7] have demonstrated an anastomosis between the lymphatic vessels and the veins, especially in the thyroid, kidney, and liver. Blalock and coworkers[8] demonstrated the presence of numerous connections between the lymphatic vessels and the inferior vena cava, the azygous and other veins, especially after ligation of the thoracic duct. Pressman et al.[9] demonstrated the existence of a communication between the lymph nodes and the blood vessels by injecting air into the lymph nodes of animals; the air was seen in both the lymphatic vessels and the veins. Wallace and associate[10] demonstrated direct lymphatic-venous communications in the normal individual, found most frequently in the cervical region and to a lesser extent in the upper extremity, and the communications were more abundant in those individuals with lymphatic obstruction.

It is not surprising to note these connections between the lymphatic and

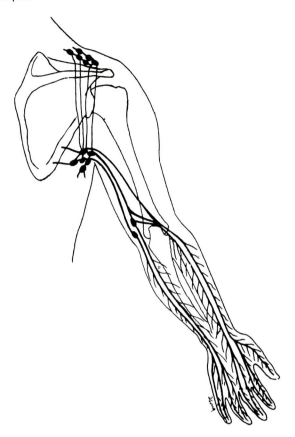

Fig. 29-5. Lymphatic vessels and lymph nodes of upper extremity. Note communications from axillary to supraclavicular lymph nodes. (Reproduced with permission from Arch. Surg. 94:117, 1967.)

venous systems, inas much as embryologically the lymphatic sacs are formed by a process of "budding" from the blood vascular endothelium. Budding sacs from the anterior cardinal veins give rise to the lymphatic vessels of the head and neck. Sprouts from the mesonephric vein develop paired sacs which become the precursors of the skeletal lymphatics; two additional sacs are derived from the mesonephric vein, one later becomes the cisterna chyli and the lower thoracic duct, and the other forms the lymphatic vessels of the abdominal viscera.

EFFECTS OF METASTASES—ALTERED LYMPHATIC DYNAMICS

Metastases in Lymphatic Vessels

The lodgement of tumor implants within either the lymphatic vessels or the lymph nodes may produce an alteration in the normal lymphatic dynamics often determined by the location and degree of obstruction. The blockage of a lymphatic vessel in either the leg or the arm may produce one or a combination of the following alterations in collateral lymphatic flow.

1. The anterior compartment may be completely blocked, shunting the lymphatic flow into the posterior compartment.
2. The anterior chain may be incompletely blocked, producing a partial shunt into the posterior compartment, resulting in function of both compartments.
3. Both compartments may be functional without evidence of block.

Accordingly, a cancer located on the dorsum of the foot may spread to the popliteal lymph nodes due to either an anatomic shunt to the posterior lymphatic chain or an obstruction in the anterior lymphatic chain.

Popliteal Lymph Nodes

When present, the popliteal nodes drain the lesser saphenous lymphatic system and may drain the greater saphenous system as well. Therefore, cancer cells may, and do, lodge in these nodes. Accordingly, for a malignant neoplasm in the location of drainage into the popliteal nodes (i.e., directly inferior to the popliteal space, the lateral aspect of the foot, the heel), the nodes should be included in the therapeutic plan.

It has been stated: "Metastasis to the popliteal nodes is so rare that the possibility of its occurrence should not enter into the discussion of the management of melanoma of the lower extremity inferior to the condyles."[11] We disagree with this premise, for we have seen many instances of metastases of melanoma and other cancers (epidermoid carcinoma and sarcoma) to the popliteal and epitrochlear lymph nodes. Although the popliteal lymph nodes are absent in a certain percentage of humans, they are present in others. The probability exists that these nodes undergo attrition with advancing age, as do many lymph nodes, and they are present in older individuals in a nonfunctioning, atrophic form.

Our data further suggest that if the lymphogram demonstrates a collateral route from the greater saphenous to the lesser saphenous system, the popliteal nodes should definitely be considered in the therapeutic plan. If lymphograms are not performed, at least a clinical search should be made in the popliteal and epitrochlear regions in all patients presenting either primary or secondary cancers distal to these sites.

Metastases in Lymph Nodes

When metastases in the lymph nodes have reached sufficient size, the resultant blockage will shunt the lymph into alternate channels in order to maintain the integrity of lymphatic flow. A vast network of potential, not normally functioning lymphatic vessels will be enlisted into service, and those in the immediate vicinity of the obstruction will first become functional. Figure 29-6 is the lymphogram of a patient with metastatic melanoma to the left inguinal region taken 5 days after the injection of the contrast medium. Stagnation of the lymphatic vessels was present and collateral circulation developed via the presacral chain of nodes. Eventually, metastases were demonstrated in the lymph nodes of the opposite groin. Should this adjacent network prove insufficient, new groups of lymphatic vessels become

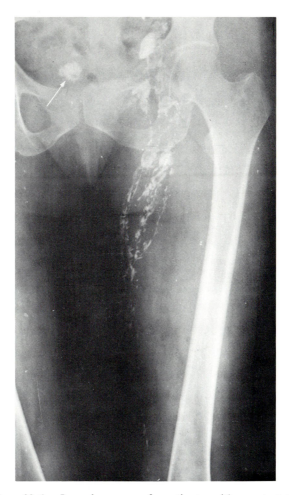

Fig. 29-6. Lymphogram of patient with metastatic melanoma to left inguinal region, taken 5 days after injection of ethiodized oil. Note stagnation of lymphatic vessels and development of collateral circulation where presacral node visualized in midline (*arrow*). Note space-occupying lesions in inguinal lymph nodes characteristic of metastases. (Reprinted with permission from N.Y. State J. Med. 68:1247, 1968.)

functional in an effort to reestablish lymphatic flow. Oftentimes an unpredictable and bizarre form of lymphatic network will assume the function of lymph transportation (and, presumably, cancer cells) for great distances uninterrupted by lymph nodes.

The nature of the collateral lymphatic vessels is often determined by the level or location of an obstruction. Obstruction in the paraaortic lymphatic vessels may produce an atypical collateral network which may extend into the visceral lymphatics. Obstruction at the level of the porta hepatis may produce such stagnation of the lymphatic system distal to the blockage that the lymph nodes may be compressed and destroyed by the back pressure. Wallace et al.[10] demonstrated that obstruction at the thoracic duct produced by posterior mediastinal lesions hindered the normal flow of lymph and induced retrograde filling of the gastrointestinal trunk as well as the intercostal lymphatics.

Those collaterals called into play after an obstruction has become extensive are so eccentric and unpredictable that they defy any effort at interpretation, and the application of therapeutic modalities is nearly impossible. This was demonstrated in an obstruction in the iliac nodes secondary to a carcinoma of the cervix which produced a lymphatic collateral chain in the anterior abdominal wall to the axilla where a metastatic cancer was encountered.[12]

Perivascular Lymphatics

The existence of potential spaces in perivascular locations was recently described by Wallace and his colleagues.[10] These spaces were successfully demonstrated by the investigators as an additional collateral route for the transport of lymph and tumor cells. They liken these perivascular spaces to the perineural or endoneural spaces which have been amply demonstrated to play a major role in the dissemination of tumor emboli. Although Wallace et al. have observed these perivascular spaces, they have been unable to establish their exact anatomy. Are they actual potential spaces between the vessel wall and its surrounding membrane, or do they constitute an integral part of the lymphatic system? However, these authors have shown conclusively the existence of a direct connection between the lymphatic system and these potential spaces to which lymph is transported, and which offers a possible route for the unopposed transport of tumor cells. These spaces, located within the perivascular sheath, have been seen in patients with and without edema.

Stagnation of Lymph

When radiopaque material is injected into a lymphatic vessel, normally it will have emptied from the lymphatics in 4 to 24 hours. In the presence of obstruction, stagnation ensues and the injected material remains within the lymphatics for long periods—as long as 2½ months, as determined by the authors, and perhaps longer, but measurements have not been made.

Clinically, a stagnant lymphatic state may be manifest by the appearance of edema. An impediment to the free flow of lymph causes an increase in lymphatic pressure with the resultant deposition of lymph within the interstitial spaces of the extremities producing edema; however, stagnation of lymphatic flow has been observed without resultant edema. We interpret stagnant lymphatic flow as presumptive evidence of the existence of an obstruction either in the proximal chain of lymph nodes or within the proximal lymphatic vessels.

Figure 29-7 is the lymphogram of a patient with metastases in the axilla from a primary melanoma of the left lateral chest wall. This patient manifested a direct lymphatic connection between the axillary and supraclavicular lymph nodes, illustrating a route for the passage of tumor emboli from the axilla into the supraclavicular region. The lymphogram showed the presence of metastases within the lymph nodes of the axilla; it demonstrated the retention of dye within the lymphat-

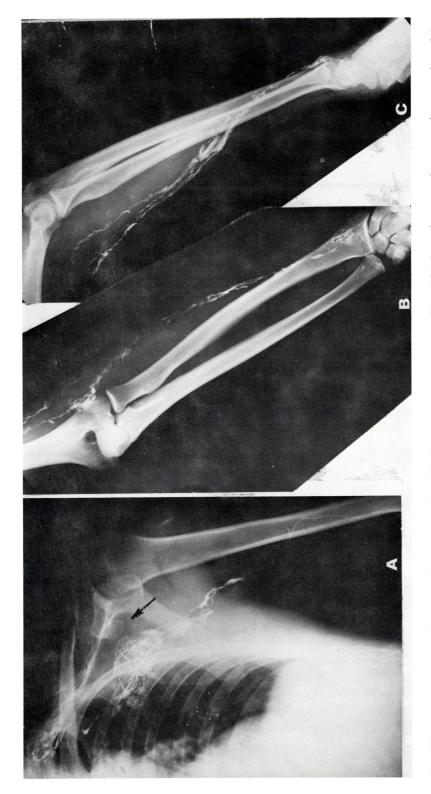

Fig. 29-7. Lymphograms of patient with metastases in axilla from primary melanoma of left lateral chest wall. (**A**): Note defect in lymph node characteristic of space-occupying lesion or metastasis (*arrow*). Also note filling of supraclavicular lymph nodes which also contain metastases. (**B** and **C**): Lymphograms demonstrating retention of dye within lymphatic vessels 3 days after its injection. Note tortuous course, irregular contour, and variation in caliber of vessels. (Reprinted with permission from N.Y. State J. Med. 68:1247, 1968.)

ic vessels 3 days after the performance of the lymphogram, indicative of stagnation in the lymphatic flow. In some instances, metastases within the lymph nodes may be of such small size as to go undetected lymphographically. For example, the stagnant state of the distal lymphatics in one patient prompted the excision of a groin lymph node for histologic study which revealed the presence of metastases.

Lymphatic stagnation with ensuing edema may be only temporary providing the development of collateral circulation is adequate. Should this occur, then the free flow of lymph within the lymphatics will be reestablished and the edema will subside. However, if an adequate collateral circulation has not developed, the edema will become more pronounced as the lymphatic pressure is increased.

Blocker and colleagues[13] have demonstrated that the normal intralymphatic pressures are subatmospheric in the lower extremity (0 to -16 mm H_2O) with a decreasing gradient upward to the thoracic duct. With blockage, the intralymphatic pressure in the lower extremity is positive, going as high as 60 to 80 mm H_2O. One patient with an inferior vena cava syndrome due to a mediastinal tumor with generalized edema from the nipple inferiorly had the extremely high intralymphatic pressure of 400 mm H_2O in the lower extremity.

Reversal of Flow

After a period of failure to establish satisfactory collateral circulation, a reversal in lymphatic flow occurs with the development of a functional superficial chain of dermal lymphatic vessels. In such instances, subsequent regurgitation of lymph occurs distally into a network of dermal lymphatic vessels (Fig. 29-8).

Lymphaticovenous Anastomosis

Previous comments have been made regarding the normal existence of lymphaticovenous anastomoses. In the presence of obstruction under the pressure of metabolic necessity, potential nonfunctioning lymphaticovenous openings become functional, and certain new communications develop in the need to mobilize a collateral circulation for the stagnant lymph, present under an increased head of pressure resulting from obstruction.[14,15,16] Under such circumstances, the transport of tumor cells from the lymphatic into the vascular circulation is probably facilitated.

Lymphatic Circulation Time

We have observed, as have Stehlin and associates,[17] that in the presence of obstruction and following isotopic administration into a lymphatic vessel of the foot, there is a delay in the time it takes for the isotope to reach the inguinal lymph nodes. To ascertain the lymphatic circulation time from foot to groin, a Geiger counter is placed over the groin as the endolymphatic administration of ^{131}I-Ethiodol is begun into a foot lymphatic vessel, and the first recording is taken as the isotope reaches the groin. In six patients without evidence of obstruction, the time averaged 5 minutes and varied from 3 to 8 minutes. In the presence of clinically detectable metastases in the lymph nodes, the time averaged 9 minutes and varied from 5 to 15 minutes.

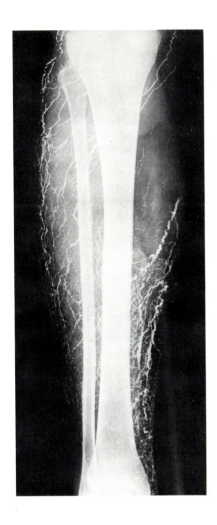

Fig. 29-8. Marked lymphedema following radical groin dissection for melanoma with development of extensive network of dermal lymphatic vessels. (Reproduced with permission from Am. J. Roentgenol. 91:1187, 1964.)

Table 29-1
Comparison of Survival Rates of Patients with Malignant Melanoma Receiving Different Treatments

Stage	Surgical Excision Alone*		Endolymphatic Radioactive Isotopes and Surgical Excision	
	No. of Patients	5-Year Survival Rate (%)	No. of Patients	5-Year Survival Rate (%)
I	37	40.5	22	82.0
II	199	14.1	11	28.5

(Reproduced with permission from Mulholland J. H., Ellison E. M., and Freison S. R. (eds.), Current Surgical Management. Philadelphia, W. B. Saunders, 1957.)
*Wide local excision and mode dissection.

329

^{131}I-Ethiodol Concentration in the Blood

When 10 ml Ethiodol containing 30 mCi ^{131}I has been injected, the concentration of ^{131}I in the blood could be considered an index of lymphatic-vascular communication. The data are presented in Table 29-1 and demonstrate a significantly increased quantity of ^{131}I in the blood of patients with metastases in the inguinal lymph nodes. Some of this may have been due to spillover via the thoracic duct into the circulation; however, the small volume injected (10 ml) minimizes this possibility.

EFFECTS OF DISCONTINUOUS LYMPH NODE DISSECTION ON LYMPHATIC DYNAMICS

Hazards of the Operation

We have demonstrated that the performance of a discontinuous operation for melanoma is not without hazard.[3,4] The following sequence of events occurs after the performance of a groin dissection:

First, there is an extensive escape of lymph through the severed lymphatic vessels resulting in the formation of a lymphocele (Fig. 29-9). A lymphogram was performed 3 days after the radical groin dissection for a malignant melanoma; a drain was left in situ. Salient in this instance is the observed escape of lymph and Ethiodol from the lymphatic system into the free tissue spaces of the dissection site, because the innumerable lymphatic vessels severed during the dissection were not patent permitting the leakage; the drain functions as a suction apparatus for the lymph and Ethiodol. When the drainage tube is removed, the Ethiodol is retained within the free tissue spaces with the formation of a tract along the course of the tube.

Cancer cells in transit within the lymphatic vessels are deposited into the free tissue spaces where they may seed and grow, presenting as metastases.

Herman, Benninghoff, and Schwartz[5] have demonstrated that a lymphocyst will subsequently become an integral part of the newly formed lymphatic system with the formation of afferent and efferent communicating vessels. However, this is a function of time; the lymph, and presumably cancer cells, will remain in the free tissues for a prolonged period.

The second major event after a groin dissection is a sealing-off of the lymphatic vessels at the incisional site. As a result, one or all of the following mechanisms occur:

1. The lymphatic vessels may seal off and block the incisional region with the resultant retention of lymph in those lymphatic vessels distal to the operative site.
2. Reestablishment in continuity may take place by regrowth of the severed lymphatic vessels.
3. The blocked lymphatic vessels may form collateral channels with adjacent lymphatic vessels with the subsequent reestablishment of lymphatic flow (Fig. 29-10).

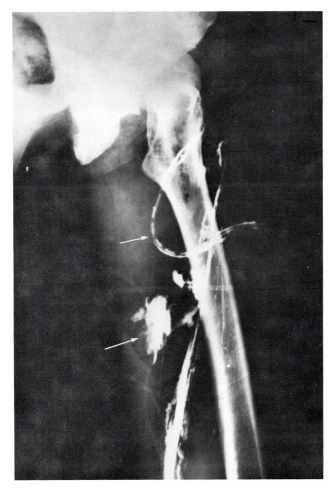

Fig. 29-9. Lymphogram taken 3 days after performance of radical groin dissection for melanoma. Note injected ethiodized oil removed by means of Hemovac (*upper arrow*) within wound site. Note lymphocele (*lower arrow*). (Reprinted with permission from N.Y. State J. Med. 68:1247, 1968.)

4. Due to lymphatic blockage, and in the presence of an inadequate development of collateral circulation, a regurgitation of lymph occurs within the subsequently functional superficial or dermal lymphatic channels. As a result, edema of the extremity may occur.

SATELLITOSIS OF MELANOMA

It is not uncommon to find the development of dermal satellite metastases involving the skin of the leg following extensive metastases to the lymph nodes of the groin, or, subsequent to the surgical excision of these nodes. Satellite cancers

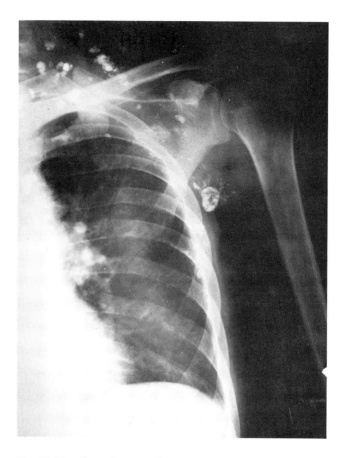

Fig. 29-10. Lymphogram demonstrating reconstituted lymphatic circulation. Regenerated lymphatic vessels communicate freely with supraclavicular lymph nodes; new collateral circulation developed with internal mammary chain of lymph nodes. Note residual lymph node in axilla harboring metastatic melanoma. Left radical axillary dissection for melanoma performed 2 years previously elsewhere.(Reprinted with permission from N.Y. State J. Med. 68:1247, 1968.)

have been noted to occur in those regions of expansive dermal lymphatic development secondary to an obstruction. It is believed that tumor emboli become implanted within the subcutaneous tissue and/or dermis via these dermal lymphatic vessels. Figure 29-11 is the lymphogram of a patient with metastatic melanoma in the left inguinal lymph nodes taken 4 days after the injection of the contrast medium, and demonstrating lymphatic stagnation. A partial groin dissection had been performed 2 years prior to the development of numerous satellitoses which involved mainly the medial aspect of the thigh. The lymphogram shows the extensively developed collateral lymphatic circulation with its large number of dermal vessels arising from the deeper lymphatic vessels and extending to the skin at sites of the satellite lesions. This patient was treated by the intralymphatic administra-

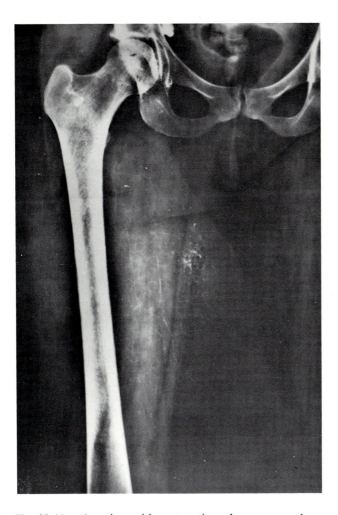

Fig. 29-11. A patient with metastatic melanoma, on whom partial groin dissection was performed 2 years before lymphography, developed extensive satellitosis. The lymphogram demonstrated extensive collateral lymphatic circulation and showed a large number of dermal vessels arising from deep lymphatic vessels at sites of satellitoses. Five years after groin dissection, and 2 years after therapeutic lymphogram, there was complete disappearance of satellitoses. (Reproduced with permission from Arch. Surg. 94:117, 1967.)

tion of radioactive isotopes, given at the time of the lymphogram, and she remains well 3 years after treatment; the satellite metastases have disappeared and new lesions have not developed.

Malignant melanoma may spread either by direct infiltration or via lymphatic channels into the adjacent tissues, with the resultant deposition of cancer cells in the regional lymph nodes. Stehlin et al.[17] have applied the epigraph "in-transit metastases'' to those cancer cells within the lymphatic vessels. This term serves to emphasize the fact that "cancer cells are conveyed via the lymphatic vessels to the regional lymph nodes." Stagnation of lymphatic flow, possibly attributable to proximal obstruction, hinders transportation, and the stalled cancer cells implant and multiply to become a fixed metastatic deposit. The latter should be differentiated from the "floating cell" in transit within the lymphatics. Metastases may be found within the deep lymphatic vessels as well as in the newly developed dermal and subcutaneous lymphatic network. Accordingly, satellitoses may be considered the result of cancer cells presumably traveling in a retrograde manner within the tiny dermal lymphatic vessels, developed in consequence of lymphatic obstruction with failure to promote adequate routes of collateral lymphatic flow; at least this is one mechanism in their development.

Stehlin and colleagues[18,19] have described the lymphatic route as being responsible for satellitoses, but have neglected to call attention to the reversal of flow, with the functionally developed network of superficial dermal lymphatic vessels as a probable mechanism attendant to the development of satellite dermal metastases.

Metastases within the lymphatic vessels of the extremity may be present at any depth, and this should be considered in any planned attack on malignant melanoma of an extremity. Consequently, melanoma cells may be found within the lymphatic vessels as (1) floating cells en route to the regional lymph nodes, (2) cells fixed within the deeper lymphatic vessels where they remain and grow, or (3) cells within the dermal lymphatic vessels transported in retrograde fashion, and come to a standstill to grow, presenting as satellitoses.

Indications and Results of Treating Malignant Melanoma with Intralymphatic Radioactive Isotopes

INTRODUCTION

The proper method of treating malignant melanoma has not been devised, although the surgical extirpation of this form of cancer is the best method at present. When a malignant melanoma is located juxtaposed to the primary chain of lymph nodes draining that region, the best method is to perform a monobloc resection of the primary cancer, the intervening lymphatics, and the lymph nodes to which the melanoma may spread. The problem arises when a melanoma is located at a great distance from the lymph node basin to which metastases may occur. For example, if a malignant melanoma is located on the foot or lower leg, the question of how to treat the lymph node-bearing area remains problematical.

A natural development from diagnostic lymphadenography was the administration of chemotherapeutic agents and/or radioactive isotopes into the lymphatic vessels as a means of delivering a large dose of irradiation to the lymph nodes.

This is a report of our results to date in the overall treatment, using endolymphatic isotopes, of patients with malignant melanoma.

TECHNIQUE

The technique of Kinmoth[20] and Taylor was utilized, and the isotope used in this investigation was ^{131}I-Ethiodol—a special preparation of radioactive Ethiodol in oil which contains 37 percent iodine in organic combination with ethyl esters of the fatty acids of poppy seed oil. A certain portion of the stable iodine has been replaced by the [131]I. This isotope has a maximum beta energy of 0.6 mev and an estimated maximum penetration in tissue of 3mm. The major therapeutic effect is from the beta rays with very little, if any, obtained from the gamma rays. The isotope has a half-life of 8.5 days, which permits protracted irradiation, and the ^{131}I-Ethiodol has a further advantage of being both diagnostic and therapeutic. Other radioactive nuclides which have been utilized are radioactive [198]gold (Jantet et al.,[11] Schwartz et al.[21], ^{90}Y microspheres (Ariel et al.[22], chromic phosphates, and ^{32}P-Lipiodol.

This presentation is limited to the results obtained with ^{131}I-Ethiodol. Radioactive chromic phosphates and ^{90}Y microspheres produced problems of administration, and the radioactive gold was found to be unsuitable because it could not be combined with the Ethiodol, and a fair amount of the administered gold was concentrated in the liver. We have abandoned their use.

The radiation factors, including distribution of the isotope, radiation doses, excretion, etc., have been described.[12] The results herein presented were those obtained by ^{131}I-Ethiodol. We are now using ^{32}P-Lipiodol. It is more readily obtained, has a more desirable radiation spectrum, and its use permits comparative evaluation with the studies being performed in England by Edwards[14,23] and his group. These results shall be reported later.

TREATMENT POLICIES

Indication for Endolymphatic Isotope Therapy

Certain treatment policies evolved as the study progressed, and the results obtained are best described by presenting the data according to the clinical staging of malignant melanoma. All melanomas were of the invasive type.

Stage I melanomas indicate that the regional lymph nodes are clinically and roentgenographically negative for evidence of metastases. Stage II indicates patients whose regional nodes contain metastases. Stage III means that satellites, i.e., deposits of melanoma throughout the skin of the involved extremity, have formed, or there is other evidence of melanoma involving the extremity, such as subcutaneous or deeper nodules. Stage IV indicates distant metastases.

STAGE I MELANOMAS

The treatment policy for this grade of cancer consists of a wide, tridimensional resection of the primary melanoma. If the melanoma is adjacent to a lymph node-draining area, an en bloc surgical dissection of the melanoma, the intervening lymphatics, and the first echelon of lymph nodes is performed. If an en bloc dissection cannot be performed, i.e., where the lymph nodes are distant from the primary melanoma, only the primary lesion is radically excised.

Within 3 to 4 weeks after the resection of the primary melanoma, a therapeutic lymphadenogram is performed. Immediately after the isotope is administered and again 24 hours later, diagnostic roentgenograms are made. When possible, the lymphatic vessel isolated is just proximal to the line of resection. In a few instances we have injected in different areas to assure filling all lymphatic vessels. The injections in the posterolateral aspects of the foot permit filling of the popliteal chain of lymph nodes.

If the roentgenogram of the lymph nodes is considered negative for evidence of metastases, no further treatments are given, but the patient is followed carefully, and repeat roentgenograms of the lymph nodes are taken. If a defect that might be considered a metastasis exists within the lymph nodes, the patient is subjected to a dissection of the lymph node-bearing region; if metastases are discovered, he is placed in the category of stage II.

Dosage and Volume

The dose of ^{131}I-Ethiodol varies from 40 to 50 mCi in 4 ml for the lower limb and 30 to 40 mCi in 2 ml for the upper limb. Smaller doses are sometimes given if clinically indicated. For example, older patients have an attrition of lymph nodes, and there is a freer flow of the isotopes to high regions in such instances. Since a certain amount of the isotope reaches the lungs, patients with pulmonary diseases are given smaller doses as well as smaller volumes. Measurements performed on the nodes regarding the radioactivity have revealed that such dosages will deliver from 50,000 to 100,000 rads beta to the lymph nodes.

In the past, we gave 10 ml to the lower extremities and 5 ml to the upper. We have reduced this to a maximum of 4 ml to the lower and 2 ml to the upper extremities. With these smaller volumes, less than 10 percent of the administered dose reaches the lungs. Repeated scannings have revealed that the isotope is rapidly eliminated from the lungs. Long-term studies, including pulmonary function tests, to date have demonstrated no untoward pulmonary reactions.[24]

STAGE II MELANOMAS

In these patients the primary melanoma is treated in the same way as with stage I. Staging is determined either by clinical examination of the patient or by the lymphogram, if it reveals a space-occupying defect in one of the lymph nodes; the node is then excised for histologic study. The overall treatment policy consists of a wide resection of the primary melanoma just as for stage I, endolymphatic administration of isotope, and 3 weeks later en bloc dissection of the lymph nodes. The delay before performing the surgical resection of the lymph nodes permits deterioration of the isotope; this results in a beneficial radiation effect to the tissues and allows the isotope to reach a dose safe for the operating team. The Atomic Energy Commission recommends a dose of 5 mCi to be safe for the operating team, and inasmuch as the biologic half-life of ^{131}I-Ethiodol is approximately 6 days, a delay from 2 to 3 weeks permits maximum irradiation to the tissues and maximum protection to the operating team. The effect of the endolymphatic isotope therapy does not contribute to any increased technical difficulties for the surgeon. The tissue is adherent, which sometimes makes it slightly more difficult to dissect the nodes free from the vessels, but in other instances makes it easier to dissect the lymph nodes. We have encountered no unusual complications resulting from the preoperative internal irradiation.[25]

STAGE III MELANOMAS

We have treated 10 patients suffering from satellitoses of their extremities by the endolymphatic administration of radioactive isotopes. Each of these patient had been treated previously by resection of the lymph nodes, and the satellitoses developed subsequently. The mechanism for this is believed to be a regurgitation of lymph carrying cancer cells as a result of blockage caused either by tumor or by the surgical procedure, described by Ariel and Resnick. Two of these patients have demonstrated complete disappearance of the satellites, and one patient remains clinically free of melanoma 5 years after such treatment. In two patients the nodes involving the inner aspects of the thigh, i.e., the distribution of the lymphatic vessels, disappeared, whereas those involving the lateral aspect of the thigh did not change in appearance. The remaining patients manifested no benefit.

STAGE IV MELANOMAS

No beneficial clinical response was observed in 10 patients treated by ^{131}I-Ethiodol delivered via the lymphatics of the feet. Metastases to the lungs, liver, or other sites existed, and irradiation to the pelvic and periaortic lymph nodes had no demonstrable clinical effect. All patients died from disseminated melanoma. We have abandoned endolymphatic isotopes for this group of patients.

RESULTS

We have previously marked shrinkage of lymph nodes[26] and destruction of malignant melanoma following ^{131}I-Ethiodol administration endolymphatically.[20]

In our series of 120 patients treated by this technique, 22 patients in clinical stage I were treated over 5 years ago. A survival rate (free of melanoma) of 82 percent was obtained (Table 29-1). A 5-year survival rate of 28.5 percent for the 11 patients in clinical stage II was obtained.

Table 29-1 compares the clinical accomplishments of endolymphatic isotope therapy with surgical excision in treatment malignant melanoma. The data for those patients treated by surgical resection alone, reported by Pack, Scharnagel, and Morfitt,[27] represent patients treated by the same technique and for the most part by the same group of surgeons. An index of improvement is noted in those patients who received ^{131}I-Ethiodol endolymphatically. This treatment appears promising and warrants further clinical trial.

DISCUSSION

Animal Experiments

As a means of determining the reliability of endolymphatic isotope therapy, Edwards[23] and his coworkers described experimental work performed on VX2 tumor in a host animal—the rabbit. They analyzed their results according to the lymphographic appearance of the lymph nodes, microscopic findings on autopsy, and survival time of the animals.

Lymphograhic findings. Serial lymphadenograhpic examination revealed that, in the animals in whom the isotope was administered over 4 weeks after the tumor was implanted, the nodes were heavily infiltrated with cancer. Inasmuch as the maximum range of the particle of ^{131}I has a maximum penetration in tissue of 20 mm with a mean range of 0.3 mm, the expectation of destroying large metastatic deposits is nil. In a group where the isotope was administered shortly after the transplant, lymphograms revealed a marked shrinkage of the treated nodes.

Macroscopic and microscopic findings. There was a marked difference in the appearance of these two groups, in which the treated nodules were markedly smaller than those of the control group. They state that the microscopic evaluation of the effects of therapy was difficult in nodes that contained a great deal of tumor. However, in minimally involved lymph nodes, due to a short transplantation-treatment interval, the radiation changes of the tumor cells due to ^{131}I-Lipiodol could be found even to the complete destruction of the tumor and the lymph nodes.

Survival time. There was a marked increase in survival times of the treated animals. Only in the animals with nodes involved with microscopic metastases was the survival markedly increased, and 25 percent of these rabbits were cured. Other treated animals eventually died, but far outlived those rabbits who were treated as controls.

Edwards obtained a 5-year survival rate of 80 percent for 45 patients with stage I melanoma and a 28.5 percent 5-year survival for patients in stage II classification treated for malignant melanoma by similar techniques (surgical excision and endolymphatic isotope therapy). The only significant difference in techniques is that Edwards used ^{32}P-Lipiodol whereas we used ^{131}I-Ethiodol. Edwards (Table 29-2) evaluated the results from *surgical ablation alone* at the St. Thomas Hospital, London, where he performed his investigations, and he was able to show that in stage I cancer, the 5-year survival rate was 58.9 percent, and in stage II, the survival rate was 12.5 percent. He further believes that a more relevant comparison of the efficiency of the endolymphatic form of therapy versus that of surgery alone is the recurrence rate in lymph nodes. In 31 patients treated by surgical resection and endolymphatic therapy, 9.7 percent developed recurrences in the region of the lymph nodes and eventually died. In those treated by surgical excision alone, of 42 patients, 15 developed recurrences in the lymph node region, and 14 died.

Table 29-2

Five-Year Survival Rates in Patients with Melanoma

Stage	Surgical excision		Endolymphatic therapy	
	No. cases	Survival rate (%)	No. cases	Survival rate (%)
I	51	58.9	45	80.0
II	8	12.5	28	21.4

(Adapted from data presented by J. M. Edwards at International Cancer Conference, Sidney, Australia, 1972.)

We have observed that approximately 40 percent of the patients in clinical stage I eventually develop metastases to the lymph nodes. We are accordingly convinced that the policy of watchful waiting is not justified.

Fortner, Booher, and Pack[28] described complications following groin dissections for melanoma. Three patients had serious complications—cardiac arrest with death, a severed ureter and bladder, and a tear in a major vein. Local complications consisted of necrosis of skin flaps necessitating skin grafts. Moreover, a significant number of patients had swelling of the affected limb, severe at times. The incidence of satellitoses varied from 9 to 25 percent.

The complications following isotope therapy have been minimal. We have an 8 percent failure rate to administer a proper therapeutic dose due to technical problems. At first, we had difficulty with the healing of the incision site, but pouring a liter of saline solution over the wound after the removal of the catheter and before the wound is sutured closed has completely eliminated this complication. One patient developed a transient rash, possibly due to a sensitivity to iodine. Five percent of the patients had a mild cough for 1 to 3 days. No pulmonary complications have been observed.

SUMMARY

The treatment of malignant melanoma by a combination of surgery and endolymphatic isotopic therapy is based on experimental evidence that the dose of irradiation delivered by this route will destroy microscopic deposits of cancer. In lymph nodes bearing cancer, there is marked destruction of melanoma in the lymph nodes after the endolymphatic administration of 40 mCi of ^{131}I-Ethiodol. This has been accomplished with no demonstrable interference to lymph flow due to marked differences in sensitivity to irradiation of the lymph nodes and the lymphatic vessels. The lymph nodes are radiosensitive, and the lymphatic vessels are radioresistant.

Endolymphatically administered ^{131}I-Ethiodol delivers sufficient irradiation to the lymph nodes in humans to destroy microscopic deposits of melanoma cells lodged within the nodes. The primary melanoma is treated by orthodox surgical techniques. Patients classified as clinical stage I receive no additional surgical intervention, but receive ^{131}I or ^{32}P endolymphatically and are thus spared the trauma of a radical axillary or groin dissection and their ensuing complications. A 5-year survival rate without evidence of residual or recurrent melanoma by 18 of the 22 patients followed 5 years or longer is encouraging.

Patients with stage II melanoma are treated by a combination of endolymphatic isotopes and surgical removal of the primary melanoma and the lymph nodes. The penetration of the irradiation from the administered isotope is not sufficient to destroy the cancer. In such instances, irradiation of lymph nodes outside the field of surgery, irradiation of any nodes inadvertently left behind, and irradiation to cancer cells within the lymphatics offer an additional dimension in the treatment of these patients. A 5-year survival rate of 28.5 percent in a small group of patients is better than that obtained with surgical excision alone.

Several patients with satellitoses have markedly benefited from endolymphatic isotopic therapy.

Patients with distant metastases so treated have shown no improvement, and endolymphatic isotopes are not indicated for such patients.

Level of Amputation for Patients with Soft Tissue Sarcomas of the Extremities as Determined by Isotopic Lymphangiography[1]

INTRODUCTION

When an amputation is necessary for a soft tissue sarcoma, particularly of the extremities, the decision of the site of amputation is often problematic. It is axiomatic that the amputation should be performed above the origin of the muscles which are involved in the given sarcoma. A factor which is not often evaluated in considering the level of amputation is the problem of metastases to the lymph nodes. In the old literature it was taught that carcinomas spread by the lymphatic system to the lymph nodes and sarcomas metastasize via the bloodstream. This is not true because many sarcomas metastasize directly to the lymph nodes (Table 29-3).

In a patient with a sarcoma of an extremity which has a proclivity to metastasize to lymph nodes, it is mandatory that the lymph nodes be considered in the treatment regime. The following case report exemplifies the problem at hand and illustrates the manner in which the performance of a lymphangiogram by means of Lipiodol to which radioactive phosphorous was attached helped to arrive at a decision and permitted a more conservative amputation than was recommended by other surgeons who had also seen this patient.

CASE REPORT

The patient, C.A., is a 24-year-old female who had a mass superior to the right popliteal space in June of 1972. The lesion, which has been slow growing

Table 29-3

Incidence of Metastases to Regional Lymph Nodes
of Soft Tissue Sarcomas*

Angiosarcomas	45.0
Rhabdomyosarcomas	22.0
Synovial sarcomas	20.0
Fibrosarcomas	5.0
Adenomyosarcoma of the kidney (Wilms' tumor)	30.0
Cystosarcoma phylloides	1.0
Dermatofibrosarcoma protuberans	0.0
Malignant histiocytoma	23.0
Malignant neurilemmoma	0.0
Kaposi's hemorrhagic sarcoma	0.0
Liposarcoma	0.0

*Author's series of 1000 cases.

since 1970, was a tender mass which produced pain that radiated down to the foot. A wide excision was performed by one of us (J.H.) in July of 1972, and a diagnosis by Drs. Howard Dorfman and Raffaele Lattes of synovial sarcoma was established. Subsequent to the wide local resection of this mass which measured 5 cm in diameter, the symptoms disappeared completely. However, on 10/1/73, the patient began to notice insidious pain at the local site which radiated posteriorly to the foot. On 10/16/73, physical examination was nonrevealing except for exquisite pain and tenderness at the site of the operation radiating down to the foot. No masses could be palpated. The question of recurrence was uppermost in our minds, but as nothing could be palpated, we suggested that an exploration of this site should be made and decision of therapy made depending on the operative and biopsy findings. An arteriogram was performed which was considered negative.

If a recurrent sarcoma should be found, a consideration which merited evaluation consisted of the possibility of metastases to the lymph nodes, and several courses of action were possible: (1) a wide local resection and a discontinuous groin dissection; (2) a midthigh amputation with discontinuous groin dissection; (3) a conservative hemipelvectomy; and (4) a hemipelvectomy (which had been the suggestion of one of the consulting oncologic surgeons).

It was decided to perform an isotopic lymphangiogram whereby an ultrafiltrate of Lipiodol was injected into a lymphatic vessel of the foot. To the Lipiodol was attached the radioactive isotope ^{32}P. The administration of the dye would give a presumptive diagnosis as to whether metastases were present. However, even if the lymphangiogram were negative, the possibility of occult metastases in the lymph nodes remained a problem. The amount of radioactive phosphorus administered endolymphatically would deliver to the femoral and inguinal nodes a dose of irradiation equal to between 50,000 and 100,000 rads beta. This has been shown to be destructive to cancer, including malignant melanoma.

On 1/30/74, the site was explored and a biopsy was taken which confirmed the clinical impression that a recurrence had taken place. The cancer was found intimately attached to the popliteal nerve and vessels and precluded any attempt at local resection. On 2/4/74, an isotopic lymphangiogram was performed with the administration of 3 ml of ultrafiltrate of Lipiodol to which was attached 4 mCi of radioactive phosphorus. The interpretation of the lymphangiogram was that it was negative from the standpoint of metastases. Accordingly, on 2/6/74, a right mid-thigh amputation was performed. The pathology report of the biopsy specimen was synovial sarcoma.

The patient made an uneventful recovery, has a well-functioning prosthesis, and remains free of evidence of recurrence 3 years and 5 months after amputation.

DISCUSSION

Older teachings have stressed that whereas carcinomas spread via the lymphatic vessels, sarcomas spread by the vascular system and seldom by the lymphatic system. This has been shown to be a misconception, for certain of the sarcomas arising from the soft somatic tissues do metastasize to lymph nodes. The worst culprit in this field are the angiosarcomas which metastasize in 45 percent of the patients studied. Rhabdomyosarcomas metastasize in 22 percent. On the other hand, fibrosarcomas metastasize in only 5 percent of the cases. We have had no instance of metastases to lymph nodes from a malignant neurilemmoma.

It thus becomes manifest that in dealing with a sarcoma whose histogenic features have demonstrated a proclivity to metastasize to lymph nodes, the overall design of the therapeutic procedure should include the eradication of those lymph nodes. Thus, for a sarcoma of the hamstring muscle, a resection of the musculature should be accompanied by a radical lymph node resection. Where amputation is indicated, rather than a hip joint disarticulation with radical node dissection, we prefer a conservative hemipelvectomy in which the pubes and ischeum are removed with the subjacent extremity, thus removing all of the femoral, inguinal, and deep iliac lymph nodes, as well as the obturator lymph nodes.

In the patient herein presented, it became essential to consider the lymph nodes of the groin in the overall treatment. She was seen by other consultants who advocated a hemipelvectomy. She begged for a midthigh amputation. By utilizing the procedure which we have described, a lymphangiogram was performed which tends to be diagnostic for the presence of gross metastases. If gross metastases had been observed, then it would have been necessary to eradicate these nodes surgically. Inasmuch as the lymphangiogram was considered negative and because approximately 20 percent of patients with synovial sarcomas have demonstrated metastases to the lymph nodes, the preparation of the radiopaque Lipiodol had attached to its molecules radioactive phosphorus.

We have performed this procedure on 12 patients to date, with initial gratifying results. The longest follow-up period in all of these patients has been 4 years. No long-term claim can be made regarding the reliability of this concept in the treatment of sarcomas, depending on the isotopic lymphangiogram to destroy occult metastases and thus perform a more conservative amputation.

SUMMARY

It is stressed that a significant number of soft tissue sarcomas metastasize to the lymph nodes, and the eradication of these lymph nodes represents an integral part of the treatment policy. A case presentation demonstrates the technique whereby an isotopic lymphangiogram (i.e., the endolymphatic administration to the involved extremity of a dye which is radiopaque, permitting roentgenologic interpretation, and to which is also attached a radioactive isotope, ^{32}P, which permits the administration of a large dose of irradiation delivered exclusively to the lymph nodes) aids materially in helping to determine whether metastases to the lymph nodes have occurred; and if occult metastases are present, they would be eradicated by the large dose of irradiation (50,000 to 100,000 rads beta) delivered internally by the technique herein described. The adoption of this technique in a young girl with synovial sarcoma whose lymph nodes are at significant risk for harboring metastases permitted the performance of a midthigh amputation instead of a hemipelvectomy. It is obviously too early to evaluate the long-term result of this concept.

Treatment of Malignant Lymphomas by the Intralymphatic Administration of Radioactive Isotopes

INTRODUCTION

Internal irradiation of the lymph nodes by the intralymphatic administration of radioactive isotopes is theoretically an ideal method of treating malignant lymphomas. This is particularly true for lymphosarcoma in its various forms, inasmuch as lymphosarcoma is a primary disease of the lymph nodes and the injected material is distributed throughout the entire lymph node including all of the disease process. In Hodgkin's disease, however, in many instances the lymph node is partially replaced by abnormal cells within the lymph node, whereas in other instances the lymph node is replaced by fibrous tissue. In the latter case the endolymphatic administration of isotopes has but limited utility.

In the series herein recorded, 74 patients with various forms of malignant lymphoma were treated by endolymphatic isotopes. Some patients presented evidence of their disease primarily in the cervical region or in the mediastinum. Those patients were treated by orthodox external radiation therapy in that they received a mantel form of cobalt therapy. They were given an average of 40 mCi of ^{131}I-Ethiodol or 5 mCi of ^{32}P-Ethiodol into the lymphatics of both lower extremities. This was done as part of a combined diagnostic and therapeutic regime. If it was considered that the lymph nodes were clinically free of evidence of disease, dependence was placed on the internal irradiation to control any possible occult involvement below the diaphragm.

In another series of patients, the disease was heralded by lymphadenopathy involving a groin lymph node. In such instances, after a biopsy had been taken, the involved side was treated by the administration of 40 mCi of ^{131}I or 5 mCi of ^{32}P into the involved extremity. The opposite side was left free for control purposes, and was not treated endolymphatically, but was treated by external means as part of an inverted Y port to the periaortic lymph nodes as well as the iliac and inguinal lymph nodes of the opposite side. Dependence was not placed on the internal irradiation from the endolymphatic isotope in these instances, because it has been demonstrated that there is a decreasing concentration of lymph nodes the higher one goes in the lymphatic chain into the periaortic nodes. Accordingly, inasmuch as it was necessary to limit the volume, most of the irradiation would be delivered to the inguinal, iliac, and lumbar lymph nodes with lesser amounts of irradiation being delivered to the lymph nodes in the region of the ciliac plexus.

In another series, patients who manifested stage IV disease and who presented evidence of involvement of the liver, spleen, lung, or other parenchymal organs, and who also presented evidence of adenopathy above and below the diaphragm, were treated by the endolymphatic administration of the radioactive isotope to note what would happen in the eventual course of the overall disease by an intralymphatic form of irradiation to the pelvic and intraabdominal lymph nodes. The material is presented according to the type of lymphoma from which the patient suffered.

NODULAR LYMPHOSARCOMA (GIANT FOLLICULAR LYMPHOBLASTOMA)

Eight patients in this series were treated (Table 29-4), and of the eight who were treated, three remain alive from 2 to 8 years after therapy. Five others have died of their disease, the median life span being 3.4 years, and ranging from 1.5 to 7 years. In all instances where death occurred, recurrence demonstrated a histiocytic type of lymphosarcoma, showing that the nodular lymphosarcoma is not a disease entity unto itself, but rather part of the generic disease of lymphosarcoma. There were four males and four females, and the average age was 48 years, ranging from 21 to 71 years.

One young male, 24 years of age, presented with an axillary lymph node. He received the radioactive isotope into a wrist lymphatic and remains free of any evidence of disease 8 years later. This was his only form of therapy.

A 43-year-old man manifested lymphadenopathy of his right groin. He was treated by the administration of the isotope into the right leg, after which he received an inverted Y course of therapy to the left groin and to the periaortic lymph node. He remained completely free of evidence of disease until he developed an enlarged lymph node in the left axilla, which on resection revealed a

Table 29-4
Nodular Lymphosarcoma* (Giant Follicular
Lymphoblastoma) 8 Patients†

Group	Median Survival	Survival Range
Patients alive (3)	7.6 years	2–8 years
Patients dead (5)	3.4 years	1.5–7 years

*In each case of death, recurrences demonstrated histiocytic lymphosarcoma.

†Four males, four females. Median age 48 years; range 21–27 years.

histiocytic reticular lymphoma. He was treated with additional external radiation therapy and combined chemotherapy, but his condition deteriorated and he died. It is interesting that this patient developed lymphadenopathy 5 years later in the right inguinal region, the site where he had received approximately 50,000 rads beta from the ^{131}I-Ethiodol endolymphatically.

Lymphadenopathy has been noted after varying doses of irradiation to the lymph nodes, and such cases emphasize the need for continued, prolonged observation of the lymph nodes for many years after radiation therapy. The effect of the internal irradiation in patients with nodular lymphosarcoma remains doubtful from the data herein presented.

Diffuse Lymphosarcoma

This treatment group consisted of 28 patients (Table 29-5), 15 male and 13 female. The median age was 47.8 years, ranging from 14 to 74 years. Four patients received prophylactic treatment. That is, their lymphadenopathy was supradiaphragmatic, and they received the endolymphatic isotopes below the diaphragm. All of these patients remain completely well an average of 6.5 years after therapy.

Eight patients were treated as part of the primary therapy. That is, the endolymphatic isotopes were given into the involved leg if groin lymphadenopathy was the primary site of the disease, or into the wrist lymphatics if axillary lymphadenopathy was the primary disease. Six of these patients remain alive, an average of 7 years postoperatively. Only two have died, an average of 2.2 years following therapy. It would seem that this form of therapy is a beneficial type of treatment in this group of patients.

Thirteen patients were treated as part of their total therapies. These people usually had evidence of dissemination of their disease process with involvement above and below the diaphragm and involvement of one or another of the parenchymal organs. Two such patients are alive an average of 8.5 years, but eleven patients in this group have died, an average of 3.3 years post-therapy. The use of internal irradiation is questionable for this group of patients.

Histiocytic Reticular Lymphoma

Ten patients in this group were treated (Table 29-6), all of them as part of their total therapy. All of these patients have died of their disease, an average of 8

Table 29-5
Diffuse Lymphosarcoma in 28 Patients*

Treatment	No. of Patients Alive (avg. survival)	No. of Patients Dead (avg. survival)
Prophylactic	4 (6.5 years)	0
Primary	6 (7.0 years)	2 (2.2 years)
Part of total treatment	2 (8.5 years)	11 (3.3 years)

*Fifteen males, thirteen females. Median age 47.8 years; range 14–74 years.

Table 29-6

Histiocytic Reticular Lymphoma (Reticulum Cell Sarcoma)
in 10 Patients*

Treatment	No. of Patients Alive	No. of Patients Dead (avg. survival)
Prophylactic	0	0
Primary	0	0
Part of total treatment	10	10 (8 months)

*Three males, seven females. Median age 54.3 years; range 40–62 years.

months post-therapy. The use of internal irradiation is questionable in patients
with histiocytic reticular lymphoma. Whether it would be of any value as part of
primary treatment or as prophylactic therapy remains questionable.

Hodgkin's Disease

Twenty-eight patients with Hodgkin's disease were treated by this form of
therapy (Table 29-7). There were 16 males and 12 females, and the median age was
49.8 years, varying from 16 to 65 years. Four patients were treated prophylacti-
cally, of whom three remain alive, an average of 5.1 years post-therapy. One
patient has died 1 year post-therapy. Seven patients were treated as part of the
primary treatment. Six of these patients remain alive without evidence of disease,
an average of 7.5 years post-therapy. Only one patient in this series has died, an
average of 1 year post-therapy. In this series was a young girl who presented
inguinal lymphadenopathy and was treated only by the endolymphatic administration of the isotope into both groins. This was her only form of therapy, and she
remains alive without any evidence of disease 8 years after treatment. Her only
untoward effect was that she did not develop normal-sized breasts. All studies
including a complete hormone survey were entirely normal. A plastic surgeon
placed inserts in her breasts which satisfied her immensely, and she became a
well-groomed, very attractive young lady with no evidence of disease.

There were 17 patients who received this form of therapy as part of overall
treatment. Only one such patient remains alive and well and has survived an
average of 11 years post-treatment. The other 16 have all died, an average of 2.1
years following therapy.

Table 29-7

Hodgkin's Disease in 28 Patients*

Treatment	No. of Patients Alive (avg. survival)	No. of Patients Dead (avg. survival)
Prophylactic	3 (5.1 years)	1 (1 year)
Primary	6 (7.5 years)	1 (1.0 year)
Part of total treatment	1 (11.0 years)	16 (2.1 years)

*Sixteen males, twelve females. Median age 49.8 years; range 16–65 years.

DISCUSSION AND CONCLUSION

These data indicate that when a patient has evidence of lymphoma supradiaphragmatically, the administration of endolymphatic isotopes for a means of treating the infradiaphragmatic therapy as part of the overall diagnostic and therapeutic problem could be indicated. If the patient is to receive a diagnostic lymphangiogram, the attachment of radioactive iodine or radioactive phosphorus to the diagnostic radiopaque material would give a good course of irradiation to these lymph nodes. There have been no untoward effects, nor any abnormal hematologic results of this therapy.

The endolymphatic administration of radioactive isotopes appears indicated as part of the primary treatment in patients with either lymphosarcoma or Hodgkin's disease. This is particularly true if the disease presents itself in the groin where a good distribution of the isotopes can be obtained and the patient can receive 50,000 to 100,000 rads beta to the inguinal and iliac lymph nodes but lesser amounts of irradiation as one ascends the lymphatic chain. In such instances it is recommended that this be part of the primary treatment, and that the patient receive in addition a routine course of external radiation therapy. The internal radiation has in no way affected the response nor the anticipated results from a complete course of external therapy in this series.

In patients who have dissemination of their disease process with involvement above and below the diaphragm plus involvement of one or another of the visceral organs, the endolymphatic administration in an effort to deliver a cancericidal dose of irradiation to certain groups of lymph nodes appears to have no beneficial effect on the overall process. Its use in such instances is strongly questioned.

REFERENCES

1. Fischer, H. W., Thornbury, J. R.: Lymphography in the diagnosis of malignant neoplasms. In: Progress in Clinical Cancer, Vol. 1, I. M. Ariel (ed.). New York, Grune & Stratton, p. 213, 1965.
2. Koehler, P. R., Wohl, G. T., Schaffer, B.: Lymphangiography—a survey of its current status. Am. J. Roentgenol. 91:1216, 1964.
3. Baum, S., Bron, K. M., Wexler, L., et al.: Lymphangiography, cavography and urography. Radiology 81:207, 1963.
4. Brom, K. M. Baum, S., Abrams, H. L.: Oil embolism in lymphangiography. Incidence, manifestations, and mechanisms. Radiology 80:194, 1963.
5. Herman, P. G., Benninghoff, D. L., Schwartz, S.: A physiologic approach to lymph flow in lymphography. Am. J. Roentgenol. 91:1207, 1964.
6. Rouvier, H.: Anatomy of the Human Lymphatic System, translated by M. J. Tobias. Ann Arbor, Michigan, Edwards Brothers, 1938.
7. Rusznyak, I., Foldi, M., Szabo, G.: Lymphatics and Lymph Circulation. Physiology and Pathology. New York, Pergamon Press, 1960.
8. Blalock, A., Robinson, C. S., Cunningham, R. S., et al.: Experimental studies on lymphatic blockage. Arch. Surg. 34:1049, 1937.
9. Pressman, J. J., Simon, M. B., Hand, K., et al.: Passage of fluids, cells, and bacteria via direct communications between lymph nodes and veins. Surg. Gynecol. Obstet. 115:207, 1962.

10. Wallace, S., Jackson, L., Dodd, G. D., et al.: Lymphatic dynamics in certain abnormal states. Am. J. Roentgenol. 91:1187, 1964.

11. Jantet, G. H., Edwards, J. M., Gough, M. H., et al.: Endolymphatic therapy with radioactive gold for malignant melanoma. Br. Med. J. 2:904, 1964.

12. Fischer, H. W.: Intralymphatic therapy for lymph-node metastases of carcinoma of the cervix. Cancer 18:1059, 1965.

13. Blocker, T. G., Jr., Lewis, S. R., Smith, J. R., et al.: Lymphodynamics. Plast. Reconstr. Surg. 25:337, 1960.

14. Edwards, J. M.: Malignant melanoma endolymphatic therapy. Melanoma and skin cancer. Proceedings of the International Cancer Conference, Sidney, Australia, 1972.

15. McNeer, G., Das Gupta, T.: Routes of lymphatic spread of malignant melanoma. Cancer 15:168, 1965.

16. Seitzman, D. M., Wright, R., Halaby, F. A., et al.: Radioactive lymphangiography as a therapeutic adjunct. Am. J. Roentgenol. 89:140, 1963.

17. Stehlin, J. S., Jr., Smith, J. L., Jr., Jing, B. S., et al.: Melanomas of the extremities complicated by in-transit metastases. Surg. Gynecol. Obstet. 122:3, 1966.

18. Stehlin, J. S., Jr., Smith, J. L., Jr., Clark, R. L., Jr.: Malignant melanoma: diagnosis and current treatment. Surg. Clin. North. Am. 42:455, 1962.

19. Stehlin, J. S., Jr., Clark, R. L., Jr., Smith, J. L., Jr., et al.: Malignant melanoma of the extremities: experiences with conventional therapy: a new surgical and chemotherapeutic approach with regional perfusion. Cancer 13:55, 1960.

20. Kinmoth, J. B.: Lymphangiography in man. A method of outlining lymphatic trunks at operation. Clin. Sci. 11:13, 1952.

21. Schwartz, S. I., Greenlaw, R. H., Rob, C., et al.: Intralymphatic injection of radioactive gold. Cancer 15:623, 1962.

22. Ariel, I. M., Resnick, M. I., Orpeza, R.: The intralymphatic administration of radioactive isotopes for treating malignant melanoma. Surg. Gynecol. Obstet. 124:25, 1967.

23. Edwards, J. M.: Malignant melanoma: treatment by endolymphatic radio-isotope infusion. Ann. R. Coll. Surg. Engl. 44:237, 1969.

24. Ariel, I. M., Resnick, M. I.: Altered lymphatic dynamics following groin and axillary dissection; its relationship to treatment policies for malignant melanoma. Surgery 61:210, 1967.

25. Ariel, I. M., Resnick, M. I.: Altered lymphatic dynamics by cancer metastases. Arch. Surg. 94:117, 1967.

26. Ariel, I. M., Resnick, M. I., Orpeza, R.: Effects of irradiation (external and internal) on lymphatic dynamics. Am. J. Roentgenol. 99:404, 1967.

27. Pack, G. T., Scharnagel, I., Morfitt, M.: The principle of excision and dissection in continuity for primary and metastatic melanoma of the skin. Surgery 17:849, 1945.

28. Fortner, J. G., Booher, R. J., Pack, G. T.: Results of groin dissection for malignant melanoma in 220 patients. Surgery 55:485, 1964.

ADDITIONAL READINGS

1. Ariel, I., Bale, W. E., Downing, V., et al.: The distribution of radioactive isotopes of iodine in normal rabbits. Am. J. Physiol. 132:346, 1941.

2. Ariel, I. M., Hartley, J.: Level of amputation for patients with soft tissue sarcomas of the extremities as determined by isotopic lymphangiography. Bull. Hosp. Joint Dis. 37(1):34, 1976.

3. Ariel, I. M., Resnick, M. I., Galey, D.: The intralymphatic administration of radioactive isotopes and cancer chemotherapeutic drugs. Surgery 55:355, 1964.

4. Ariel, I. M., Resnick, N. J.: Treatment of lymphomas with radioactive isotopes, in Pack, G. T. and Ariel, I. M. (eds.): Treatment of Cancer and Allied Diseases, vol. 9. Scranton, Penn., Hoeber Medical Division of Harper & Row, 1964, pp. 73–94.

5. Burger, R. H.: Lymph node response to high-dose intralymphatic injection of radio-chromic phosphate. Bull. N.Y. Acad. Med. 40:142, 1964.

6. Chiappa, S., Galli, G., Palmia, C.: Observations on lymphatic radiotherapy and general chemotherapy. Clin. Radiol. 15:202, 1964.

7. Fuchs, W. J., Book-Henderstrom, G.: Inguinal and pelvic lymphography. A preliminary report. Acta. Radiol. (Stockh.) 56:340, 1961.

8. Healy, R. J., Amory, H. I., Friedman, M.: Hodgkin's disease; a review of two hundred and sixteen cases. Radiology 64:51, 1955.

9. Hine, G. J., Brownell, G. L.: Radiation Dosimetry. New York, Academic Press, 1956.

10. Kaplan, H. S.: Presentation at the Symposium on Hodgkin's Disease, French Academy of Hematology and Radiology, Hospital St. Louis, Paris, February 23, 1965.

11. Molander, D. W., Ariel, I. M., Pack, G. T.: Hepatic gammascanning as an aid in the management of patients with malignant lymphomas. Am. J. Roentgenol. 99:851, 1967.

12. Olsen, G.: Removal of fascia—cause of more frequent metastases of malignant melanoma of the skin to the region? Cancer 17:1159, 1964.

13. Pack, G. T., Ariel, I. M.: Treatment of malignant melanoma by adequate (radical) surgical resection and radical amputation when indicated. In: Current Surgical Management, J. H. Mulholland, E. M. Ellison, and S. R. Freison (eds.). Philadelphia, W. B. Saunders Co., pp. 438–446, 1957.

14. Seitzman, D. M., Halaby, F. A., Flanagan, P., et al.: Intralymphatic radioisotope therapy. Surg. Gynecol. Obstet. 118:52, 1964.

15. Siegel, P., Liebner, E. J.: Intralymphatic radioactive therapy for pelvic cancer. Am. J. Obstet. Gynecol. 91:122, 1965.

16. Tubiana, M.: Presentation at the Symposium on Hodgkin's Disease, French Academy of Hematology and Radiology, Hospital St. Louis, Paris, February 23, 1965.

Edgar D. Grady

30
Adjuvant Therapy for Colon Cancer by Internal Radiation to the Liver

Last year 9800 Americans died of cancer in the liver (H. E. Talmadge, *personal communication*). The greatest single source of lesions was metastases from the colon. Many were present as sublinical foci at the time of colon resection. In order to prevent the development of clinical liver cancer from occult metastatic cancer after colon resection, it was supposed that internal radiation therapy (in an appropriate dose) to the liver would be effective. Such an adjuvant therapy to the liver soon after colon resection, where the probability of liver metastases is calculated to be high, would seem likely to prevent the development of gross tumor.

It would, of course, require homogeneous intrahepatic distribution of the material, with acceptably small spillover to vital areas, especially the bone marrow. The liver would have to tolerate the radiation without significant immediate or late side effects. Finally, the incidence of later established liver cancer would have to be reduced sufficiently.

MATERIALS AND METHODS

To demonstrate a procedure to be effective, and acceptable to the FDA, it was necessary to establish an animal model first. The best methodology had to be developed and the effective remedy demonstrated in the animal. The following materials and methods were tested and eliminated as not qualified in the rat:[1]

1. Yttrium-90 resin spheres injected into the portal vein did not give homogeneous distribution.
2. Phosphorus-32 colloid introduced into a peripheral vein gave a satisfactory distribution in the liver, but too much radiation to the bone marrow.
3. Phosphorus-32 colloid administered into the portal vein showed streamlining and nonhomogeneous distribution to the liver, but spared the bone marrow.
4. Phosphorus-32 colloid injected into the arterial supply of the gut passed on through the gut and came back thoroughly mixed in the portal circulation to give an even distribution in the liver, sparing the bone marrow.

The last method was selected to test in the animal model.[2]

A suspension of Walker-256 tumor cells was introduced in the portal vein of the Sprague-Dawley rat; 2 days later in the animals to be treated, ^{32}P-chromic phosphate colloid was injected into the abdominal aorta in a temporarily isolated segment containing the origin of the celiac and superior mesenteric arteries. The dose of 100 μCi was calculated to deliver 5000 rads to the liver. Control animals were given tumor cells only.

RESULTS

Of 101 control animals, 53 died of cancer; whereas of 102 animals treated with ^{32}P-colloid, 25 died of cancer. Therefore, 52 percent of control animals developed cancer, but only 25 percent of treated animals did so. Follow-up on survivors for over 1 year failed to show adverse systemic hematological effects. There was no apparent liver damage. Twenty-five such rats had autopsies upon sacrifice after 1 year. There was no microscopic evidence of liver necrosis or scar and no evidence of induced neoplasm. Two of these, however, contained minimal residual cancer lesions seen microscopically only in the liver.

CLINICAL PROTOCOL

The following clinical protocol was proposed.

We will select patients to be treated, on the basis of probability that they have occult cancer in the liver, after the primary lesion has been resected. We will consider all patients who survive the operation without significant complications, whose gastrointestinal function has returned to normal, and whose abdominal wound is apparently healing 1 week after the operation. Every such patient who has a pathology report showing one or more mesenteric lymph nodes containing metastatic cancer (and who has no other apparent metastases) will be considered in the study.

Alternate patients will then be treated. Each patient included will have the following procedures (between 7 and 14 days postoperatively): liver scan, carcinoembryonic antigen (CEA), BCP (SMA-20), and complete blood cell count (CBC); selective catheterization of the superior mesenteric artery and of the celiac artery; and arteriogram with radiopaque contrast material to verify locations of catheters and to see anatomy of circulation.

With catheters still in place, half of the dose of ^{32}P-chromic phosphate colloid is injected (slowly, over at least 2 minutes) via a shielded syringe into each catheter so that the liver will receive 5000 rads. Calculate dose as follows:

$$\text{Dose (rads)} = 73.8 \times T \times E \times \text{Amount } (\mu\text{Ci/g})$$
$$\text{Dose in tissue} = 6.82 \ \mu\text{Ci/g},$$

where T is the half-time (days), and E is the average beta ray energy (MeV).

The average size of the liver is about 2 percent of body weight, varying from about 1200 to 1600 grams. Usual dose would then be, for a 1200-gram liver, 8.2 mCi to give 5000 rads if 100 percent was absorbed.

Since the animal measurements show that only 70 percent is absorbed by the liver, the dose for a 1200-gram liver would be 11.4 mCi divided equally between the superior mesenteric and the celiac arteries.

Follow-up of all cases (treated and untreated) would be as follows. Record complications due to arterial catheterization and/or treatment. Record duration of stay of patient both treated and untreated after primary operation (and after catheter arterial injection in the treated patients).

Repeat every 3 months in all patients (treated and untreated): CBC, CEA, BCP, and clinical evaluation. Repeat liver scan and x-ray of the chest every 6 months in all patients. Reports will be collected at the end of each year after surgery, for treated and untreated patients.

After FDA approval to begin clinical trials, three volunteer patients with Dukes C colon cancer had ^{32}P injected a short time after colon resection. The case reports of the three patients follow.

CASE I: L.M.H.

A 62-year-old-man had a right hemicolectomy on 1/31/76 for a carcinoma of the midascending colon. Pathology reports showed a 10×6 cm cancer, moderately well-differentiated adenocarcinoma, invading the full thickness of the muscle wall and extending into immediately adjacent lymph nodes (Dukes C). Liver appeared normal at time of surgery. CEA preoperatively was 2.5 (normal is 0 to 5); SMA-20 preoperatively was normal, except for a slightly elevated CPK to 135 (normal is 10 to 125).

It was intended to give him adjuvant internal radiation therapy to his liver as soon as he recovered from the operation; however, approval by the FDA was delayed. On 3/22/76, he was treated with 15 mCi of ^{32}P-colloid; 7.5 mCi was delivered into each of the celiac and superior mesenteric arteries by selective femoral artery catheterization. A "road map" arteriogram was first done to show that there was normal circulation.

There were no side effects until a month later, when he developed jaundice, hepatomegaly (with liver being down three fingers), and a gradual change in liver enzymes. He was never clinically ill, but on May 25, the bilirubin was 4.1, alkaline phosphatase rose to 379, and the SGOT to 68. WBC dropped from 4900 to 3600. Hemoglobin stayed up at 14.9 grams. By June 6, bilirubin had gone to 11.3 and other enzymes remained about the same. Some ascites developed and therapy was begun with prednisone 20 mg/day and furosemide (Lasix®) 40 mg/day. All findings gradually improved in the next 6 months. By 8/20/76 bilirubin was 1.9, alkaline phosphatase 273, SGOT 68; other enzymes remained normal. On the last follow-up, 2/21/77, he was asymptomatic. There was no ascites, bilirubin was 1.4, alkaline phosphatase 229, LDH 231, SGOT 48. Today he is clinically well. WBC is staying at 3800 with a hemoglobin of 13.9 grams. Liver scan, x-ray of the chest, barium enema, and sigmoidoscopy are all normal now.

CASE II: E.B.

A 70-year-old-man had a right hemicolectomy with terminal ileum included on 1/5/76 for a carcinoma involving the ileocecal valve, cecum, and base of the appendix. Pathology report showed an 8-cm tumor mass of adenocarcinoma infiltrating the muscularis and into the mesenteric fat with metastasis to several lymph nodes including the one in the highest point of the mesentery. The liver appeared normal at the time of surgery.

There was a complication of hematuria from a kidney stone and possibly a pulmonary embolus 6 weeks after surgery. The latter was not confirmed, although chest x-ray and lung scan both were compatible with small emboli. Because of the hematuria, he was treated only with dextran, and both problems were solved. CEA preoperatively was 4.4, SMA-20 preoperatively showed normal CPK, SGOT, LDH, and alkaline phosphatase. The patient did well, and on 3/23/76 he was treated with 15 mCi ^{32}P-colloid (7.5 mCi into each of the celiac and superior mesenteric arteries by selective femoral artery catheterizations). Normal arterial anatomy again was demonstrated prior to the selective catheter placement. The patient had absolutely no side effects from the procedure, nor in the immediate follow-up.

Serial hematological and SMA-20 evaluations demonstrated no significant changes. WBC was stable at 5000 to 6000 (on 11/9/76 the lowest WBC was 4700, but it was back up to 9100 a month later).

SMA-20 has had no enzyme change except an alkaline phosphatase that went up to 155.

By August 10, 1976, the patient had evidence of bilateral lung disease, but the CEA remained normal. Treatment with methyl-CCNU, 5-FU, and vincristine failed to control the lung disease; and in February 1977, he had brain metastasis. He died on 2/28/77. Autopsy showed 18 small tumor nodules in the liver, normal liver between nodules, massive bilateral lung metastases, and brain metastases.

CASE III: N.L.

This 52-year-old woman had, on 7/18/75, a low anterior sigmoid colon resection for an adenocarcinoma 6.2 × 4 cm with invasion through the full thickness of the muscle wall and metastasis to a single lymph node. The liver was normal at the time of surgery. The patient had no postoperative complications.

On 3/23/76, selective catherization of the superior mesenteric and celiac arteries was done and 7.5 mCi of ^{32}P-colloid was injected into each artery for internal radiation therapy to the liver. There was no symptomatic reaction; however, there was some evidence of bone marrow suppression. The WBC gradually decreased from the preoperative level of 5200 to 4400 on 4/2/76, 3700 on 4/12; 2600 on 5/7, 2900 on 5/22, 3600 on 6/24, and it has persisted at about this number since then, being 3100 on 1/5/77. The CEA has remained below 5. There have been no abnormal enzyme changes on the SMA-20 except a transient elevation of the LDH to 270 on 6/26/76. The barium enema and the liver scans remain normal. Sigmoidoscopy done a few days ago again is normal.

SUMMARY

A safe and statistically effective method of internal radiation therapy to the liver using ^{32}P-chromic phosphate colloid has been demonstrated in the Sprague-

Dawley rat. Rats with occult liver cancer, untreated, went on to die of progressive liver tumor. Those treated usually had their disease controlled.

Three patients in a pilot study, having Dukes C colon cancer (positive nodes), were treated with ^{32}P-colloid into the arterial supply of the gastrointestinal tract, giving radiation to the liver. There has been, for 12 months now, no apparent liver cancer in two patients. One who died of brain and lung metastasis did show minimal tumor in the liver. This is much less tumor than would have been expected in the organ. One patient (free of disease now) had post-therapy radiation hepatitis, but apparently recovered without much liver damage. The third had no significant sequelae; she, as well as one other patient, had a drop in the white cell count to about 3200. The method seems effective with acceptable side effects, considering the apparent benefits.

REFERENCES

1. Nolan, T. R., Grady, E. D., Crumbley, A. J., et al.: Internal hepatic radiotherapy: I. Am. J. Roentgenol. 124:590–595, 1975.
2. Grady, E. D., Nolan, T. R., Crumbley, A. J., Internal radiotherapy: II. Am. J. Roentgenol. 124:596–599, 1975.

Irving M. Ariel

31

Treatment of Metastatic Cancer to the Liver from Primary Colon and Rectal Cancer by the Intra-Arterial Administration of Chemotherapy and Radioactive Isotopes

INTRODUCTION

Approximately 25 percent of all patients who die from any cancer have metastases to the liver at postmortem examination. This value increases to approximately 50 percent in patients who die whose primary cancer is located in the gastrointestinal tract.[1] Not infrequently, when the patient is subjected to a celiotomy for resection of a cancer from the colon or rectum, metastases to the liver are observed. The problem of treating such patients is a great one and various modalities have been advocated, ranging from radical extirpation of the lobe containing the metastases to a ''hands-off policy.''

This chapter details the results of our continuing investigations obtained by the administration into the hepatic artery of the combined course of a cancer chemotherapeutic agent, 5-fluorouracil, and a radioactive isotope in the form of [90]yttrium microspheres.*

The usual route for metastases to reach the liver is via the portal system (less frequently by the lymphatic vessels or by direct extension from exogenous organs). In most instances, metastatic cancers to the liver receive their nutrient supply by way of the hepatic artery. Thus, to administer anticancer agents via the hepatic artery is logical.

Republished with modification from J. Surg. Oncol. 10(4), 1978.

Assisted by Grants-in-Aid from the Arnold P. Rosen Cancer Research Fund, the Harold S. Brady Memorial Cancer Fund, and the Foundation for Clinical Research, New York, New York.

*Obtained from the 3M Company, St. Paul, Minnesota. Now available from Georgia Technical University, Atlanta, Georgia.

SELECTION OF PATIENTS

Two groups of patients are analyzed in this series. The first group consists of those patients who were asymptomatic but whose metastatic cancers to the liver were discovered at the time of operation. Twenty-five patients of this group were treated.

Forty patients were referred for treatment with symptoms resulting from metastatic cancer to the liver. They presented either a large liver, a sense of distention with abdominal pain, loss of weight with inanition, certain blood chemical findings demonstrating hepatic dysfunction, evidence of hepatic defects as noted on Scintillation scans, or angiographic evidence of hepatic lesions.

At the onset of the study, three patients demonstrated signs of hepatic coma with marked increase in blood ammonia. These patients harbored far-advanced cancers and should not have been entered into the course for therapy. They are included in this series, but patients with far-advanced hepatic dysfunction were excluded from further celiotomy and hepatic artery infusion by the technique herein described.

METHOD AND MATERIALS

All patients are hospitalized and the catheter is inserted by means of a laparotomy performed under general anesthesia. A polyethylene catheter is inserted retrograde into the right gastroduodenal artery and is threaded into the hepatic artery and anchored in place to the artery by means of 5–0 vascular sutures. The catheter is inserted into the main hepatic artery in all instances, even when either lobe contains obvious metastases. This is done in the belief that occult metastases may be resident within the other lobe. The position of the catheter is often determined by the intraarterial injection of a 5 percent solution of sodium fluorescein (Fluorescite®). When the liver is viewed under ultraviolet light, a characteristic discoloration is noted. An adapter is applied to the polyethylene catheter and a two-way stop cock is placed in position. Saline solution to which has been added a small amount of heparin is then injected to maintain the patency of the catheter and to prevent clotting. The catheter is exteriorized through a tiny stab wound and anchored to the skin through 3–0 silk sutures. The abdominal wound is closed by continuous sutures of chromicized catgut for the peritoneum and interrupted 2–0 silk for the fascia and interrupted 3–0 silk for the skin. No drains are left within the abdomen. When the patient reaches his room, the catheter is attached to a Fenwall pump to which has been added the 5-fluorouracil. The ^{90}Y microspheres are administered to the patient while he is in his room. Photoscans of the abdomen, using bremsstrahlen from the yttrium, reveal the distribution of the administered radioactive isotopes. This has been described.[2]

The drug dosage consists of 1 gram of 5-fluorouracil every 24 hours for an average of 15 days. Thus, the average patient receives 15 grams of 5-fluorouracil. Considering an average weight of 70 kg per patient, this results in approximately 3.2 g/kg for the total course of therapy. The dosage, of course, varies. In some instances where the 1 gram is well tolerated, it is increased to 1.5 grams of

5-fluorouracil per day, whereas with other patients, gastrointestinal symptoms or abdominal pain develops and the dose is decreased to 750 mg a day or even to 500 mg a day. There is tremendous variation in the tolerance of the patients to the 5-flurouracil.

The drug is diluted with 1 liter of 5 percent dextrose solution, in a sterile plastic bag containing approximately 5000 units of heparin. The insert is placed in a Fenwall bag and pumped to a pressure of 200 mm Hg to propel the solution. A valve regulates the flow to vary between 12 and 20 drops per minute. At the completion of the contents of one insert, a new insert containing the drug is placed within the Fenwall bag, thus maintaining a closed system throughout.

At the completion of therapy the catheter is removed by simply pulling it through the stab wound. No untoward reactions have occurred. The patient is kept in the hospital for 2 to 3 additional days, at which time hematologic and liver function blood studies are performed. No further therapy is administered for 2 weeks. If after 2 weeks the hematologic findings are normal, the patient is placed on a course of maintenance systemic therapy consisting of 500 mg of 5-fluorouracil given intravenously, ususally twice a week.

If there is a depression of the white blood count below 3000 cells per cubic millimeter, therapy is stopped until an increase in the white blood count is noted, after which the drug is given at a slower rate. If undue vomiting or nausea occurs, an effort is made to control these by administration of medication for symptomatic purposes. If these fail, the rate of drug administration is reduced or temporarily stopped.

After completing the course of therapy, approximately 50 percent of the patients had a sense of listlessness, a sense of ill-feeling which they could not adequately describe. The administration of steroids in such patients often had a pronounced symptomatic beneficial effect.

COMPLICATIONS FROM INTRA-ARTERIAL CATHETER INFUSION

The complications encountered from the administration of the therapeutic agents into the hepatic artery are summarized in Table 31-1. In 10 patients there was technical difficulty resulting from massive cancers obstructing the hepatic artery. These patients were usually treated either by the interstitial administration

Table 31-1
Complications Encountered from Intrahepatic Artery
Infusion—75 Patients

Complication	No. of Patients
Technical inability to catheterize the hepatic artery	10
Displacement of catheter before treatment terminated	8
Leaking catheter	6
Gastrointestinal bleeding	5
Hepatic coma	3

of radioactive sources into the cancer[3] or by an umbilical vein catheterization.[4] They are not included in this series as they were not subject to intrahepatic arterial therapy. In eight cases the catheter was displaced before treatment was terminated. The displacement was usually determined by means of angiographic studies. If the displacement occurred within 5 days of the drug administration, the patients were not included in this series (three patients). If it occurred after 5 days, the patients were included. In six patients a leaking catheter was observed, but angiographic studies demonstrated that despite the leak, a significant amount of the drug was delivered into the liver via the hepatic artery. No unusual untoward reactions occurred from this leaking catheter. Five patients manifested bleeding from the upper intestinal tract toward the end of the treatment. This was believed to be due to gastritis, and therapy was stopped.

The dose of ^{90}Y miscrospheres varied from 100 to 150 mCi. This does has been estimated to administer approximately 10,000 rads to the liver.[2] No untoward effects occurred from the ^{90}Y microspheres. There was no evidence of extrahepatic escape of the nucleodes as determined by scanning. No clinical symptoms or signs (either hepatic or extrahepatic) occurred. The only abnormality that was observed was a transient increase in the hepatic SGOT.

RESULTS

Clinical Evidence of Favorable Response

The criteria of Watkins et al.[5] were adopted; namely, that a significant decrease in the size of the liver in addition to relief of symptoms and return of results of biochemical tests of liver function to normal or near normal values had to be accompanied by an improvement in functional capacity for normal life activities and had to be prolonged for more than 3 months to be classified as a favorable response.

Table results (Table 31-2) were further divided into two groups: (1) objective response, in which there was a significant decrease in the size of the liver and/or a significant improvement of any of the hepatic function tests; and (2) subjective response, in which there was a decrease in the symptoms accompanied by a sense of well being. When results did occur, they were marked and left little doubt as to the efficacy or lack of efficacy of therapy. Oftentimes, a liver that had reached

Table 31-2
Response to Intraarterial Chemotherapy and
Isotope Therapy for Metastatic Cancer to the
Liver*

	Patients Responding	
No. of Patients	Objective	Subjective
40	40%	60%

*All patients had clinical evidence of cancer.

below the umbilicus shrank so much that it could no longer be palpated. A slight shrinkage was not considered of any demonstrable benefit. Some patients who came in extremely weak with severe malaise and anorexia with clinical evidence of jaundice enjoyed a clearing up of the jaundice and a sense of well being.

Only the 40 patients who had clinical evidence of cancer are included in the analysis of response. (The other patients, whose cancers were asymptomatic but were discovered at the time of operation, are not evaluated inasmuch as they had neither subjective symptoms nor objective signs.)

Forty percent of the patients manifested an objective response. In 60 percent, a significant subjective improvement occurred. The duration of improvement varied greatly from individual to individual.

Longevity

Table 31-3 reports the results of duration of life after the course of intraarterial therapy. Of the 25 patients who had asymptomatic metastases to the liver, the average duration of life was 26 months, and varied from 9 to 60 months. In contrast, among the 40 patients who had clinical evidence of cancer, the average duration of life was 12 months and varied from 4 to 54 months.

Toxic Reactions to Individual Hepatic Artery Infusion

Of the 65 patients treated, 30 suffered some degree of nausea and vomiting (Table 31-4). These were usually controlled by antiemetics, but in some patients the nausea and vomiting were so severe that therapy had to be stopped. Ten patients developed diarrhea which was interpreted to be the result of the infusion of the drug into another artery. The diarrhea was usually not severe and could be readily controlled by constipating medications.

Stomatitis was a complaint of 40 patients. This gradually developed as the therapy progressed. Applying gentian violet or gargling with lido-caine (Xylocaine®) viscous produced relief. Abdominal pain was a complaint of 30 patients, but it was never severe enought to stop therapy and could be controlled with analgesics. In only 5 patients was a significant leukopenia observed, with a drop in the white count below 2000 cells/mm^3. No severe bacteremia or septicemia occurred, nor were there any other complications resulting from the leukopenia. The patients usually complained of weakness during the immediate post-treatment period.

Table 31-3

Longevity after Intrarterial Therapy for Patients with
Metastatic Cancer to the Liver from the Colon and Rectum

	25 Patients Without Clinical Evidence	40 Patients with Clinical Evidence
Avg. duration life	25	40
after treatment (months)	26	12
Range (months)	9 to 60	4 to 54

Table 31-4
Toxic Reaction to Intrahepatic Artery
Infusion—65 Patients

Toxic Reaction	No. of Patients
Nausea and vomiting	30
Diarrhea	10
Stomatitis	40
Abdominal pain	30
Leukopenia (WBC < 2000)	10

DISCUSSION

Metastasis in the liver from any cancer usually carries with it an ominous prognosis. In our ongoing study regarding the efficacy of different modalities in the treatment of hepatic cancer, it is to be noted that in a series of 27 patients who had surgical resections of their metastases, the average duration of life was only 10 months.[6] This is not significantly different from the results reported by Pestana et al.[7] in a series of 353 patients who received no treatment whatsoever for their hepatic metastases and who survived an average of 9 months.

Systemic 5-fluorouracil has no significant effect on longevity.[8] In 35 patients so treated, the average survival was 9 months. In a series of 20 patients who received this drug via the umbilical vein, the results were similar to those of patients who had received the drug systemically, with an average survival of 8 months.[4]

Forty patients with metastases from colon and rectal cancer were treated by the intraarterial administration of 5-fluorouracil.[9] Their average survival was 12 months. In a previously reported series of patients with inoperable cancer treated by the administration of 5-fluorouracil and the isotope directly into the aorta, the average duration of life of the 59 patients was 5.6 months. The material was administered directly into the aorta at the level of the celiac axis. This has since been found to be an improper method and has been abandoned.[10] In the present series, all patients received their drugs directly into the hepatic artery (Table 31-5). This report analyzes the effects of giving a cancer chemotherapeutic agent supplemented by radiation therapy in the form of ^{90}Y microspheres.

The use of intraarterial radioactive isotopes has been previously reported.[2] Briefly, the irradiating microspheres represent a method for internal irradiation whereby a radioactive isotope is attached to an inert carrier. The spheres are made of ceramic or plastic material, are completely inert chemically and physiologically, and measure from 10 to 200 μm in diameter. We have utilized 15-μm microspheres. They have a melting point in excess of 1500°C and are insoluble in inorganic and organic solvents. The isotope of yttrium, namely, ^{90}Y, has a rather good radiologic spectrum for systemic clinical therapeutic application. It is a 2.18-mev pure beta ray emitter with a half-life of 2.5 days; it has a maximum penetration of about 8 mm in tissue, thereby limiting radiation to the vicinity of the microspheres. Its average penetration is about 5 mm.

Studies in utilizing the combined parameters of gamma ray scanning and

Table 31-5

Duration of Life* after Treatment of 201 Patients with Metastasis to the
Liver from Colon and Rectal Cancer

Method of Treatment	No. of Patients	Average Duration of Life (months)
No treatment (Pestana et al.[19])	353	9
Surgical resection	27	10
Systemic 5-FU	35	9
Umbilical vein 5-FU	20	8
Intraarterial HN$_2$	14	5
Intraarterial 5-FU	40	12
Intraarterial 5-FU and ^{90}Y microspheres	65	19
Without clinical evidence of cancer	25	26
With evidence of cancer in the liver	40	12

*From the time of diagnosis.

angiography have revealed that the larger metastases have largely outgrown their blood supply with the maximum of the blood supply remaining in the outer periphery, but the middle portion is devoid of a blood supply. In such instances effects from chemotherapy are limited, and the use of the radiating microspheres, which are completely dependent on an adequate blood supply to the locus for irradiation, makes such large lesions unsuitable for internal irradiation.

The patients who respond best are those with multiple small metastases with an adequate blood supply. Patients whose metastases were discovered at the time of operation for a primary cancer were the ones who responded best from the standpoint of longevity. Inasmuch as they had no symptoms, one could not determine either objective or subjective improvement. In approximately 50 percent of the patients, there was a transitory increase in the SGOT which returned to a normal level in 5 to 7 days, even while the patients were receiving 5-fluorouracil intraarterially. This was the only observed untoward effect of the internally administered irradiation to the liver.

Watkins et al.[5] have practiced elective intrahepatic artery catherization: 82 patients were treated with the Watkins chromametric pump and received treatment varying from 3 to 6 weeks after which there was a period of rest and then the intraarterial therapy was continued. The drug used by these authors was fluorodeoxyuridine. The effects on longevity are presented in Table 31-6.

Ansfield and his group[11] at the University of Wisconsin have had extensive experience with intrahepatic arterial chemotherapy. They treated 293 patients with various types of cancers by percutaneously placing the catheter into the hepatic artery, threading it into the hepatic artery via the brachial artery. These investigators have used 5-fluorouracil exclusively for metastases from the GI tract. Their results are presented in Table 31-6.

The intraarterial administration of the combined cancer chemotherapy and isotope therapy, in the 65 patients herein reported, was accomplished by insertion of the catheter into the hepatic artery via the gastroduodenal artery. No effort was made at localization as was practiced by Watkins et al. We administered 5-fluorouracil, an average of 1 gram a day, for 15 days for a total dose of 15 grams.

Table 31-6
Longevity of Patients Treated by Intraarterial Chemotherapy as Reported by Different Authors

Author	Technique	Drug Used	Average Total Dose	Duration of Treatment Dose	Average Longevity
Watkins et al.[22] Met Ca from colon & rectum. 82 patients.	Selective intrahepatic artery catheterization. Patients treated on outpatient basis by means of Watkin's chromametric pump.	Fluorodeoxyuridine	20 mg/day × 3–6 weeks; Total: 420–840 mg	3–6 weeks, then rest; Total: 3–6 months	15 months from onset of symptoms. Average of 4.3 months before treatment. (Untreated control group survived average of 4.2 months.)
Ansfield et al.[1] All cancers. 293 patients.	Percutaneous placement into hepatic artery via brachial artery.	5-Fluorouracil	25 mg/kg × 4 days = 6000 mg; 20 mg/kg/day × 4 days = 4800 mg; 15 mg/kg/day × 17 days = 2600 mg; Total: ± 13.5 g	3 weeks	Mean survival of those who improved: 161 patients, 11.6 months. Mean survival of those who did not improve: 132 patients, 5.6 months.
Ariel. Met Ca from colon & rectum. 65 patients.	Operative placement of catheter into hepatic artery via gastroduodenal artery.	5-Fluorouracil & 100 mCi ^{90}Y microspheres	1 g/day × 14 days Total: 14 g	2 weeks	Asymptomatic patients: 25 patients, average survival 26 months. Symptomatic patients: 40 patients, average survival 12 months. Total average survival, 19 months.

The average survival of all patients in our series was 19 months. Twenty-five patients who were asymptomatic survived 26 months, whereas those whose cancers had produced clinical signs and symptoms survived a shorter period of 12 months. These results are slightly better than those reported by others and would suggest some added improvement for the internal irradiation derived from the ^{90}Y microspheres. The data, however, do not permit a categoric conclusion regarding the beneficial effects of the internal irradiation supplementing the cancer chemotherapy. A series of patients are now being evaluated who receive a smaller dose of 5-fluorouracil (average 5 grams) combined with the internal irradiation. This will be presented in a subsequent report.

SUMMARY

Sixty-five patients with metastases to the liver from primary cancers of the colon and rectum were treated by a combination of a chemotherapeutic agent (5-fluorouracil) and internal irradiation in the form of ^{90}Y microspheres delivered into the hepatic artery.

They received an average dose of 1 gram of 5-fluorouracil each day for a total of 15 days and an average dose of 100 mCi ^{90}Y microspheres, calculated to administer approximately 10,000 rads beta to the liver.

The overall survival of all patients was 19 months. Forty patients referred for treatment because of symptoms from the hepatic metastases survived an average of 12 months. The 25 patients whose metastases were discovered at the time of the original operation and were asymptomatic from the standpoint of the metastases to the liver survived an average of 26 months.

Toxic reactions were not severe and consisted of nausea and vomiting, stomatitis, abdominal pain, and leukopenia.

Patients with far-advanced cancer causing severe hepatic dysfunction did poorly. Three such patients developed hepatic coma. Intraarterial chemotherapy and/or isotope therapy is considered contraindicated for such patients.

Of the 40 patients with symptoms, 40 percent exhibited objective evidence of response and 60 percent were subjectively improved.

Smaller tumors have a richer vascular supply than large ones. The blood supply is essentially from branches of the hepatic artery. Intrahepatic artery administration of anticancer agents offers the best logistics for administration of the agents. Large masses have virtually outgrown their blood supply and hence do not respond to this form of therapy as well as similar tumor deposits.

The administration of the radioactive isotope ^{90}Y offers a means of supplying internal irradiation as a supplement to chemotherapy, with no observed complications.

REFERENCES

1. Pack, G. T., Islami, A. H.: Metastatic cancer to and from the liver. In: Tumors of the Liver, G, T. Pack and A. H. Islami (Eds.). New York, Springer-Verlag, pp. 72–84, 1970.

2. Ariel, I. M.: Treatment of inoperable primary pancreatic and liver cancer by the intra-arterial administration of radioactive isotopes (^{90}Y radiating microspheres). Ann. Surg. 162:267–278, 1965.

3. Ariel, I. M.: Treatment of metastases to the liver with interstitial radioactive isotopes. Surg. Gynecol. Obstet. 11:739–745, 1960.

4. Ariel, I. M.: Hepatic metastasis from rectal and colon cancer treated by infusion of 5-fluorouracil into the umbilical vein. N.Y. State J. Med. 72:2629–2632, 1972.

5. Watkins, E., Jr., Khazei, A. M., Nahra, K. S.: Surgical basis for arterial infusion chemotherapy of disseminated carcinoma of the liver. Surg. Gynecol. Obstet. 130:581–605, 1970.

6. Miller, T. R.: End results in the surgical treatment of liver tumors. In: Tumors of the Liver, G. T. Pack and A. H. Islami (Eds.). New York, Springer-Verlag, pp. 293–298, 1970.

7. Pestana, C., Reitemeter, R. J., Moertel, C. G., et al.: The natural history of carcinoma of the colon and rectum. Am. J. Surg. 108:826–829, 1964.

8. Ariel, I. M.: Systemic 5-fluorouracil in hepatic metastases from primary colon and rectal cancer. N.Y. State J. Med. 72:1041–1044, 1972.

9. Ariel, I. M., Pack, G. T.: Intra-arterial chemotherapy for cancer metastatic to liver. Arch. Surg. 91:851–862, 1965.

10. Ariel, I. M., Pack, G. T.: Treatment of inoperable cancer of liver by intra-arterial radioactive isotopes and chemotherapy. Cancer 20:793–804, 1967.

11. Ansfield, F. J., Davis, H. L., Jr., Ramirez, G., et al.: Further clinical studies with intrahepatic arterial infusion with 5-fluorouracil. Cancer 36:2413–2417, 1975.

ADDITIONAL READINGS

1. Ariel, I. M.: Treatment of primary and metastatic cancer of the liver. Surgery 39:70–91, 1956.

2. Ariel, I. M., Pack, G. T.: Treatment of inoperable cancer of the biliary system with radioactive ^{131}Rose Bengal. Am. J. Roentgenol. 83:474–490, 1960.

3. Ariel, I. M., Lehman, W. B.: Five-year control of an "inoperable" obstructing carcinoma metastatic to the porta hepatis in a 79-year old male. J. Am. Geriatr. Soc. 9:786–790, 1961.

4. Ariel, I. M.: An aid for determining treatment of liver cancer by combined hepatic gamma-scanning. Surg. Gynecol. Obstet. 121:267–274, 1965.

5. Ariel, I. M.: Continuous intra-arterial chemotherapeutic infusion utilizing a portable syringe. Cancer 18:1489–1492, 1965.

6. Ariel, I. M., Molander, D., Galey, D.: Hepatic gammascanning: an aid in determining treatment policies for cancer involving the liver. Am. J. Surg. 118:5–14, 1969.

7. Ariel, I. M.: Treatment of inoperable retroperitoneal and hepatic cancer with alkylating agent having a half-life of 4 1/2 seconds. Proc. Am. Assoc. Cancer Res. 13:106, 1972 (Abst. #424).

8. Miller, T. R. and Griman, O. R.: Hepatic artery catheterization for liver perfusion. Arch. Surg. 81:423–425, 1961.

9. Nolan, T. R., Grady, E. D., Crumbley, A. J., et al.: Internal hepatic radiotherapy: I. Am. J. Roentgenol. 124:590–595, 1975.

10. Sullivan, R. D., Norcross, J. W., Watkins, E., Jr.: Chemotherapy of metastatic liver cancer by prolonged hepatic artery infusion. N. Engl. J. Med. 270:321–327, 1964.

11. Watkins, E., Jr.: Chronometric infusor; an apparatus for protracted ambulatory infusion therapy. N. Engl. J. Med. 269:850–851, 1963.

R. J. Blanchard

32
Precautions in the Use
of ^{90}Y Microspheres

Based on our observations of safety and effectiveness of ^{90}Y microspheres in treating VX-2 carcinoma in rabbit liver, and encouraged by reports from other centers, we have embarked on a clinical trial in which the criteria for selection of patients have been uniform and strict. We are including only those patients with vascular metastases, in whom the primary tumor has been controlled, and who are not receiving other therapy. Treatment has been a single dose of 50 mCi of ^{90}Y via percutaneous transfemoral Seldinger catheter in the hepatic artery. *No adjuvant treatment has been given as we want to observe the effect of the microspheres per se.* Since September 1976, we have treated six patients. Ten others were excluded from treatment either because angiograms failed to show vascular tumors or because of inability to manipulate the catheter into the artery. In all six treated patients, there has been objective evidence of tumor regression.

One patient received an anomalous treatment as follows. This 55-year-old man was treated on a Linac 4, with two opposed fields, to the left lower lobe of the lung and the mediastinum for oat cell carcinoma in July 1976. Total dose was 2400 to 2600 rads. On August 11, 1976, liver enlargement and altered liver functions were observed. By September 14, his liver was down to iliac crest, there was edema of legs, and he was unable to lie down. Serum bilirubin was 5.6, alkaline phosphatase 1120 IU, SGOT 370 IU, LAD 1400 IU, and serum albumin 3.1 grams. On September 21, 1976, he received 30 mCi ^{90}Y. The low dose was due to delays in shipping.

After an initial regression in liver span from 25 cm to 19.5 cm and a drop in liver enzymes, progress slowed and he was given a single dose of 60 mg adriamycin on October 7 (Fig. 32-1). On October 25, he received a second infusion of 60 mCi of ^{90}Y. There was profound reduction in liver size and further lowering of liver enzymes, and leg edema disappeared. He was walking 2 miles per day. Then on November 3, he developed respiratory insufficiency which progressed rapidly until he died on November 7.

The chest x-ray in September 1976 showed no unusual features (Fig. 32-2, *top*). However, the chest x-ray on October 30 showed pulmonary edema or fi-

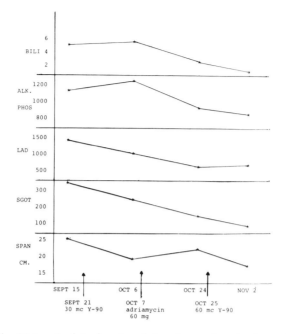

Fig. 32-1. A plot of various laboratory values in the patient as a function of time.

brosis especially in the left lower lobe which progressed to bilateral extensive infiltrates by November 4 (Fig. 32-2, *bottom*).

Was this due to spillover of ⁹⁰Y microspheres into the lung? Unfortunately, we did not have a lung scan, by use of the bremstrahlung, post-treatment. Liver bremstrahlung was strong.

At autopsy there was pulmonary fibrosis and very low radiation levels in the lungs. An autoradiograph of a 1.5-cm thick slice of lung showed evidence of radioactivity only after 7 days of exposure. The liver, on the other hand, showed numerous hot spots after only 2½ days' exposure with adjacent relatively cold areas. By superimposing a tracing of the liver slice with tumors marked, we observed that the hot spots corresponded moderately well with sites of tumor; liver free of tumor was not radioactive (Fig. 32-3).

These liver autoradiographs confirm, in a human, the localization of ⁹⁰Y in metastases we had observed in rabbits. The very low levels of radiation in the lungs seem insufficient to explain the severe pulmonary insufficiency and the necrosis seen at autopsy. However, it is evident that some shunting had occurred. In addition to the ⁹⁰Y spillover, the patient had received external radiotherapy to the lung and a dose of adriamycin (which is known to cause pulmonary fibrosis in some patients). Perhaps the first dose of ⁹⁰Y and/or the adriamycin caused partial necrosis of tumor, stimulating development of shunts greater than 15 μm thereby permitting some of the second dose to pass through into the lungs.

Because of this possibility we wonder whether repeated infusions are safe. In such patients, and in patients with tumors that may have large anteriovenous shunts such as hepatic tumors, we now plan to perform a preliminary infusion of albumin Tc 99m microspheres, followed by a scan of the lungs, to detect whether

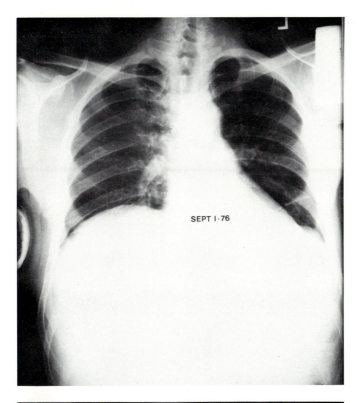

SEPT 1·76

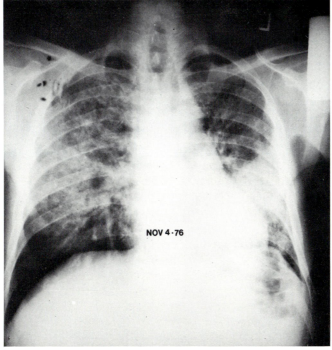

NOV 4·76

Fig. 32-2. Chest radiographs of the patient.

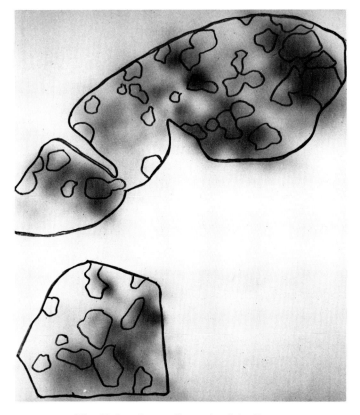

Fig. 32-3.   Autoradiograph of the liver.

spillover has occurred. We did this in a patient with hepatic cell carcinoma and no shunting was observed. Treatment of this tumor with ^{90}Y resulted in 50 percent regression and marked clinical improvement. Besides the risk of shunting into the lungs, there is a danger of exposing the upper gastrointestinal tract to ^{90}Y if the catheter is not placed beyond the gastroduodenal artery.

One patient had a large solitary central metastasis from the colon. The left lobe was supplied from the celiac artery and the right lobe from the superior mesenteric artery. The tumor received all its blood supply via the celiac artery. During infusion, the catheter was dislodged proximal to the gastroduodenal artery and the patient developed symptomatic gastroduodenitis which subsequently subsided. The tumor seems to have disappeared on follow-up angiography.

Although the method had apparent beneficial effect, not all patients are suitable due to avascular tumors, and precautions need to be taken to avoid exposing the gastrointestinal tract and lungs.

33
A Discussion of the Presentations

Dr. I. R. McDougall. I will take a minute to show the most recent results of ^{125}I therapy for hyperthyroidism. These are described by McDougall and Greig in *Annals of Internal Medicine* (85:720–723, 1976). Dr. Greig and I carried out a large study treating 355 patients with hyperthyroidism and diffuse goiters. Of the total group, 63 percent became clinically euthyroid. One-third of the patients are hypothyroid. Three percent were still hyperthyroid (49 months average follow-up). Hypothyroidism was lowest in the group given 6 to 10.5 mCi of ^{125}I (23 percent). In those receiving over 20 mCi, the incidence of hypothyroidism was 63 percent. The frequent occurrence of thyroid underactivity after ^{125}I therapy shows that ^{131}I is still the radionuclide of choice when treating hyperthyroidism.

Dr. H. Atkins. It is commonly accepted that particle emitters would be preferable for therapy with radionuclides and that those radionuclides which are primarily gamma emitters are to be avoided. However, it is not necessary to restrict one's consideration of potential sources to beta and alpha emitters for delivery of radiation dose with unsealed sources. This is based on two factors: (1) High-energy gamma emitters have been successfully used as sealed sources in the interstitial radiation therapy for malignancy. Their efficacy is based on the rapid falloff in dose outside the treated volume in accordance with the inverse square law. (2) There are no "pure" gamma emitters. There is either associated beta minus emission, or in the case of radionuclides undergoing decay by isomeric transition or electron capture, there are associated conversion and Auger electrons, which, in fact, make the major contribution to organ dose.

In support of the major role of conversion and Auger electrons in radiation dose, consider ^{99m}Tc. In the thyroid, the ratio of dose from photons (including x-rays) to the dose from nonpenetrating radiation is 0.19. Of course this will change for different sized organs. In the liver the ratio will be 0.93 because of the greater absorbed fraction of the photons in the organ.

For effective therapy with radionuclides the radiation dose should be concentrated in the region of interest, and nontarget tissues should receive the lowest possible dose. The limiting factor in treatment of malignancy is the radiation dose to the red marrow. If we set our limit of dose to the marrow as 50 rads and the desired target organ dose is 5000 to 10,000 rads, a ratio of target organ/red marrow dose between 100 and 200 is required. Furthermore, a dose limit of 500 rads to any nearby organ is reasonable. This would require a target/nontarget ratio of about 10 to 20.

In order to assess the efficacy of various radionuclides as unsealed therapy sources, let us look at several possibilities. Consider the following: ^{22}Na ($\beta+$, high energy), ^{60}Co ($\beta-$, high energy), ^{99m}Tc (low energy, conversion and Auger electrons), and ^{125}I (low energy, conversion and Auger electrons). Doses to pancreas (target organ), spleen (nontarget organ), and marrow are considered. Table 33-1 illustrates the effect of using these radionuclides.

In each instance, despite the presence of high-energy photons in the case of ^{22}Na and ^{60}Co, the criteria for a useful radionuclide are met although this is borderline in some cases, and obviously some nuclides appear more favorable than others.

If the target organ is large, e.g., liver, the ratios are less satisfactory. For example, with ^{60}Co the liver/marrow dose ratio is only 38.75, which means 129 rads to marrow for 5000 rads to liver. In this case the liver/pancreas ratio is 9.25 resulting in a pancreas dose of 541 rads.

If the subcellular distribution of dose is important (e.g., ^{125}I and the thyroid), then the energy and type of emission are important and the above discussion is irrelevant.

Although particle emitters would be optimal for most conceivable applications, particularly where the metabolic uptake of the radioactive material is used to deliver the radionuclide to the target, concentration on beta and alpha emitters is unnecessarily restrictive. Other factors are more important. These are the maximum possible selective concentration of radionuclide in the target area and the effective time over which the radiation is delivered.

It must be acknowledged that shielding requirements are much reduced with nonphoton sources. In such situations, radiation protection of personnel and the patient's family is simplified.

Table 33-1
Ratio of Doses of Target Organ to Nontarget Organs
for Various Radionuclides

		^{22}Na	^{60}Co	^{99m}Tc	^{125}I
Dose	Pancreas*/Spleen	26.4	18.3	30.5	52.7
Dose	Pancreas*/Marrow	284.6	196.4	207.1	1128.6
Dose	Pancreas†/Marrow	219.5	156.2	164.7	554.8

*All the radionuclide in target organ.
†Radionuclide distributed 80 percent target organ, 20 percent total body.

Dr. A. Friedman. The reason people discuss alpha emitters is not the range so much, but the tremendous ionizing capabilities of the alphas. They destroy far more tissue along their path.

Dr. H. Atkins. That is true, but they destroy normal tissue as well as tumor tissue. It depends on the specific localization. If as good localization can be achieved with a gamma ray emitter, the dose falls off sharply from the treatment volume. I doubt that using a particle emission, for example, will make much difference.

Dr. F. Hosain. That is correct, unless intense uptake of a beta emitter in a tumor can be obtained. That would provide a point source with little extra tumor radiation.

Dr. S. J. Adelstein. We heard a little about the problems of microdosimetry and that microdosimetry is important with internal conversion electrons and Auger electrons. The microscopic distribution of radioactivity is extremely important. This is best demonstrated experimentally with iodine 125 purines or pyrimidines. The material is actually located within the target (that is, it is in the DNA). Here it is highly toxic, unlike extracellular ^{125}I. Now this is even more important when you want to think about linear energy transfer. The low-energy electrons are a low LET radiation. But a cell nucleus has a small volume, probably less than 50 nm. The LET is very high, and indeed is higher than that of alpha radiation. Dr. Chan, whose name has been mentioned several times today, has been working with a related system, and with some commonly employed radioactive nuclei. She finds that she cannot obtain a concentration of technetium pertechnetate that will actually sterilize cells. We cannot bring enough in to the laboratory to do that. Hence location as well as the low-energy electrons are of importance. On the other hand, selenium 75 selenomethionine is extremely toxic to cells in culture. I think it is important, even with some of the diagnostic radionuclei, that we pay some attention to microdosimetry. The question that I throw out has to do with extending some of the TDF concepts from a therapeutic field to the diagnostic field.

Dr. R. Bigler. Perhaps we are overestimating some of our diagnostic dosimetric concepts at the present moment, because we are not making TDF calculations. However, we will have to extrapolate results. The microdosimetry would have to be examined.

Dr. I. Ariel. I would like to address a question to Dr. Beierwaltes. He attributes a good radiation response to thyroids which are highly differentiated and often do not show pickup on scans. I should like to hear his opinion on stimulating these cancers with the use of TSH or other stimulants as mentioned by Dr. Spencer.

Dr. W. Beierwaltes. We take patients off thyroid hormone for 6 weeks prior to the radioiodide studies. The first reason for this is that if the patient has enough functional metastases, he will not become hypothyroid and therefore will not be uncomfortable. Indeed that is one way to tell whether a patient has functional metastases. If 6 weeks after a total thyroidectomy the patient is euthyroid, radioiodide scans of the lungs are indicated since there may be functioning metastases. The second aspect is that of endogenous TSH secretion versus exogenously administered TSH. A recently published article described a series of patients without thyroids who were given TSH injections (10 units a day); there was a peak each day. The maximum peaks did not approach those occurring when we take patients off thyroid hormone and follow them for 6 weeks. (I think the top peak in the series was approximately 150 μU/ml). In children TSH levels rise to very high levels (350 to 400 μU/ml). Jim Sission studied 45 of our adult patients; we were disturbed to find that 15 of the adults had relatively low serum TSH levels after being off thyroid hormone for 6 weeks. Our criterion now is that unless the patient has many functional metastases after being off thyroid hormone for 6 weeks, serum TSH levels must be over 90 before we consider treatment. In other words, monitoring serum TSH levels will indicate whether the patient has really been off thyroid. Therefore, you won't maximize the effect of the dosage given. Many times investigators from other universities have said they had a patient with well-differentiated thyroid carcinoma metastatic to lung without iodine uptake. I asked how they knew the metastases were well differentiated; they answered, by lung biopsy. They also stated that they were positive the patient had been off thyroid hormone for 6 weeks. I saw these patients. I remember the first one. When I asked her if she was really off all thyroid hormone, she said, "Oh no, I just stopped the thyroxin, but they told me I could continue T_3 up until 2 or 3 weeks before the time of the uptake study." I said, "Stop all pills and come back in 4 weeks and we will repeat your lung scan." She had visible lung metastases by x-ray. Four weeks later she had a high serum TSH. Radioiodide scan showed uptake throughout both lungs; we then treated her. We have also had that happen in our own institution. Dr. Sission had been very careful; finally he went to a lung biopsy and proved that the patient had well-differentiated metastatic thyroid cancer in the lungs. After another 20-minute discussion, the patient finally admitted taking thyroid hormone. We told the patient to take no pills and come back in 5 weeks. At that time the patient had beautiful uptake in the lungs. We then treated him with radioactive iodine. It is difficult to tell whether or not the patient is really off thyroid hormone without serum TSH levels.

I have seen 1 patient, out of 447, with well-differentiated thyroid carcinoma, proved in lymph nodes, that did not concentrate radioactive iodine. The patient was off thyroid hormone and was reliable. The TSH values were high. The only explanation for that related to the time when we were doing a contract for the Atomic Energy Commission (studying iodine uptake in the fetal thyroid and in the mother's thyroid). We had specimens of the fetal thyroid from 3 weeks on up. We put them on large posters. The morphology of this woman's well-differentiated thyroid carcinoma (with follicles) was very much like that of the fetus of about 4 weeks. I think it is a medical curosity that the patient's neoplasm had reverted to a near primitive state, even though it showed differentiation.

Dr. R. Spencer. Is there a possible role for TRF in preparing these patients for radioiodide therapy?

Dr. W. Beierwaltes. Dr. Thomas Haynie and coworkers wrote an article in which they could see no advantage in giving TRF over having the patient off thyroid for 6 weeks. You cannot override the effect of thyroid with TRF.

Dr. S. Spraragen. Dr. Beierwaltes, what dose of radioiodine do you use when you are searching for reccurrence of thyroid carcinoma?

Dr. W. Beierwaltes. We routinely use 300 μCi of radioiodine, and I would not argue with anyone who wanted to use more. We did try relatively large tracer doses, such as 5 to 15 mCi, in searching for metastases. One of my associates at that time asked why we did not use more. We tried 5 mCi, and then I suggested that we use 200 mCi for a tracer dose and scan the patient before he goes home. After a year of this (about 15 to 20 patients) in only one patient had we found a metastasis with 200 mCi of radioiodide that we had not seen with 300 μCi. I think it is entirely possible and very reasonable to use 1 to 2 mCi if you want to.

Dr. E. Kaplan. Do you have any experience in the clinical behavior of post-radiation thyroid carcinomas versus spontaneously occurring thyroid tumors?

Dr. W. Beierwaltes. I think there is a very high incidence of multicentricity in spontaneous thyroid carcinomas, particularly those of small size. There is no convincing evidence that the radiation-related thyroid carcinoma is overwhelmingly multifocal (more so than the spontaneously occurring disorder). This may come as a surprise to a lot of people. I think basically that most of the data on "radiation-induced thyroid carcinoma" is confused by the fact that a great majority are the so-called occult carcinomas, which were originally defined as under 1.5 cm. At the University of Chicago conference last September, the group decided to call them 1 cm or under. That's a whole different world. We have decided that occult carcinomas are not to be treated like clinical cancers at all; they just behave differently. Several investigators have shown that if the thyroid gland is sectioned at 3-mm intervals and each section is examined under a dissecting microscope, and then three microscopic sections are prepared on each abnormality seen, there are some very disturbing and exciting findings. First, in such investigations there has been no incidence of thyroid carcinoma under 13 percent of the people studied. They come to autopsy from burns, gunshot wounds, and so forth. Certainly some of the little things you think are cancer turn out to be scars. Some of the scans contain calcospheroids, which suggests there has been a papillary carcinoma of the thyroid and that it has regressed. Thirdly, in the small cancers, there may be a much higher incidence of occult sclerosing carcinoma. I think Samson has evidence that 5 out of something like 19,000 people that had occult carcinoma went on to develop clinical cancer. Furthermore, I predict that this same technique, when applied to lung, would give 13 to 25 percent incidence of carcinoma of the lung.

Dr. E. Kaplan. What is your feeling on the main problem of treating verified carcinoma?

Dr. W. Beierwaltes. That is a common question. We have no inviolate routine. In other words, we do not give the treatment dose of 150 mCi to everyone who shows any uptake. In many patients the main desire is to wait for a year and see what happens. You may recall that I listed several conditions under which treatment should be begun immediately, such as in the person past 40, if the primary was removed surgically if very rapidly growing (the prognosis is very poor), and if the primary is 5 cm in diameter (always ablate the thyroid because there is a terrible prognosis). Another criterion is that if the tumor is locally invasive, the death rate rises markedly. Generally speaking, we have treated all good remnants in patients unless the primary was under 1.5 cm and if none of those bad prognostic factors were present. A dose of 150 mCi was used. This has been worked up to gradually over the years. My first treatment dose for thyroid carcinoma was 5 mCi. I found myself penny wise and pound foolish. In order to save the person some radiation, I gave them 50 mCi the first time and the next time 100 mCi. Finally, 200 mCi was given to ablate the remnant. The most common causes of failure of radioiodine treatment are (1) inadequate surgery, (2) failure to keep patient off thyroid hormone for 6 weeks or longer, and (3) giving treatment doses of under 150 mCi. What you do is like giving pencillin to someone with a bacteremia that is penicillin insensitive. The first dose kills "the best." You saw evidence that fractionated doses are less effective. You tend to decrease the storage space and increase the turnover rate with each dose. Dr. David Becker has evidence that 15 percent of patients with Grave's disease are extremely resistant to treatment with radioiodine. They do a 2-week uptake study on Grave's disease. He has found these unusually resistant patients have a very short transit time. You decrease the transit time of radioiodine in the carcinoma each time you treat them. Therefore, there is a marked decrease in the radiation dose. I prefer to accomplish everything I am going to accomplish on the first dose and have no cause to regret it.

Dr. J. W. Turner. Have you had any metastases become necrotic and bleed after radioiodide therapy?

Dr. W. Beierwaltes. No. A case was described in the literature with a tumor metastatic to the brain. I am very concerned about the metastases to brain. I used to follow patients with malignant melanoma, 13 of whom I followed to their death. In following these 13 patients I was intrigued that one day they would have one lung metastasis on chest x-ray and 24 hours later they would have six metastases. All solid tumors tend to develop necrosis and hemorrhage, even without radiation. Hot thyroid nodules also develop hemorrhage.

Dr. G. Burrow. A comment in regard to the question of using antithyroid drugs in the treatment of pregnant women. We did some follow-up studies in the offspring, directed toward determining the effect on intelligence and development. Looking at children who had been exposed to propylthiouracil, and comparing them to their siblings who had been born when the mother was not receiving propylthiouracil, we were unable to find any differences; in fact, the two smartest youngsters in the group had been born while their mothers were on propyl-thiouracil. One of my reluctances in giving radioactive iodine to women in the child-bearing age reflects my 2 years with the Atomic Bomb Casualty Commission. There may be genetic problems which, if they occur today, would not be shown until the F2, F3, or F4 generations. The data that are used are for the F1 generation.

Dr. W. Beierwaltes. A common statement is that we may not observe any harmful effects now, but first of all, radiation is harmful. Second, wait until the F4 generation rolls around. But of course the children we are treating for thyroid cancer are important. The average patient in such cases is a child who has a good pediatrician who says, "If you are going to do something with this patient it has to be finished within 3 months, because the child will be dead from lung metastases in 3 months." At that point, the parents are not worrying about the fourth generation.

Question. I would like to bring up the question of low-dose ^{131}I therapy. The people who seem to be against it claim that the low dose does not do much good. I believe Dr. Atkins showed there was a marked delay in development of hypothyroidism. Now it may not have cured patients, but it may have stopped hypothyroidism.

Dr. H. Atkins. In the present state of the art, the low-dose therapy is preferable to high dose because you have that many more years before hypothyroidism develops. I think the theory for a high dose is that if the patient is not properly instructed, and myxedema develops gradually, it can lead to serious complications. It is then difficult to treat because it has gone on for such a long time. The other thing you have to weigh against it in the low dosage is continued hyperthyroidism in many patients. I doubt that that is the real problem these days, with propranolol and antithyroid drugs to handle the situation.

Dr. W. Beierwaltes. I am only going to emphasize what has been said earlier. I think I can clarify this. We published our article in 1966 or 1967, on 826 patients treated for hyperthyroidism with radioiodine, as compared to 142 treated by surgery. As part of the national center follow-up, everybody looked at our initial rise in hypothyroidism within 1 year and said obviously the problem was that they used too large a dose. If you examine that article carefully, it is impossible to relate hypothyroidism to dose. As was said this morning, the lowest incidence of hypothyroidism occurred when the patients with thyroid overactivity received over 100 mCi (there were 11 of them). The highest incidence of hypothyroidism occurred in persons who received 10 mCi or less. In between all these dose levels there was no absolute, but a good linear correlation. It is not a simple problem of dose. As Dr. Atkins said, it is logical. Guess who received 100 mCi? Patients with huge multinodular goiters. Guess who received 10 mCi? Young people with small thyroids. As a result of those data you saw here, even people who were given 3 mCi eventually (after 1 year) developed a rising incidence of hypothyroidism. As a surprise to me, I found an article published 4 or 5 years ago, from the University of Wisconsin, in which exactly the same thing was described. That shows the constantly rising incidence of hypothyroidism. I think the final answer to your question of what are you going to do tomorrow is summarized by Chapman in an editorial in the *New England Journal of Medicine*. He said that young people with almost no enlargement of the thyroid, and no nodules, are given a mean dose of 3.5 mCi. That article states that the patients on whom the low dose was used *excluded* patients with multinodular goiters. In other words, that is a very biased statistical group. However, the reason for getting by without the first year rise was that young people without nodules were included. The reason we had the rise, I am sure in retrospect, is that we see principally patients with multinodular goiters at the University of Michigan. So we were treating patients with Grave's disease with the same formula.

Dr. I. Ariel. I would like to address this question to Dr. Antar. I strongly question the validity of the claim that the dose of radiation he gave destroyed the left lobe of the liver. The reason for this is that years ago we showed that external radiation to the liver was tolerated. Paul Hahn demonstrated long ago that livers irradiated with radioactive gold, if the patient was in decent shape, could tolerate massive irradiation. In a study done at Brookhaven, with Doctor James Robertson, radiation was delivered to the liver by means of different isotopes of platinum. This was tolerated. Did the slides he showed represent the immediate response to radiation, or that after a prolonged period?

Dr. M. Antar. These studies were performed during and shortly after the conclusion of radiation therapy. Hence we know the scan results as a function of the radiation dose. It is clear that when you get above 2000 R you begin markedly losing function. Some of the patients have been followed for many months. As you approach 3000 R you begin to collect evidence of lack of repair of altered RE function. We have seen, at lower doses, some function come back in a period of a year. You can permanently lose reticuloendothelial function at doses above 3000 R.

Dr. H. Atkins. The liver is not a radioresistant organ. The situation is probably similar to that in the thyroid in that radiation injury is not manifest in this organ, with a low mitotic rate, until it is called upon to undergo regenerative processes by some other injury. The conclusion of Ingold et al.[1] was that the liver was not radioresistant when irradiated in its entirety. Radiosensitivity of the liver was exceeded only by that of bone marrow, lymphoid tissue, germinal tissue, and the kidneys.

Radiation hepatitis was described by these workers and occurred in 13 of 25 patients who received radiation to the entire liver in a dose range from 1300 rads in 18 days to 5100 rads in 40 days. Three of thirteen patients with this complication died of it. They suggested a safe dose limit of 3500 rads with conventional fractionation.

Functional and histological changes in the liver following irradiation of 3000 to 11,000 rads from intravenously administered [198]Au in animals was demonstrated by Wordsworth et al.[2] A radiation dose greater than 5000 rads produced slowly developing but permanent histological damage. Radiation hepatitis has been reported following excessive administration of radiocolloid.

Dr. W. Beierwaltes. I agree with you, but was wondering if there were data which would enable you to make a statement on the child's liver. Is it more sensitive than that of adults?

Dr. H. Atkins. I have no data on that.

Dr. I. Ariel. I think we need to examine this closely. A dose of 150 mCi of ^{198}Au is a huge amount. We gave 10,000 R locally by injecting interstitial radium. We found normal inner cells. Some patients in poor metabolic state would not tolerate radiation.

At Brookhaven, when the boron study was begun, investigators were plagued with holes in the skull because of the escape of activity into the scalp and the bones of the head. Are you facing that problem at all?

Dr. G. Brownell. Yes. At Brookhaven they did not open the scalp, and that created some serious burns. In our case the technique will be, after the original craniotomy, to reflect the scalp and remove the skull bone. The collimator we use actually channels the neutrons directly into the tissue, and by means of various absorbing media prevents neutrons from going outside. Our experience with dogs has been good; the wound healed perfectly and there has been no untoward radiation effect.

Dr. H. Atkins. Dr. Bloomer indicated at the beginning of his talk that the irradiation from ^{125}I-deoxyuridine is of high LET nature. Actually it is only secondarily so because there is a difference between iodine 125 as sodium iodide and as deoxyuridine. The LET for the Auger electrons is not high. It is in the range of x-rays and electrons generally. However, there is a chemical effect of the large molecule disintegrating, as the iodine 125 undergoes transformation. In other words, there is an excessive charge locally. It is not Auger electrons per se, but the breakup of the large molecule does this. In effect, secondarily there is high LET radiation.

Dr. P. Bardfeld. I have a question and a comment for Dr. Bloomer. Do you have any data on the uptake of ^{125}I-deoxyuridine in the normal gastrointestinal mucosa? I would imagine, since that is a rapidly replicating tissue, it should accumulate the compound. Also, you might use this agent as a diagnostic test to check to see when the cyclic active chemotherapeutic agents would be most effective. I think you might be able to detect it externally.

Dr. W. Bloomer. We have seen no gross toxicity with the ^{125}I-IUDR in terms of the alimentary tract thus far. However, we have not done any bone marrow or gastrointestinal toxicity studies. There is at least one paper in which ^{125}I-IUDR was looked at as a diagnostic agent.

Dr. J. Bateman. A question for Dr. Bloomer and a comment for Dr. Brownell. In sequence, I was fascinated with the survival curves with the ^{125}I-IUDR. I have done work with fast neutrons and was intrigued with the possible implications with regard to the presence or absence of dose-rate effect. In regard to Dr. Brownell, I was interested in the presentation since I was involved peripherally with work at Brookhaven. We did, in fact, raise bone flaps but became somewhat disenchanted with the rather marked falloff of dose with depth. What this meant was that peripheral regions of the operative site and the ears were suffering rather high doses merely from the thermal neutrons. They did lose pieces of ears and tissue in this area.

Dr. W. Bloomer. With regard to the dose rate, we have no real information about this. One way to look at that of course would be to look at the ^{123}I-IUDR versus ^{125}I-IUDR; this we have not done. I would like to comment on regard to Dr. Atkins' remark. We are aware that what we are describing is a biological phenomenon that behaves like high LET. I think that these Auger electrons and conversion electrons are very densely ionizing and in fact they probably do represent a high LET type of radiation especially when they are deposited within the DNA.

Dr. G. Brownell. I think that the improvements in the technique of boron capture therapy have been on order of magnitude, at least, over the past decade or two. Mr. Fairchild is still studying this and we are working closely with him. I would simply cite again that these beagle dogs got exactly the radiation that they were supposed to get and there was absolutely no untoward effect. Other than the possibility (in the very highest dose level) of these dogs having a slight bit of brain swelling, they have been absolutely normal.

Dr. T. Haynie. My question is to alternative sources of neutrons, and what you thought about californium 252 or the neutron generators. I know the trials with californium 252 as brachytherapy were not generally very successful. Whether or not that could be enhanced by infusion of boron at the same time that the californium 252 was delivering neutrons to the tumor is unknown. Have you considered other sources of neutrons besides reactors?

Dr. G. Brownell. I think that other neutron sources, such as machines and californium 252, could be considered. However, you would want to remove the energy from the neutrons. For example, californium 252 has an average energy of 2.7 mev. The tritium-deuterium neutron generator has an average energy of 15 mev. Unless you use those in a fast-neutron therapy mode, that is, with collimation, they would effectively be a background in your radiation. They would not be boron enhanced. Only when they go to thermal energy does the boron capture enhance this radiation. I think that you would have to be somewhat ingenious. I do not think you could simply put californium 252 into a site and then expect to get the differential dose distribution. The fast neutron dose itself would probably swamp the boron level. We actually are interested in californium 252 and I think it might be possible to think of a moderator system that could be used with californium 252 to make this technique more widely applicable.

Dr. K. Mayer. I would like to ask you a question because I do think it may have some merit. It is possible with modern blood separators and processors to very quickly, in a few hours, plasmaphorese an individual totally. This can be done in an innocuous manner. If the tumor versus blood ratio is of major importance, in addition to your efforts to reduce it by chemical means, I wonder whether this might not be much enhanced by doing a thorough job of plasmaphoresis and removing the boron from this plasma.

Dr. Brownell. I think it is an interesting idea. I intend to take your suggestion back and discuss it.

Dr. B. Shapiro. It's my impression that the halogenated pyrimidines cannot be used systemically because of dehalogenation by the liver. I wonder what you were thinking of in terms of application for the ^{125}I-IUDR. Have you considered using it for malignant effusions, for example?

Dr. W. Bloomer. The halogenated pyrimidines are all rapidly dehalogenated. Usually they have a serum half-life in the order of minutes. That was one of the reasons we chose an intraperitoneal tumor and the intraperitoneal route of administration. We felt that this way we have more direct access of the drug to the tumor. I think that systemically the experience with the nonradioactive halogenated pyrimidines showed that even though they were rapidly dehalogenated, enough of the agents did get into the general circulation to cause the side effects that have been described in terms of damage to cellular systems, epilation, and loss of nails. So I think that there is a gradation. This works against you and in fact means that this particular type of agent would have to be used intraarterially or in a more directed fashion than intravenously.

Dr. K. Mayer. Some years ago we did work on radiation-protective agents. Although these never became clinically useful because of the toxicity, protection was delivered to the bone marrow. Perhaps this might be something that could be used in the future, if we get an agent which is sufficiently nontoxic to protect the bone marrow. There were sulfhydryl compounds or compounds which became sulfhydryl in the metabolic system. It might be something that could be used to protect bone marrow temporarily so that you could get your material into the tumors.

Dr. R. Spencer. I would like to ask Dr. Mayer two questions. One, could the sulfur 35 be incorporated in a certain precursor such as chondroitin sulfate that might go to the tumor but avoid bone marrow? And second, in the large tumor masses, is it possible to inject the sulfate directly into the mass, attempting to get rid of a portion of the malignant cells?

Dr. K. Mayer. These are thoughts that we have had before. We would have to do some animal work to try this out, because of the results we have had up to this time. Using a precursor substance may perhaps be an excellent approach and that way perhaps we would avoid the bone marrow. It is conceivable that it is probably the same mechanism, the same precursor may also go into megakaryocytes. Sulfur 35 was one of the first agents used to measure platelet survival because it does in fact go into megakaryocytes and go into platelets. We have had many other thoughts. For example, it may be possible to suppress megakaryocytosis by massive platelet transfusions. This can be done in animals. That would be the order of magnitude of 100 units of platelets, to any of these individuals, administered by transfusion. Of course, that would stop platelet production completely. It is conceivable that then the megakaryocytes would be protected. On the other hand, we do not really know where the damage is being done, whether it is in fact in the early megakaryocyte or in some stem cell that is ill-defined at this time.

Dr. I. Ariel. I would like to comment on Dr. Mayer's remarks pertaining to autotransplants. A number of years ago we utilized this technique in the treatment of malignant melanoma with lethal doses of phenylalanine mustard. We took bone marrow out of the sternum. We found out that we could not store it (with the techniques we used at that time) any longer than 6 hours. This was satisfactory because the phenylalanine mustard was cleared from the bloodstream within 6 hours. Then by injecting the bone marrow back intravenously, we found that the bone marrow selectively went back to the marrow spaces and set up colonies. This worked satisfactorily in those cases with huge otherwise lethal doses of phenylalanine mustard in the treatment of malignant melanoma.

Dr. S. J. Adelstein. I think we have been very confused about one matter, and I'm going to tell it the way I understand it. Two important things happen with Auger cascade. One, you are left with a number of electrons in a very small volume. Some of them have a short range as Dr. Bloomer showed in his chart this morning. Second, the resulting tellurium atom has an enormous charge. The charge has been measured carefully in the gaseous phase and seems to be an average charge of about +9. There are two kinds of effects that can happen. One is that the rapid production of a high electrostatic charge can be very destructive. In the gaseous phase with methyl iodide or ethyl iodide, you can see the molecules literally blow apart. But in the condensed phase, and you and I are both condensed phases, it is not clear that that is what happens at all. This charge may be dissipated without doing any damage. We do not know. We only know that if what happens after the disintegration or decay of the iodine in IUDR is measured, the thing that you are left with is deoxyuridine. Only the iodine or the tellurium has left, and the charge has been dissipated in some nondestructive fashion. So it seems unlikely at this stage that that is the mechanism where all the damage is done, although it is possible that in a nucleic acid it could be more complicated. That leaves us with the possibility that what you are dealing with is the highly localized ionization produced by these electrons. In very small volumes, the specific ionization is greater by calculation than it is from an alpha track. In that particular volume, this is high LET radiation. Once it gets out of that volume (for example, out of the thyroid follicle and into the cell), then it is probably spread out so that you are really dealing with low LET radiation. I think there are two possible effects, but right now my money is on the high specific ionization. By the way, there is little recoil from the ^{125}I atom.

Dr. S. Wong. There is an interesting paper from Germany studying the chemistry and the aftereffects of the ionization of ^{125}I-IUDR. They also used an extensive source of gamma radiation to irradiate the IUDR in order to study the aftereffects. The conclusion was, and a lot is theoretical, that ^{125}I-IUDR may suffer fragmentation from coulombic explosion.

Dr. S. J. Adelstein. There is no conclusive evidence that the *aromatic* molecules are blown apart in the condensed phase.

Dr. R. Bigler. I would like to comment on Dr. O'Mara's paper, and the use of ^{32}P-diphosphonate in therapy. In collaboration with Proctor and Gamble, we studied the tissue distribution of ^{32}P-diphosphonate in patients with osteosarcoma. It pointed out a possible prophylactic use of the radiopharmaceutical in such cases. The rationale is that uptake of the diphosphonate is a surface phenomenon. In the patients with osteosarcoma we had a 4 to 1 radioactivity ratio between primary tumor and spongy bone, and an 18 to 1 ratio between cortical bone and spongy bone. The calculations I showed in my talk were obtained from this study. In metastatic nodules taken at thoracotomy, we found extremely high concentrations of ^{32}P, equal to that in primary tumor. In this case we have a calcifying metastatic tumor with uptake of radioactive diphosphonate. The other key is that the bone tumor (in lung) to normal lung ratio of uptake was 26 to 1. A further view is that high-dose methotrexate and external radiation may sterilize osteosarcoma (but external radiation cannot be used to the lung in high doses, since pulmonary fibrosis might result). The diphosphonate uptake, however, may allow us to give radiation to metastatic osteosarcoma in lung. Going along with the previously discussed TDF concept, we obtain a TDF of about 2.7. This is right at the upper level of what the bone marrow can tolerate in dogs. Above this we are in the dangerous area, discussed by Dr. Mayer for ^{35}S. In osteosarcoma, which acts as a concentrating factor for the labeled diphosphonate, we are going to localize only about 5 percent of the radioactivity. That would be 5 percent additive to the effects of chemotherapy. It might allow us to destroy the tumor at an earlier stage.

Dr. I. Syed. I have a question for Dr. McDougall on the radiolabeled vesicles. I understand that it is useful to add therapeutic radionuclides inside the vesicle, since tumor cells have a large pinocytic activity. However, I do not see how these vesicles can be used for diagnostic purposes. The biological behavior is mainly of the vesicle and not that of the radionuclide (unless the vesicle is ruptured). The biological behavior is not influenced by the radiopharmaceutical. A worker in Oregon delivers chemotherapeutic agents by means of vesicles. She has found that vesicles make good "packages" for chemotherapeutic agents because there are no side effects; the target to nontarget ratio is high. Are there any comments on this?

Dr. I. McDougall. I would agree with you that it probably makes little sense to put a diagnostic agent inside of the vesicle, because the distribution obtained is not of the diagnostic agent but of the vesicle. Some people in Britain have looked at indium bleomycin inside vesicles, but it does not make sense to me. In relation to the increased pinocytosis of tumors, I think some tumors have it although others do not. The few patients in which this has been carried out (injecting the vesicles into patients with tumors) have shown quite variable results. Sometimes the tumors take up the vesicles in large quantities, sometimes they do not. We cannot rely entirely on the pinocytosis because it is not always there.

Dr. I Syed. The second question is to Dr. Burns. I have found that it is easier to make a pharmaceutical than a radiopharmaceutical in one sense. Just to label with an iodine radionuclide is easy. We call it iodination, but it is often not specific (some specific examples such as iodocholesterol are known). The important point is that it is difficult to use desirable radionuclides such as technetium 99m. We have not seen anybody labeling technetium 99m to cholesterol or other lipids.

Dr. H. D. Burns. As far as being easy to iodinate things is concerned, I am sure that Dr. Beierwaltes would be glad to point out that making 19-iodocholesterol is not a simple iodination. It involves a large number of steps and a great deal of synthetic organic chemistry. Incorporating iodine into a radiopharmaceutical is not always a simple process. I think that incorporating technetium into molecules such as lipids can be accomplished eventually, and that is one area I'm spending most of my time working on. I do not feel that enough is known about the chemistry of technetium to do it now. Molecules such as this have been designed with other transition metals. For example, a cobalt complex (which is a structural analogue of cholesterol) has been developed which inhibits cholesterol synthesis, and an osmium complex which is an analogue of curare has also been prepared. Both of these are transition metal complexes just as the technetium complex would be; they both behave as analogues of these other organic molecules.

Dr. E. Grady. I want to address a question to Dr. Puri about the interstitial administration of radioactive materials for therapy of lesions. Have you utilized large amounts of nonradioactive carrier to make it stay in the lesion longer? In rabbit tumors I used yttrium chloride mixed with two forms of yttrium, yttrium 89 as a nonradioactive carrier in about a million to one ratio with the yttrium 90. The yttrium chloride is in solution at pH 3.5. It precipitates when you get above that (as it would when injected into tissue). Such a mixture has an excellent effect on the rabbit tumor so that it is localized and does not "spill out." Good retention is obtained in the tumor by injecting it interstitially that way. What about the ^{32}P that you talked about?

Dr. S. Puri. As far as ^{32}P is concerned, we have used the insoluble chromic phosphate by injecting directly into the tumor's center. I cannot say whether distribution within the tumor is uniform or not. I think that it was not uniform; therefore, we were considering giving multiple injections. We did not use any added carrier. We are now trying to use this beta emitter or other particulates by injecting interstitially along with pharmaceuticals, to see if we can get a "double effect." We want to take advantage of the antitumor effect of the cold pharmaceutical with the added radiation effect. Work with antitumor agents which have been emulsified prior to local administration has been very intriguing to me, and it has been to my interest to go further.

Dr. E. Grady. I have made a transcutaneous gun which will vary the distribution of pharmaceuticals by varying pressure and distance. A more even distribution of the material can be achieved by using this gun; it is another approach that might help.

Dr. R. Spencer. I think you are forced to go here with short-lived radionuclides if you think about it. If you are successful in treating a lesion, it will start shrinking. Materials will escape from it to the bloodstream or the lymphatics. Hence, away goes some of your radioactive material. Unless you have a short-lived material, you will eventually be delivering some radioactivity to the remainder of the body. Perhaps then we should be going to shorter lived energetic emitters, trying to deliver radiation locally before it escapes systemically.

Dr. J. Smith. I want to thank you for organizing this meeting. You are bringing together the new directions in nuclear medicine. Not only are the therapeutic implications here, but also the implications for the identification of disease processes by identifying changes in function rather than simply changes in anatomy or changes in shape. Dr. Burns said something of great importance: he pointed out that we probably should take another look at things called "artifacts." Throughout the history of science it is more often than not the anomaly rather than the routine observation that leads to the new things.

REFERENCES

1. Ingold, J. A., Reed, G. B., Kaplan, H. S., et al.: Radiation hepatitis. Am. J. Roentgenol. 93:200, 1965.
2. Wordsworth, O. J., Dykes, P. W.: A functional and morphological study of liver radiation injury following intravenous injection with colloidal gold (^{198}Au). Int. J. Radiat. Biol. 14:497, 1969.

Moderator: Henry N. Wagner, Jr.
Panelists: Gerald A. Bruno, Stephen P. Bartok,
Irving M. Ariel, Ervin Kaplan,
and Edgar D. Grady*

34

Therapeutic Implications of Nuclear Medicine: Significance and Problems

Dr. H. Wagner. First of all, thank you for inviting me to come to this meeting, and secondly for having the idea that it would be important to take a new look at radioisotope therapy with the assumption that it may germinate into something really interesting, important, and exciting. During this meeting I formed a series of hypotheses that are not necessarily true but hopefully can be rules for action. I think one of the things that Dr. Spencer and all of us tried to do at a meeting like this was not just to get a good feeling in communicating ideas (Lewis Thomas says that to communicate with each other is among the favorite activities of human beings), but also to try to take something away in terms of actions that would follow from having attended this meeting. I hope that in the course of discussion with the panelists, whom I will introduce in a minute, we can come up with some possible actions that could be taken.

It seems to me that as I have seen and heard the papers that have been presented over the last few days, perhaps radioisotope therapy is moving from the inorganic era to the organic era just as diagnostic nuclear medicine is so moving. We all recognize that most of the good things that can be gotten from elements have really been obtained in diagnostic nuclear medicine. We have to become much more sophisticated as we make further progress. A group of very good chemists are now working in the field of nuclear medicine, and I think they are on the verge of producing a whole series of important diagnostic agents. Although it may not be too humble to say so, I think the paper that Dr. Burns gave is a good example of that, and I think that Dr. Burns and people like him (who are organic chemists and synthetic chemists) are the chemists of the future in the field of nuclear medicine. It is equally important to look at the therapeutic capabilities of these labeled compounds just as it is important to look at the diagnostic capabilities. So I agree with Dr. Burns that what we think of is sort of a triangle with stable pharmaceuticals and radioactive pharmaceuticals as two corners and the third corner being both diagnosis and therapy.

---

*With comments by symposium participants.

There is, and has always been, a close relationship between nuclear medicine, pharmacology, and physiology. The more strictly "structurally" oriented modalities such as ultrasound or diagnostic radiology have always seemed to me to have been more closely related to surgery. Because of its chemical and physiological orientation, since the beginning of nuclear medicine, there has been an orientation toward drug therapy. Dr. Spencer's thought in having this type of meeting certainly brings that forward. The advances in inorganic nuclear medicine, both diagnostic and therapeutic, need not stop. For example, thallium 201 is a good example of an inorganic substance that is useful in diagnostic nuclear medicine. The developments in inorganic nuclear medicine will continue, but by far the greatest strides will be made in the synthesis of organic compounds labeled with a variety of radioactive tracers.

I would like to ask the panel what they believe it will take to make things happen in the field of therapeutic nuclear medicine. Ashley said that there are four types of people who make up the world: those who make things happen, those to whom things happen, those who watch things happen, and those who do not realize that things are happening. Perhaps we should ask ourselves how can we make things happen in the field of the application of radioactive tracers in therapeutic nuclear medicine. We must have the proper blending and harmonizing of the people in the field with the events in the field. I will call on the others to comment and then perhaps to respond to any questions or comments that you have.

We now need sponsorship for research in the field of nuclear medicine. We can take advantage of the fact that there is now reorganization of the government, with ERDA being blended into the department of energy. We can really take the bull by the horns and point out to both the executive and legislative branches of the government that it would be a shame not to continue the excellent type of work that was sponsored by the Atomic Energy Commission. We can point out both in the therapeutic and the diagnostic field that it would be worthwhile to "pull together" (with new legislation) the types of activities that we have all become used to with respect to the atomic energy developments. Certainly, the development of the field of nuclear medicine was a blending of the efforts of individual people with events such as the Manhattan Project in providing radioactive materials that came from their reactors. It was absolutely essential for nuclear medicine to develop to the point that it has today, and probably with the right amount of effort we can convince the legislative and executive branches of the government that it would be worthwhile to take a new amalgamated approach toward advancing the use of radioactive materials in medicine.

I have been asked by Dr. Jim MacIntyre, the President of the Society of Nuclear Medicine, to be chairman of the committee that will report to the Society on a plan for generating research support in the field of nuclear medicine. If you have any suggestions or ideas along these lines, please send them to me. They will be looked at carefully by me and by the committee and hopefully can be incorporated into a program for developments in this field.

I would like now to introduce the panel. Dr. Stephen P. Bartok from the Food and Drug Administration is on the far left. Next to him is Dr. Ervin Kaplan. Dr. Gerald Bruno from E. R. Squibb is in the middle. Dr. Irving Ariel you have met before, and Dr. E. Grady you have also met previously. I would like to ask each of you who wishes to make a brief statement that you would like to leave with the group. Then we will run down the list and then open it up for questions and comments.

Dr. S. Bartok. Since I am working for the Food and Drug Administration, it would be rather hard for me to comment on generalities, if you ask a specific question, I would be glad to answer.

Dr. I. Ariel. I agree with what Dr. Wagner said about therapy for cancer. You can look at it with a great deal of humility. Ehrlich, after he discovered 606, started working on cancer therapy. He said he quit when he recognized that nothing would be discovered about cancer therapy until something was discovered about life itself. We have to use the modalities we have available today, and with much humility to utilize these modalities to their utmost. Further, a great deal of research (utilizing organic chemistry) is necessary to develop diagnostic and from diagnostic into therapeutic internal irradiation.

Dr. G. Bruno. In your analogy, the radiopharmaceutical industry would be in the class of people watching things happen rather than forcing things to happen because the development process for a therapeutic radiopharmaceutical is considerably more complex—for a variety of reasons—than for a diagnostic one. The higher levels of radiation create formulation and stability problems. When it comes to proving efficacy in preclinical studies, we have problems with experimental animal models matching the human model. Clinical studies take considerably longer and are more extensive. Shipping and packaging these materials are more expensive and more complex. All these factors make a therapeutic radiopharmaceutical considerably more time consuming and difficult, and consequently more expensive, to produce. Does the end use of a therapeutic radiopharmaceutical justify that great expense? There has been little activity in the development of these agents because of difficulty in answering that question. That is not to say that if an agent were discovered that justified the amount of expense involved it would not or could not be developed. It definitely could be, but the discovery would have to be made to justify that.

Dr. H. Wagner. It seems to me that by using radiopharmaceuticals one might greatly decrease the cost of development stable pharmaceuticals. The only radioactive tracer that is now widely excepted by the whole world (as a therapeutic agent) in my opinion is ^{131}I. I think you will agree that ^{131}I is used to turn down a function of the body that is too fast. Since the time of Hamilton and others, who developed radioiodine therapy, people have been searching for agents that would be useful therapeutic agents. Perhaps we should not constantly talk about what could be considered a magic bullet approach, where an agent is given that finds a tumor and kills the cell. As the field of nuclear medicine is developing, we are constantly measuring regional function. It seems to me, and to many other people I am sure, that there are a whole list of diseases that are characterized by the fact that some particular body process is "turned up too much." An example that was mentioned at this meeting is synovitis. The inflammatory response in a knee joint was "turned up" beyond what it should be. So it seems that if a diagnostic agent measures a specific function, and that particular function is accelerated (as in adrenal hyperplasia), that agent might potentially be useful as a therapeutic agent. That seems to be much more rational and efficient than using a model such as seizures in animals and testing 500,000 drugs to find out whether the number of seizures decreases (the most empirical trial and error type of approach to stable pharmaceuticals). So I think that radiopharmaceuticals, if properly blended with stable pharmaceuticals, can give much more information. Dr. Burns pointed out that this can be synergistic, and perhaps the certainty that something would be a good therapeutic agent can be increased by having a better understanding of how it behaves in vivo.

Dr. E. Kaplan. I would like to take precisely the opposite approach (of trying to turn down something that has been turned up) and instead try to turn something up that has been turned down: that is, the host defense mechanism. In the establishment of malignancy you probably all have observed numerous somatic mutations in which we've developed small lesions that probably disappear and never develop into anything because we have the means of either controlling or destroying them. It would be quite useful to heighten the bodily host defenses while trying to combat the development of a fulminating malignancy. I think that both of these approaches have validity. In other words, one has to analyze the specific situation, and in doing this one is using combination therapy (the combination therapy of heightening host resistance as well as the use of various chemotherapeutic agents). This combination might be very helpful, and this is simply a suggestion that would take the rather sophisticated multidisciplinary approach.

Dr. H. Wagner. How do you foresee that radiation can increase body function such as a defense mechanism?

Dr. E. Kaplan. I do not see radiation doing that. I see radiation doing just the opposite. But I do see things, for example, that might stimulate reticuloendothelial function prior to therapy. In other words, there are means of doing this prior to the administration of the radionuclide so that one would heighten the effect of the host defense before giving the therapeutic radiopharmaceutical. Then both the body and the external agent would be working in concert.

Dr. E. Grady. In this meeting we seem to have begun to establish the spirit of cooperation in development of radioactive materials for therapy. I hope that we can do this again and meet again next year or some time soon to present new methods and new ideas. We have just begun to explore a number of different agents that should be developed further. Certainly you can more properly utilize what you have in your own facility by expanding the use of these agents. For instance, there are many good "catheter men" in every hospital who might be able to help you put some of these things in the proper locations to see if we can control disease with better placement of radiopharmaceuticals.

Regarding the employment of the immune process to augment use of radiopharmaceuticals, I believe that radioactive antibodies have a great potential in both diagnosis and treatment. Radioactive antibodies to normal tissue may improve the methodology of scanning. Radioactive antibodies at therapeutic

levels may certainly carry agents into the needed place and be the "silver bullet."
I look forward to hearing other people develop new methods of utilizing these
antibodies for both diagnosis and therapy.

Dr. H. Wagner. There seems to be a tremendous need in this area. In all the
things that have been mentioned, such as ^{32}P for bone treatment (or for intraarticular or intralymphatic injections), controlled clinical trials must be instituted. As
Dr. Ariel pointed out, one characteristic that is essential in working in any of these
innovative areas is humility. The studies must be designed to indicate whether or
not the therapy used is effective. If there are no controlled trials, this question will
not be answered.

To illustrate the difficulties, I will mention a study that Dr. Tom Chalmers
reported. There was an extensive controlled study of portocaval shunting in the
treatment of cirrhosis of the liver. The most effective treatment for cirrhosis of the
liver (that is, for bleeding esophageal varices due to cirrhosis) was found to be in
the group that was selected to have a portocaval shunt and then elected not to
have it. That really illustrates how difficult it is to prove these things. We should
always keep in mind that very intelligent people, people who were at least as smart
as us, carried out blood letting for 150 years on the assumption that it really was
helpful.

Another story gives me a great sense of encouragement, but it illustrates how
difficult it is to make progress. I recently read a letter that Thomas Jefferson wrote
in 1806 to Edward Jenner. The President congratulated Jenner on his fantastic
achievement in inventing vaccination. In the last sentence Jefferson said that
although William Harvey's discovery of the circulation of the blood was a great
contribution to knowledge, he (Jefferson) could see that it really had resulted in no
great alleviation of human disease. All of us would admit that Thomas Jefferson
was pretty smart, yet even he could not see how knowing about the circulation of
the blood could be translated into improving human health.

If we really want these techniques to be accepted, the burden of proof is on
the person that says the technique is worthwhile. The greatest need in any of these
therapeutic efforts in 1977 is to have well-controlled and well-designed studies.
They have to be constructed so that it is possible to show that the technique is not
effective, just as it is possible to show that the technique is effective.

Dr. T. Hazra. I would like to reemphasize the importance not only of controlled clinical trials but also of group controlled trials. Very few centers will have
a sufficient number of cases to obtain any meaningful results. These trials must
involve the nationally surgical groups, or those in radiotherapy or chemotherapy if
they are to be done on a regional or national basis. Anecdotal incidents are
interesting, but they may have limited application. Dr. Kaplan, do you think that
once a clinical manifestation of malignancy has occurred, most of the in vivo and
in vitro data show that the immune system has failed? Most of the modalities of
treatment that are used—including surgery, radiation, and chemotherapy—
depress the immune system. Do you think it would be better to give an immune
stimulant prior to the treatment or after the treatment when the body tumor cell
burden has been reduced?

Dr. E. Kaplan. If one is dealing with a failing immune system, there are two options. One option is to stimulate the immune system with an appropriate agent (for example, the BCG trials). On the other hand, certain humoral agents being studied rather intensively will aid a failing immune system. One group of such substances is the α_2-globulins. The opsonic proteins may very well be harvested and administered as a means of "jacking up" the host ability to deal with foreign agents. For example, in the development of a malignancy, there is some evidence that the host defense is stimulated by the presence of the opsonic proteins that are "stimulating the appetite" of the macrophages that go to work on the tumor. This is simply one example. In order to develop this thesis, one could study many other aspects including the specific development of antibodies.

Dr. H. Wagner. Perhaps Dr. Bruno can carry the gallium story back to Squibb as an example of synergism between diagnostic radiopharmaceutical development and stable drug development. As Dr. Burns pointed out, when it was discovered that gallium accumulated in neoplasms, people began to investigate whether stable gallium might have some kind of an antineoplastic effect, perhaps similar to that of platinum. Radiopharmaceuticals are not a stepchild that is relatively worthless in terms of dollar volume and therefore can be developed outside of industry. We certainly know the contributions that industry has made to stable pharmaceuticals, and we hope that industry can make the same contribution to radiopharmaceuticals.

Dr. Bartok, we are all aware that there are many government-sponsored clinical trials at the present time, such as that of low-dose heparin. What is the relationship between the National Institutes of Health and the Food and Drug Administration with respect to controlled clinical trials, in terms of responsibility?

Dr. S. Bartok. If I can answer briefly: technically none. The National Cancer Institute has much of the funding for future use in the development of radiopharmaceuticals. A good part of the National Cancer Institute budget could potentially be given for therapeutic use of radionuclides in cancer. However, the FDA has no relationship with NIH or any other agency other than a regulatory one. We would encourage them, but the only thing we do is to enforce the law and to act on drug applications within as short a time as possible.

Dr. H. Wagner. What I meant was that if somebody applies for an Investigational New Drug (IND) application, does the Food and Drug Administration look at the quality of the study to see whether it is a scientific study rather than just an uncontrolled trial? Does the FDA look at the protocols or do they simply say whether or not a drug can be used in human beings?

Dr. S. Bartok. The current regulations and the law require us to look at every IND. We can put a new IND on "hold" only if there are questions of clinical safety. At that point we do not get involved with the efficacy of the drug.

Dr. H. Wagner. What about scientific merit? When an investigator submits an Investigational New Drug application, does the Food and Drug Administration look at the scientific merit of the proposal as well as the safety and efficacy?

Dr. S. Bartok. Directly no, indirectly yes. We do require well-controlled studies and we have minimum standards, but we do not get involved with the scientific merits as such and we do not comment on it.

Dr. R. L. Meckelenberg. Jefferson was like all politicians: while lauding Jenner, he also sent some letters to his son in college warning him to stay away from physicians. I ask that your committee contact some of the oncology groups because these groups now control the cancer patients. Until about 3 years ago we had treated about 90 ovarian carcinomas with the instillation of ^{32}P. When the protocols came out, all these patients were effectively removed from receiving this type of therapy because the radiopharmaceuticals were not written into the protocols. The people in the institutions of course follow the protocols completely. At the present time, in order to get back into this field, it is absolutely mandatory that we have these procedures written into the protocols. This is the only way those in the different hospitals can stay active with their main groups. I suggest that our efforts be directed toward the different cooperative groups, to try to get them to include radiopharmaceuticals. This would be an opportune time because we have had 2 or 3 years' experience, particularly on the ovarians tumors. They have likely accumulated enough data to show where they stand. We could ask them to put in several other agents (such as radiopharmaceuticals), and they might be responsive to these suggestions.

Dr. H. Wagner. Dr. Hazra, following up on that question, could you comment on (generally speaking around the country) the relationship among three things—chemotherapy, radiation therapy, and radioisotope therapy—in terms of an organizational sense.

Dr. T. Hazra. As was just mentioned, there are large groups, some of which are "site oriented," such as the prostate-oriented groups. There are also the national cooperative groups: for example, the acute leukemia group, obstetrics-gynecology group, and various others. These groups, and the national breast study group, are probably the most vocal. Most of these groups initially set up a protocol which has an input from surgeons, radiotherapists, and chemotherapists. The three of them are asked to write a proposed protocol. Naturally, when three people meet, the person who gets most in is the one who can make his point the best. The National Cancer Institute, which funds most of these controlled trial groups, is coming out strongly where the key word is *multidisciplinary approach.* You really have to make an input, not just a token input. You really need a tremendous input from all the groups to get any funding. A recent example is the Cancer and Leukemia Group B which involves most of the New York and New England including Maryland and Virginia. They were criticized because they were basically dealing with chemotherapists. They were told that they would have to get surgeons and radiotherapists into the discussions. If we want new radiopharmaceuticals to be used, that is the way to go. If there are patients to be treated, then somebody has to propose a protocol and try to sell it.

Dr. H. Wagner. How many people here are radiation therapists? Please raise your hands. One. How many people are radiologists? Seven. How many are internists? Fourteen. Probably it is not unpredictable that internists tend to have a greater interest in therapy than do most radiologists. Those of us who believe that the field of nuclear medicine is greatly strengthened by the idea that it is multidisciplinary can take the fact that one big area where internists can continue to make an important contribution is in therapeutic uses. They can help in making certain that any potential therapeutic advances that might be made are in fact made. That is a useful derivative of this meeting. Perhaps many of us can agree that radioisotope therapy has been too long neglected. I would not try to revive old methods for ^{32}P treatment in bone pain or try to convince as many people as possible to use intraarticular injection of microspheres. It should be recognized that this is an important scientific, academic, and clinical part of the field. We should try to obtain real support to ensure that if anything of value can be developed, that it will be developed.

Dr. T. Hazra. One reason most radiologists have gone away from treatment of cancer is because they have found that although they were able to deliver radiation, they were really not keeping up with, or did not have the knowledge of, the biology of cancer. Anybody dealing with any form of therapy, including radiation with radiopharmaceuticals or even with immunotherapy, must receive training and have an interest in the biology of cancer. These persons must be interested basically in the biology of cancer, and secondarily in the use of radiopharmaceuticals as one of the modalities of treatment. There is a need for a "cure training" prior to learning chemotherapy or radiation therapy.

Dr. H. Wagner. Because his orientation is so different, the average radiotherapist is unlikely to make an important advance in the use of radioactive materials and therapy. People oriented toward nuclear medicine will have to come up with an advance in the therapeutic studies. The radiation therapist is so concerned with external irradiation that he does not think much about the chemistry of the body, and how processes can be hyperplastic.

Dr. T. Hazra. That does not necessarily follow. The initial contributions, at least from the old centers, were all by radiotherapists. Most people, especially young people training in any form of cancer of therapy, need a basic interest in cancer biology. I feel that to have "modality training" now, whether it be for a surgeon, radiotherapist, or chemotherapist, is wrong.

Dr. H. Wagner. Why such an interest in cancer? I think that the most valuable use of radioactive iodine is in the treatment of hyperthyroidism. Perhaps 98 percent of the value of radioisotope therapy has been derived from therapeutic radioiodine use in hyperthyroidism (not in cancer of the thyroid).

Dr. T. Hazra. Yes, but I am not specifically making my remarks for the nonneoplastic disease.

Dr. H. Wagner. That is a good example of the orientation of a radiation therapist. In my opinion it is wonderful and I am not criticizing it. I am saying that because of such orientation, advances in the field of therapeutic nuclear medicine will probably not come from radiation therapists.

Dr. T. Hazra. I think labeling people as surgeons, radiotherapists, or internists is not the issue. The issue is what is their basic interest and work. A pathologist might come up with the answer if he has an interest, a natural interest.

Dr. M. A. Antar. I would like to follow on the comments about support for research. I think the basic question has to go back to research support. As you are aware in the last few years "the politicians" have been reluctant to support basic research. They want to see some things happening. I would like to hear some of your comments.

Dr. H. Wagner. I think everyone would agree that before any advances can be made, a firm foundation of basic sciences is necessary.

Dr. I. Ariel. A great deal of work must be done in basic research, but the minute a little bit is done in basic research it is immediately carried over into clinical investigation with great claims made about the accomplishments. I know nothing that is really beneficial from the standpoint of immunology that is going to help the patient suffering today from cancer today. No one can deny the tremendous importance of immunology as it pertains to cancer, but what are you going to do for the patient now?

Dr. E. Kaplan. A journey of a thousand miles begins with a single step. You need to develop the basic information. Perhaps your patients today will not benefit, but perhaps someone's grandchildren will.

Dr. S. Puri. In regard to Dr. Kaplan's statement about enhancing the immune response before we treat these patients with radioisotopes, I think that's an ideal situation. Unfortunately, in real life in patients with tumors the immune response is not that good. Giving BCG before treatment is going to be filled with problems. In those situations, delivering the radiopharmaceutical directly into the tumor might help. Maybe when the tumor burden is small, the immune system will respond in a better fashion. The fact that the body's immune response is not good should not be disheartening. We might still treat these patients with radiopharmaceuticals by local injections or by delivering them directly into the vessels leading to the area.

Dr. E. Kaplan. I agree with what you pointed out. I do feel that there is hope in immune stimulation of one sort or another.

Dr. Meckelenberg. I have a couple of suggestions. When we inject these beta emitting isotopes for therapy, we should follow them and localize them more accurately if we also use a gamma emitter. For the past 3 years, whenever I use ^{32}P therapy for an ovarian tumor, I also inject 5 mCi of technetium sulfur colloid. I do this before I inject the ^{32}P so that I can tell if there is good distribution. If there is not, then the instillation of ^{32}P is avoided. In two instances this avoided what could have been a serious subcutaneous infiltration. I suggest that Dr. Grady do the same: when he has his catheter in the artery, before he injects the therapeutic radionuclide into the liver, he can easily inject ^{99m}Tc-MAA and see exactly where it is going. The other suggestion is one I made to Dr. James Smith and Dr. E. Kaplan in the past. That is, using the V.A. to study ^{32}P in a polyphosphate of some type, in carcinoma of the prostate. In the V.A. system there must be 10,000 patients right now with cancer of the prostate. Many of them are miserable and I think could be helped by treatment with a ^{32}P-tagged pyrophosphate. I think it just needs someone, and Dr. Kaplan would be in a perfect position to do this. He has that first publication, and he is well known in the V.A. Dr. Wagner said it is better actually to do something rather than just sit on the side. I think a good cooperative study in the V.A. of the use of ^{32}P polyphosphate is a natural thing to do.

Dr. E. Kaplan. Let me point out that in the early sixties we actually set up such a cooperative study within the V.A. We combined it with the ongoing study of carcinoma of the prostate which was evaluating estrogens and orchiectomy. Two things happened. The protocol was accepted on merit by a good review committee. We started the study and the two study groups were competing for patients. In other words, the only patients that we could get while working this way were the rejects of the initial group. This went on for several years. It ceased to be productive. I agree with you that it is essentially a good idea to do this; perhaps it should be reinstituted. Almost all of the ^{32}P therapy has been done in terminal patients. It might be a good idea to deal with people with early involvement of metastasis to the bone because the prognosis of bone metastasis is not really brilliant even in early lesions, and perhaps some of these may be much more responsive.

Dr. H. Wagner. It just occurred to me that a very good example about the interfacing of radiopharmaceutical development with stable pharmaceutical development is the development of DOPA at Brookhaven. The early study on the distribution of substances such as gold in the brain took them into the topic that did result in this tremendous advance made in DOPA treatment at a National Laboratory under AEC sponsorship.

Dr. E. Grady. The FDA has a number of regulations that we respect. But what do we do when we see a regulation that is of no benefit? How do we go about changing it? For instance, before new radiopharmaceuticals are used in patients we need a rabbit test for pyrogenicity. The limulus tests are superior to the rabbit ones, but we cannot give up the rabbit test because it is in the book. In some cases the regulations said we had to give such a large amount of material that we would kill the rabbits. Hence it would be of no value to use that for testing for pyrogens. I asked permission to wait until the radioactive material had decayed to do the rabbit test and it would be a retrospective pyrogen test. Now it seems to me we ought to have some way of throwing that regulation out, but how do we go about it?

Dr. S. Bartok. That is an easy question to answer. The pyrogen testing by the limulus method instead of the rabbit method is done under USP auspices. It is not an FDA regulation.

Dr. H. Wagner. What is the FDA's position on limulus testing right now?

Dr. S. Bartok. I do not know how much I can comment on it. I am an advocate of the limulus test. I have approached USP on several occasions. It is in the works and I hope that within a year we will have it under USP auspices. Dr. Grady, really the FDA does not write the rules. We are under Congressional instructions. Our regulations are published as proposed regulations. When those proposed regulations come out, this is the time for you to comment. Once they become regulations it is rather difficult to remove them. I was really disappointed in some of these hearings. Practically nobody from the public shows up. When a proposed regulation is being discussed, that is the time for the scientific community to come and voice what they feel. Because if we have to pass a regulation by default, please do not blame us for it.

Dr. G. Ammerman. One question for Dr. Wagner. I noticed the emphasis mainly on therapy. The chemotherapists have been adding one poison on another with some apparently beneficial effect. Again taking Dr. Wagner's suggestion that the stable and radioactive pharmaceuticals might lead one to another, perhaps the strategy of the radiopharmaceutical being an adjuvant to some of the chemotherapeutic regimes might add something.

Dr. F. Hosain. I would direct a comment to Dr. Henry Wagner. Many participants in oncology groups are internists who are ot familiar with therapeutic radionuclides. The contributions of the nonphysicians should be noted. He who knows the subjects will do his thing.

Dr. Meckelenberg. I would like to direct a comment to the FDA. I do not mean to be critical about this, but how many people here read the Federal Register? It comes out every day. Reading it every day is exactly what it takes to be able to know what is coming out of the government. You have 60 days to reply; if it is a really bad situation you have 90 days to reply. There needs to be education so that everybody understands exactly how these things are done. The FDA is not going to get any other feedback information if this is the only mode of announcing changes they have. It is an extremely limited mode. The Federal Register is difficult for physicians to read because it is written in "legalease" rather than in plain language. I hope that there will be some developments to overcome this because one of our biggest problems is communication. Again, I am not being critical but I think we have a big stumbling block in our way.

Dr. S. Bartok. I would like to thank you for so nicely expressing my own feelings. When I came to FDA this was one of my first questions. Under the current regulations we have no other way to go about it. My suggestion was that a proper scientific organization should somehow get organized. We would be glad to submit the necessary copies of the Federal Register to them. As the government is set up currently, we have no other way to do it. I am concerned about it. I spent 10 years in nuclear medicine in the field and I know what it means to read the Federal Register.

Dr. E. Kaplan. Dr. Wagner, would it be an appropriate function of the Society of Nuclear Medicine to abstract the nuclear medicine components of the Federal Register and circulate this into the membership?

Dr. H. Wagner. I agree absolutely. I think it is a function of the professional society to do things like this, just as other professional societies do. What this field really needs is something that is as effective as ^{131}I is in the treatment of hyperthyroidism. One innovation like that would advance the field of therapeutic nuclear medicine tremendously. We have to set the framework and develop the policies and strategies so that the possibility of that happening is at least finite. I would like to thank the members of the panel for their participation and also thank the audience.

Dr. R. Spencer. Dr. Wagner, panel members, ladies and gentlemen, we appreciate your participation. I want to thank you all for attending. By your comments it appears that there should be follow-up meetings in the not too distant future.

Index